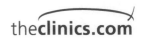

ENDOCRINOLOGY AND METABOLISM CLINICS

OF NORTH AMERICA

Molecular Basis of Inherited Pancreatic Disorders

GUEST EDITORS
Markus M. Lerch, MD, FRCP
Thomas Griesbacher, MD
David C. Whitcomb, MD, PhD

CONSULTING EDITOR
Derek LeRoith, MD, PhD

June 2006 • Volume 35 • Number 2

SAUNDERS

An Imprint of Elsevier, Inc.
PHILADELPHIA   LONDON   TORONTO   MONTREAL   SYDNEY   TOKYO

W.B. SAUNDERS COMPANY
A Division of Elsevier Inc.

1600 John F. Kennedy Boulevard • Suite 1800 • Philadelphia, Pennsylvania 19103-2899

http://www.theclinics.com

ENDOCRINOLOGY AND METABOLISM	Volume 35, Number :
CLINICS OF NORTH AMERICA	ISSN 0889-852‹
June 2006	ISBN 1-4160-3870-1
Editor: Rachel Glover	

The ideas and opinions expressed in *Endocrinology and Metabolism Clinics of North America* do not necessarily reflect those of the Publisher. The Publisher does not assume any responsibility for any injury and/or damage to persons or property arising out of or related to any use of the material contained in this periodical. The reader is advised to check the appropriate medical literature and the product information currently provided by the manufacturer of each drug to be administered to verify the dosage, the method and duration of administration, or contraindications. It is the responsibility of the treating physician or other health care professional, relying on independent experience and knowledge of the patient, to determine drug dosages and the best treatment for the patient. Mention of any product in this issue should not be construed as endorsement by the contributors, editors, or the Publisher of the product or manufacturers' claims.

Endocrinology and Metabolism Clinics of North America (ISSN 0889-8529) is published quarterly by W.B. Saunders, 360 Park Avenue South, New York, NY 10010-1710. Months of publication are March, June, September, and December. Business and editorial offices: 1600 John F. Kennedy Boulevard, Suite 1800, Philadelphia, PA 19103-2899. Accounting and circulation offices: 6277 Sea Harbor Drive, Orlando, FL 32887-4800. Periodicals postage paid at New York, NY and additional mailing offices. Subscription prices are USD 175 per year for US individuals, USD 295 per year for US institutions, USD 90 per year for US students and residents, USD 220 per year for Canadian individuals, USD 355 per year for Canadian institutions, USD 240 per year for international individuals, USD 355 per year for international institutions and USD 125 per year for Canadian and foreign students/residents. To receive student/resident rate, orders must be accompanied by name of affiliated institution, date of term, and the *signature* of program/residency coordinator on institution letterhead. Orders will be billed at individual rate until proof of status is received. Foreign air speed delivery is included in all *Clinics* subscription prices. All prices are subject to change without notice. POSTMASTER: Send address changes to *Endocrinology and Metabolism Clinics of North America*, Elsevier Periodicals Customer Service, 6277 Sea Harbor Drive, Orlando, FL 32887-4800. **Customer Service: (+1) 800-654-2452 (US). From outside of the US, call (+1) 407-345-4000; e-mail: hhspcs@harcourt.com.**

Reprints. For copies of 100 or more, of articles in this publication, please contact the Commercial Rights Department, Elsevier Inc., 360 Park Avenue South, New York, NY 10010-1710; phone: (+1) 212-633-3813; fax: (+1) 212-462-1935; e-mail: reprints@elsevier.com.

Endocrinology and Metabolism Clinics of North America is covered in *Index Medicus, EMBASE/Excerpta Medica, Current Contents/Clinical Medicine, Current Contents/Life Sciences, Science Citation Index, ISI/BIOMED, BIO-SIS, and Chemical Abstracts.*

Printed in the United States of America.

CONSULTING EDITOR

DEREK LeROITH, MD, PhD, Chief, Division of Endocrinology, Metabolism, and Bone Diseases, Mount Sinai School of Medicine, New York, New York

GUEST EDITORS

MARKUS M. LERCH, MD, FRCP, Department of Gastroenterology, Endocrinology, and Nutrition, Ernst-Moritz-Arndt Universität Greifswald, Greifswald, Germany

THOMAS GRIESBACHER, MD, Medizinische Universität Graz, Graz, Austria

DAVID C. WHITCOMB, MD, PhD, Giant Eagle Foundation Professor of Cancer Genetics, Departments of Medicine, Cell Biology and Physiology, and Human Genetics, University of Pittsburgh, Pittsburgh, Pennsylvania; Chief, Division of Gastroenterology, Hepatology, and Nutrition, University of Pittsburgh, Pittsburgh, Pennsylvania

CONTRIBUTORS

DETLEF K. BARTSCH, MD, Department of Surgery, Städtische Kliniken Bielefeld-Mitte, Bielefeld, Germany

DANIEL BIMMLER, MD, Pancreatitis Research Laboratory, Department of Visceral and Transplantation Surgery, University Hospital Zurich, Zurich, Switzerland

RANDALL E. BRAND, MD, Associate Professor of Medicine, Department of Medicine, Northwestern University, Feinberg School of Medicine, Chicago, Illinois; Section of Gastroenterology, Evanston Northwestern Healthcare, Glenview, Illinois

PHILIPPE FROGUEL, MD, PhD, Director of the CNRS UMR8090 Unit, Institute of Biology and Pasteur Institute of Lille, Lille, France; Professor of Genomic Medicine and Head of Section of Genetics, Imperial College, Hammersmith Hospital, London, United Kingdom

ROLF GRAF, PhD, Pancreatitis Research Laboratory, Department of Visceral and Transplantation Surgery, University Hospital Zurich, Zurich, Switzerland

WILLIAM GREENHALF, PhD, Lecturer in Microbiology, Division of Surgery and Oncology, The University of Liverpool, Liverpool, United Kingdom

NILS HABBE, MD, Department of Surgery, Philipps-University Marburg, Marburg, Germany

NATHAN R. HOWES, MB, ChB, MD, FRCS, Consultant Surgeon, Honorary Senior Lecturer, Division of Surgery and Oncology, The University of Liverpool, Liverpool, United Kingdom

ROSHAN S. JAHANGIR TAFRECHI, PhD, Department of Molecular Cell Biology, Leiden University Medical Centre, Leiden, The Netherlands

GEORGE M.C. JANSSEN, PhD, Department of Molecular Cell Biology, Leiden University Medical Centre, Leiden, The Netherlands

MATTHIAS KRAFT, MD, Department of Gastroenterology, Endocrinology, and Nutrition, Ernst-Moritz-Arndt Universität Greifswald, Greifswald, Germany

PETER LANGER, MD, Department of Surgery, Philipps-University Marburg, Marburg, Germany

HERMAN H. LEMKES, MD, Department of Endocrinology and Metabolic Diseases, Leiden University Medical Centre, Leiden, The Netherlands

MARKUS M. LERCH, MD, FRCP, Department of Gastroenterology, Endocrinology, and Nutrition, Ernst-Moritz-Arndt Universität Greifswald, Greifswald, Germany

BRIAN C. LEWIS, PhD, Associate Professor, Programs in Gene Function, Molecular Medicine, and Cancer Center, University of Massachusetts Medical School, Worcester, Massachusetts

RODGER A. LIDDLE, MD, Professor of Medicine, Department of Medicine, Duke University and Durham VA Medical Centers, Durham, North Carolina

HENRY T. LYNCH, MD, Chairman and Professor of Medicine, Department of Preventive Medicine/Public Health, Creighton University School of Medicine, Omaha, Nebraska

JOHANNES A. MAASSEN, PhD, Department of Molecular Cell Biology, Leiden University Medical Centre, Leiden, The Netherlands

JULIA MAYERLE, MD, Department of Gastroenterology, Endocrinology, and Nutrition, Ernst-Moritz-Arndt Universität Greifswald, Greifswald, Germany

HASSAN MZIAUT, Experimental Diabetology, Carl Gustav Carus Medical School, Dresden University of Technology, Dresden, Germany

JOHN P. NEOPTOLEMOS, MA, MB, BChir, MD, FRCS, Head of the School of Cancer Studies, Division of Surgery and Oncology, The University of Liverpool, Liverpool, United Kingdom; Professor, Division of Surgery and Oncology, The University of Liverpool, Liverpool, United Kingdom

ANTON K. RAAP, PhD, Department of Molecular Cell Biology, Leiden University Medical Centre, Leiden, The Netherlands

MICHAEL G.T. RARATY, MB, BS, PhD, FRCS, Senior Lecturer, Division of Surgery and Oncology, The University of Liverpool, Liverpool, United Kingdom

ANDRÉ REIS, MD, Institute of Human Genetics, University of Erlangen-Nuremberg, Erlangen, Germany

MANUEL RUTHENBÜRGER, PhD, Department of Gastroenterology, Endocrinology and Nutrition, Ernst-Moritz-Arndt Universität Greifswald, Greifswald, Germany

MIKLÓS SAHIN-TÓTH, MD, PhD, Associate Professor, Department of Molecular and Cell Biology, Goldman School of Dental Medicine, Boston University, Boston, Massachusetts

PETER E. SCHWARZ, III° Medical Clinic, Carl Gustav Carus Medical School, Dresden University of Technology, Dresden, Germany

PETER SIMON, MD, Department of Gastroenterology, Endocrinology, and Nutrition, Ernst-Moritz-Arndt Universität Greifswald, Greifswald, Germany

MERCEDES SINA-FREY, MD, Institute of Clinical Genetics, Philipps-University Marburg, Marburg, Germany

MICHELE SOLIMENA, Experimental Diabetology, Carl Gustav Carus Medical School, Dresden University of Technology, Dresden, Germany; III° Medical Clinic, Carl Gustav Carus Medical School, Dresden University of Technology, Dresden, Germany

ELISABETH SPILCKE-LISS, MD, Department of Gastroenterology, Endocrinology and Nutrition, Ernst-Moritz-Arndt-University, Greifswald, Germany

LEEN M. 't HART, PhD, Department of Molecular Cell Biology, Leiden University Medical Centre, Leiden, the Netherlands

MIRKO TRAJKOVSKI, Experimental Diabetology, Carl Gustav Carus Medical School, Dresden University of Technology, Dresden, Germany

STEFAN TURI, MD, Department of Gastroenterology, Endocrinology, and Nutrition, Ernst-Moritz-Arndt-University, Greifswald, Germany

MARTINE VAXILLAIRE, PharmD, PhD, Associate Researcher, CNRS UMR8090, Institute of Biology and Pasteur Institute of Lille, Lille, France

LOUIS J. VITONE, MB, ChB, MRCS, Research Fellow, Division of Surgery and Oncology, The University of Liverpool, Liverpool, United Kingdom

HENRI WALLASCHOFSKI, MD, Department of Gastroenterology, Endocrinology and Nutrition, Ernst-Moritz-Arndt-University, Greifswald, Germany

F. ULRICH WEISS, PhD, Department of Gastroenterology, Endocrinology, and Nutrition, Ernst-Moritz-Arndt Universität Greifswald, Greifswald, Germany

DAVID C. WHITCOMB, MD, PhD, Giant Eagle Foundation Professor of Cancer Genetics, Departments of Medicine, Cell Biology and Physiology, and Human Genetics, University of Pittsburgh, Pittsburgh, Pennsylvania; Chief, Division of Gastroenterology, Hepatology, and Nutrition, University of Pittsburgh, Pittsburgh, Pennsylvania

MARTIN ZENKER, MD, Institute of Human Genetics, University of Erlangen-Nuremberg, Erlangen, Germany

CONTENTS

> The pancreas is an important exocrine and endocrine organ that
> develops from the dorsal and ventral anlagen during embryogen-
> esis and arises from the endodermal lining of the duodenum within
> the first month of human embryonic life. A number of develop-
> mental disorders can either lead to anatomic abnormalities of the
> pancreas and its ducts, or can be part of complex disorders that
> affect multiorgan systems. Other genetic changes can lead to meta-
> bolic abnormalities that affect the pancreas exclusively or increase
> the lifetime risk for developing pancreatitis or pancreatic diabetes.
> This article reviews some of the developmental and metabolic dis-
> orders that can affect the endocrine and exocrine pancreas.

> The most recent elucidation of an inherited disorder of the pancreas
> concerns the Johanson-Blizzard syndrome (JBS). Positional cloning
> identified loss-of-function mutations in the UBR1 gene on the long
> arm of chromosome 15 to be the cause of JBS in more than a dozen
> patients. In patients with JBS the absence of UBR1 results in early
> prenatal destruction of the exocrine pancreas that involves

impaired apoptosis, induced necrosis, and prominent inflammation. Knockout mice with absent UBR1 expression suffer from exocrine pancreatic insufficiency and increased susceptibility to experimental pancreatitis. The UBR1 protein substrate, presumably impaired degradation of which causes JBS, is not yet known.

Polygenetic Traits in Pancreatic Disorders
David C. Whitcomb

Rapid advances in information and technology provide opportunities to discover the risks or causes for various disorders within individual patients. The availability of new data and new technology has outstripped the conceptual framework of simple disorders, however, and challenges current statistical approaches. The author addresses the issues surrounding study design and sample size for complex genetic traits with special attention to meta-analysis and systems biology. The author concludes that meta-analysis should play a limited role in evaluating studies of complex genetic diseases. Instead, systems biology-based approaches should be developed to integrate multiple, focused, and mechanistic association studies, with the goal of assisting in the risk assessment of patients on a person-by-person basis.

Trypsinogen Mutations in Pancreatic Disorders
Louis J. Vitone, William Greenhalf, Nathan R. Howes,
Michael G.T. Raraty, and John P. Neoptolemos

There are multiple PRSS1 mutations described in hereditary pancreatitis but only a minority of these are clinically relevant. The two most frequent point mutations are in exon 2 (N29I) and exon 3 (R122H), found in diverse racial populations. Both mutations result in early onset pancreatitis but the mechanism underlying this phenotype is unclear. The frequency of these mutations in such diverse populations suggests they have spontaneously occurred many times. The origin of the major mutations may be explained by gene conversions, accounting for multiple founders. The implications are discussed in terms of mechanism of action of the mutations and clinical presentation.

Germline Mutations and Gene Polymorphism Associated with Human Pancreatitis
F. Ulrich Weiss, Peter Simon, Julia Mayerle, Matthias Kraft,
and Markus M. Lerch

A wide range of mutations and polymorphisms in genes that relate to pancreatic function seem to be involved in the development of pancreatitis. Some of these genetic alterations lead to disease phenotypes with unequivocal mendelian inheritance patterns, whereas others seem to act as modifier genes in conjunction with environmental or, as yet unidentified, genetic cofactors. This article reviews germline changes in the genes for trypsin, pancreatic secretory trypsin inhibitor, the cystic fibrosis conductance regulator, lipid metabolism proteins, inflammatory mediators for cytokines, and cathepsin B.

The past decade has witnessed remarkable progress in the genetics of chronic pancreatitis. Despite these accomplishments, the understanding of the molecular mechanisms through which PRSS1 and SPINK1 mutations cause chronic pancreatitis has remained sketchy. Pancreatitis-associated gene mutations are believed to result in uncontrolled trypsin activity in the pancreas. Experimental identification of the disease-relevant functional alterations caused by PRSS1 or SPINK1 mutations proved to be challenging, however, because results of biochemical analyses lent themselves to different interpretations. This article focuses on PRSS1 mutations and summarizes the salient biochemical findings in the context of the mechanistic models that explain the connection between mutations and hereditary pancreatitis.

More than 100 years ago it was proposed that pancreatitis essentially is a disease in which the pancreas undergoes autodigestion by its own prematurely activated digestive enzymes. Why and how digestive zymogens autoactivate within the pancreas early in the disease process has been a matter of controversy and debate. Some of the mechanisms that are considered to be involved in digestive protease activation are inherited and as of recently can be tested for clinically. Here we review the most recent progress in elucidating the mechanisms involved in the onset of pancreatitis. We specifically focus on serine and cysteine proteases in the autodigestive cascade that precedes acinar cell injury and the biochemical processes involved in their activation.

This article summarizes structural and functional properties of pancreatic secretory trypsin inhibitor (PSTI), which has been identified in many species. Its prominent role is to protect the pancreas from prematurely activated trypsinogen before entry into the duodenum. In the rat there are two isoforms, one of which is PSTI-I, a 61-amino acid peptide involved in the feedback regulation of pancreatic enzymes. Independent investigations in neoplastic diseases led to the discovery of tumor-associated trypsin inhibitor, which is identical to PSTI.

diabetes during life. Enhanced aging of pancreatic β-cells, a reduced capacity of these cells to synthesize large amounts of insulin, and a resetting of the ATP/ADP-regulated K-channel seem to be the pathogenic factors involved.

The pancreas is specified during embryonic development from the gut endoderm. Among the signaling pathways required for the proper development of the organ are the notch and hedgehog signaling pathways. Both of these pathways are reactivated in pancreatic cancers, and sustained hedgehog signaling is required for the viability of most pancreatic cancer cell lines. Further, mouse models of the disease show activation of these pathways, and expression of pancreas progenitor markers. These findings indicate that developmentally regulated gene expression programs are important in the pathogenesis of pancreatic cancer.

It is estimated that 5% to 10% of pancreatic cancer cases are attributable to hereditary factors. We believe that the number of cases that are genetic in etiology are even greater, however, based not on a classic autosomal dominant pattern of inheritance but rather when one takes into account low-penetrant inherited susceptibility factors. There is also a growing recognition that the development of pancreatic cancer in pancreatic cancer-prone families is dependent not only on genetic variables but on nongenetic factors. The aim of this article is to review the challenges in identifying pancreatic cancer-prone families and how environmental factors interact with genetic factors in these families.

Hereditary pancreatic cancer (PC) is rare and extremely heterogeneous, and it accounts for approximately 2% of all PC cases. The major component of hereditary PC is the familial pancreatic cancer syndrome. Although up to 20% of hereditary PC cases are associated with germline mutations in the BRCA2, CDKN2A, PRSS1, STK11, or MMR genes, the major underlying gene defect(s) is still unknown. Although hereditary PC is rare, the data on PC families that have been collected by various study groups worldwide provide a unique opportunity to evaluate the natural history, causative gene alterations, new diagnosis and chemoprevention strategies as well as treatment modalities.

FORTHCOMING ISSUES

RECENT ISSUES

ELSEVIER
SAUNDERS

Endocrinol Metab Clin N Am
35 (2006) xv–xviii

ENDOCRINOLOGY
AND METABOLISM
CLINICS
OF NORTH AMERICA

Foreword

Molecular Basis of Inherited Pancreatic Disorders

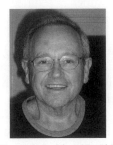

Derek LeRoith, MD, PhD
Consulting Editor

In this issue of the *Endocrinology and Metabolism Clinics of North America*, Drs. Lerch, Griesbacher, and Whitcomb have compiled several articles on the molecular basis of inherited pancreatic disorders by experts in this field of research.

In a comprehensive approach to developmental and metabolic disorders of the pancreas, Lerch, Zenker, Turi, and Mayerle describe some rare abnormalities that may result in pancreatitis. In some cases, pancreatitits is the major feature of the disorder, whereas in others it is associated with other quite serious abnormalities in other organs. Although the various disorders may be unusual, they present important challenges to pediatricians, internists, and specialists and are important conditions to be aware of.

The gene for Johansen-Blizzard syndrome has been identified as the UBR1 gene product by Zenker, Mayerle, Reis, and Lerch, who summarize the positional cloning that they used to identify the gene and the clinical findings of the syndrome. Interestingly, in addition to numerous developmental defects, there is exocrine pancreatic insufficiency, hypothyroidism, and short stature. UBR1 is a ubiquitin ligase, and it is therefore postulated that mutations in UBR1 in this syndrome may cause a prolongation of the half-life of certain proteins. The result, as far as the pancreas is concerned, is an embryonic variety of pancreatitis.

The article by Whitcomb covers the issues of complex polygenic disorders and reviews both the usefulness of meta-analyses as well as its limitations.

Although the article is largely theoretical, it is extremely useful to the reader with regard to diseases of the pancreas, as well as to other disorders not discussed in this issue, and as such is a welcome addition.

Vitone, Greenhalf, Howes, Raraty, and Neoptolemos describe mutations in the trypsinogen gene that are related to pancreatitis. The phenotypic presentation of this hereditable form of pancreatitis is extremely variable, with some individuals presenting with severe acute pancreatitis followed by chronic disease, alternatively with milder later onset of the disorder and a small but significant number not suffering from the clinical disorder. Although the hereditary form constitutes approximately 1% of all cases of pancreatitis (acquired cases being induced by alcohol or gallbladder disease), it represents a fascinating entity worthy of further study. The biochemistry and mechanistic models that explain the connection between these mutations and the clinical presentation of hereditary pancreatitis are discussed in a separate chapter by Sahin-Toth.

Germline mutations and gene polymorphisms that are associated with human pancreatitits are outlined in the article by Weiss, Simon, Mayerle, Kraft, and Lerch and then discussed in more detail in the articles by Liddle (SPINK-1) and Vitone et al (trypsinogen).

An important article that introduces the topic of pancreatitis to the less knowledgeable reader is the one contributed by Ruthenberger, Mayerle, and Lerch, who describe the cell biology of pancreatic proteases. They discuss the cellular events following ductal obstruction, pancreatitis, and autodigestion. In addition, they describe sites of protease activation and the role of various enzymes such as trypsin and cathepsin B in digestive protease activation.

Liddle describes a newly identified association between SPINK mutations and pancreatitis. SPINK-1 protects the pancreas by inhibiting trypsin, and mutations in the SPINK-1 molecule may be associated with acute and chronic pancreatitis. However, the mutation is also found in the general population without pancreatitis. This suggests that SPINK-1 mutations are not sufficient to cause pancreatitits and that other genetic or environmental factors are necessary, making it a fascinating molecule for further study. The biochemistry and biology of SPINK-PST1 is presented by Graf and Bimmler in a separate article.

Type 2 diabetes is associated with two major pathologic features: the dysfunction of beta cells and insulin resistance. There are numerous genes and proteins that may be affected in each of these pathways, leading to this common disorder. Trajkovski, Miziaut, Schwarz, and Solimena cover the most commonly known genetic disorders of beta cells that are associated with type 2 diabetes. These susceptibility genes involve beta cell glucose metabolism, insulin gene expression, and insulin secretion.

Vaxillaire and Froguel address the genetic basis of maturity-onset diabetes of the young (MODY). Six subtypes have been identified with autosomal dominant mutations in single genes. These include glucokinase; hepatocyte nuclear factors 4α, 1α, and 1β; insulin promoter factor 1; and NeuroD1. Many of the MODY patients are from large family cohorts and this has helped with the identification of the gene mutation. Presentation before the age of 25 years is usually associated with beta cell dysfunction and clinically resembles type 2 diabetes. These forms of diabetes represent less than 5% of Caucasians with type 2 diabetes.

Maassen, Tafrechi, Janssen, Raap, Lemkes, and 't Hart discuss new aspects of the molecular biology of maternally inherited diabetes and deafness syndrome, a genetic disorder with a mutation in the mitochondrial DNA–encoded tRNA. The 3243A > G mutation is associated with a propensity of beta cells of the pancreatic islets to prematurely age, which results in beta cell dysfunction leading to a 100% penetrance and the development of diabetes. In addition to the beta cell aging, there is a reduction in insulin biosynthesis and insulin secretion.

As described in the article by Lewis, the notch and hedgehog signaling pathways are important for pancreatic development, and these pathways are reactivated in pancreatic tumors. In the common form, pancreatic ductal adenocarcinoma, activating mutations in KRAS, AKT oncogenes and inactivating mutations in p16, p53, and Smad4 have been found. In this article, Lewis presents work from his laboratory on an interesting mouse model of pancreatic cancer, supporting the role of these signaling pathways as pathogenic in this disease.

Brand and Lynch's article deals with the problems of genotype/phenotype aspects of rare disorders such as familial pancreatic cancer and suggests that any model requires the inclusion of environmental factors such as smoking on a polygenic model.

Familial pancreatic cancer is a rare (∼2%) component of pancreatic cancers and is discussed in the article by Habbe, Langer, Sina-Frey, and Bartsch. The occurrence of familial pancreatic cancer is seen in situations of genetic mutations resulting in conditions such as Peutz-Jeghers syndrome, familial multiple mole melanomas, hereditary breast and ovarian (BRCA 1 and 2) cancers, and ataxia telangiectasia, among others. Screening of family members in these high-risk families offers the best answer to early detection and perhaps reasonable management.

Simon, Spilcke-Liss, and Wallaschofski summarize our current understanding of endocrine tumors of the pancreas—both those secreting hormones as well as nonfunctioning tumors. They describe the clinical presentation, criteria, and tools for making an accurate diagnosis, as well as our knowledge regarding molecular aspects of the pathogenesis. Most significantly, they address the therapeutic approaches for those tumors that are not cured by surgery.

Although the syndromes and disorders discussed in this issue are not common, they represent examples of disease entities that have enabled investigators to gain insight into critical processes, both genetic and environmental, that are causative in the development of these diseases and will certainly pertain to more common diseases. For these and other reasons, including the clarity of the articles, this issue of the *Endocrinology and Metabolism Clinics of North America* should stand as an example to editors attempting to bring this type of information to our readers.

Derek LeRoith, MD, PhD
Division of Endocrinology and Diabetes
Department of Medicine
Mount Sinai School of Medicine
One Gustave L. Levy Place, Box 1055
Annenberg Building, Room 23-66B
New York, NY 10029-6574, USA

E-mail address: derek.leroith@mssm.edu

ELSEVIER
SAUNDERS

Endocrinol Metab Clin N Am
35 (2006) xix–xx

ENDOCRINOLOGY
AND METABOLISM
CLINICS
OF NORTH AMERICA

Preface

Molecular Basis of Inherited Pancreatic Disorders

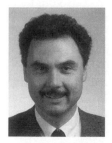   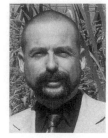   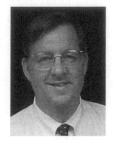

Markus M. Lerch, MD, FRCP   Thomas Griesbacher, MD   David C. Whitcomb, MD, PhD
Guest Editors

Progress in understanding the genetic basis of pancreatic disorders has been very rapid in recent years. This progress is marked by two important anniversaries. It is 20 years ago that the insulin receptor was cloned and 10 years to the day that the genetic basis of hereditary pancreatitis was solved—a discovery that has permitted research into the pathogenesis of pancreatitis in general to proceed in completely new directions. To update the current knowledge on the molecular basis of inherited pancreatic disorders affecting the endocrine and the exocrine portion of the organ, the present volume of the *Endocrinology and Metabolism Clinics of North America* was compiled.

Many of the advances involving pancreatic diseases that are detailed in this volume were organized and presented in preliminary form at the Fifth International Symposium on Inherited Diseases of the Pancreas held in Graz Austria in the summer of 2005 and sponsored jointly by the European Pancreatic Club and the North American Pancreatic Study Group. For the first time, this meeting brought together experts on endocrine disease with experts on exocrine pancreatic disorders to discuss recent developments in their fields. The meeting also provided the backdrop for the introduction of new and previously unpublished data, such as the discovery of mutations in the ubr1 gene as the cause of Johanson-Blizzard-Syndrome. One of the benefits of research into the genetic basis of pancreatic disorders is the fact that disease mechanisms identified in rare and often monogenetic disorders can lead to a much better understanding of pancreatic diseases in general.

This issue of the *Endocrinology and Metabolism Clinics of North America* is filled with practical information about the unusual as well as the common diseases of the pancreas, with a major focus on inherited forms of diabetes, pancreatitis, and cancer. Clinical and genetic aspects deal with early detection, phenotype-genotype correlation, and treatment. Also, new experimental disease models in which the pathophysiology of the respective disorders has been studied are introduced to the reader. Together, this volume represents the most important and up-to-date information on new aspects of pancreatic diseases that the editors could assemble.

The editors would like to thank all of the contributing authors for their gracious and prompt work, the speakers and contributors of the Fifth International Symposium on Inherited Diseases of the Pancreas, and the National Pancreas Foundation and Solvay Pharmaceuticals for providing unrestricted support to the symposium that served as a foundation for this volume.

Markus M. Lerch, MD, FRCP
Department of Gastroenterology, Endocrinology, and Nutrition
Ernst-Moritz-Arndt Universität
Greifswald
Friedrich-Loeffler-Str. 23A
17475 Greifswald
Germany

E-mail address: lerch@uni-greifswald.de

Thomas Griesbacher, MD
Institut für Experimentelle und Klinische Pharmakologie
Medizinische Universität Graz
Universitätplatz 4
A-8010 Graz
Austria

E-mail address: thomas.griesbacher@meduni-graz.at

David C. Whitcomb, MD, PhD
Division of Gastroenterology, Hepatology, and Nutrition
University of Pittsburgh
200 Lothrop Street, Mezzanine 2
Pittsburgh, PA 15213, USA

E-mail address: whitcomb@pitt.edu

Endocrinol Metab Clin N Am
35 (2006) 219–241

ENDOCRINOLOGY
AND METABOLISM
CLINICS
OF NORTH AMERICA

Developmental and Metabolic Disorders of the Pancreas

Markus M. Lerch, MD[a],*, Martin Zenker, MD[b],
Stefan Turi, MD[a], Julia Mayerle, MD[a]

[a]*Department of Gastroenterology, Endocrinology and Nutrition,
Ernst-Moritz-Arndt-University, Friedrich-Loeffler-Strasse 23A, Greifswald 17485, Germany*
[b]*Institute of Human Genetics, University of Erlangen-Nuremberg, Schwabachanlage 10,
91054 Erlangen, Germany*

The pancreas is an important exocrine and endocrine organ that develops from the dorsal and ventral anlagen during embryogenesis and arises from the endodermal lining of the duodenum within the first month of human embryonic life. A number of developmental disorders can either lead to anatomic abnormalities of the pancreas and its ducts, or can be part of complex disorders that affect multiorgan systems. Other genetic changes can lead to metabolic abnormalities that either affect the pancreas exclusively, as part of a multiorgan process, or that merely increase the lifetime risk for developing pancreatitis or pancreatic diabetes. This article reviews some of the developmental and metabolic disorders that can affect the endocrine and exocrine pancreas.

Development of the normal pancreas

During embryogenesis the pancreas develops from dorsal and ventral anlagen that arise from the endodermal lining of the duodenum. The dorsal anlage arises directly from the dorsal side of the duodenum before the 28th day of human embryonic life. The ventral anlage is located close to the bile duct and appears between 30 and 35 days of embryonic development. At Day 37, the ventral pancreas rotates counterclockwise around

The authors own studies are supported by grants from the DFG Le 625/7-1, Le 625/8-1, and HA 2080/5-1; Mildred Scheel Stiftung 10-2031-Le I; and Alfried Krupp von Bohlen und Halbach-Stiftung (Graduiertenkolleg Tumorbiologie).
* Corresponding author.
E-mail address: lerch@uni-greifswald.de (M.M. Lerch).

the duodenum and fuses with the dorsal pancreas. A failure of complete fusion (particularly of the ducts) results in the so-called "pancreas divisum" and a failure to rotate completely results in pancreas annulare, an abnormality that can lead to duodenal obstruction because of the resulting ring of pancreatic tissue around the duodenum. The ventral anlage gives rise to the processus uncinatus and part of the head of the pancreas, whereas the larger dorsal anlage predominantly forms the pancreatic tail [1]. The fusion of the two ductal systems is a complicated process and various different varieties of ductal anatomy can arise. The duct of the ventral anlage usually persists and forms the main pancreatic duct (duct of Wirsung) together with the distal portion of the dorsal anlage. The proximal portion of the dorsal duct may disappear or persist as the accessory pancreatic duct or the duct of Santorini [2].

Pancreas divisum

Pancreas divisum is the most common anatomic variant of the pancreas [2]. Its estimated incidence varies from approximately 4% to 14% in autopsy series and between 2% to 7% in endoscopic retrograde cholangiopancreatography studies. Because the prevalence of a pancreas divisium is the same in the healthy control population and patients with chronic pancreatitis it is no longer regarded as a risk factor for pancreatitis. Recent evidence even suggests that the prevalence of SPINK1 and cystic fibrosis transmembrane conductance regulator mutations, which are frequently associated with idiopathic pancreatitis, are just as common among chronic pancreatitis with pancreas divisum [3] as without. This suggests that chronic pancreatitis with pancreas divisum is essentially idiopathic pancreatitis with the same genetic risk factors. In pancreas divisium there is absent or incomplete fusion between the dorsal duct of Santorini and the ventral duct of Wirsung [2], resulting in most of the gland draining by the smaller duct of Santorini into the minor papilla. The pancreatic head and the processus uncinatus with less tissue mass and secretory load then drain by the duct of Wirsung through the larger papilla of Vater. Although this is usually harmless and drainage satisfactory, it can in patients with chronic pancreatitis add to the problem of impaired ductal flow. In these circumstances the question arises whether endoscopic sphincterotomy and stent insertion at the minor papilla is of benefit for the patient or can affect the natural history of chronic pancreatitis.

Pancreas annulare

The exact cause of pancreas annulare is not known but two hypotheses have been proposed. One of these predicts that the dorsal and the ventral anlage both undergo hypertrophy resulting in a complete ring around the duodenum with subsequent duodenal obstruction. A second hypothesis predicts that an abnormal adherence of the ventral duct to the duodenum before rotation causes the pancreatic ring. Roughly one half of all patients present in the neonatal period with duodenal obstruction. In this period diagnosis is often made by imaging techniques, such as CT or MRCP, but even abdominal ultrasound or a double-bubble sign on plain abdominal radiograph can be diagnostic. Patients in whom pancreas annulare becomes symptomatic later in life are sometimes diagnosed by endoscopic retrograde cholangiopancreatography. The differential diagnosis of duodenal obstruction should include duodenal atresia and intestinal volvulus. Annular pancreas is associated with other congenital anomalies in most cases. In infants these include duodenal stenosis or atresia in 40%, Down syndrome in 16%, tracheoesophageal fistulas in 9%, and congenital heart defects in 7% [4]. Agenesis of the dorsal pancreatic anlage [4], also known as "congenitally short pancreas," can also be associated with pancreas annulare.

It is expected that this disorder may be caused by a monogenic defect, the discovery of which is still pending. The short pancreas can occur as a solitary finding or in association with polysplenia syndrome, an entity in which only a pancreatic head is seen on imaging techniques and the body and tail of the organ are missing. Because most of the islet cells are located in the missing distal pancreas, patients with this anomaly have an increased risk of diabetes mellitus [2].

Ectopic pancreas

Ectopic pancreatic tissue is an aberrant focus of normally developed pancreatic tissue that lacks anatomic and vascular continuity with the main organ and can be found in various locations [5]. Autopsy studies suggest that ectopic pancreatic tissue is quite common (1% to over 13%) but its clinical manifestation is very rare [5]. Most ectopic pancreatic tissue is discovered endoscopically in the stomach (particularly antrum); duodenum; and jejunum. Other locations include the ileum, liver, spleen, biliary tract, mesentery, or umbilicus [2]. Most ectopic pancreas is anatomically located in the submucosa but some can be found in the muscularis or serosa. Ectopic pancreatic tissue can undergo similar changes as the pancreas proper, particularly cystic degeneration, pancreatic cancer formation, and even ectopic pancreatitis. The time point when patients with ectopic pancreatic tissue become symptomatic, however, is often the result of the mass effect, which can cause either obstruction of the intestinal passage where they reside or bowel intussusception.

Pancreatic agenesis

Primary agenesis of the pancreas represents a very rare disorder of the pancreatic development. Its exact incidence is not known. Absence of the pancreas does not only manifest postnatally with diabetes mellitus and malabsorption, it is also consistently associated with intrauterine growth retardation, which seems to relate to the fact that insulin is a major intrauterine growth factor. Pancreatic agenesis may occur as a monogenic condition (OMIM 260,370). A mutation in the gene for insulin promoter factor-1 (IPF1) was demonstrated in one patient affected by pancreatic agenesis [6]. Recently, an autosomal-recessive disorder comprising pancreatic and cerebellar agenesis was found to be caused by mutations in the gene PTF1A, encoding pancreas transcription factor 1α [7]. PTF1A is known to play a pivotal role in mammalian pancreatic development.

Beckwith-Wiedemann syndrome (OMIM 130,650)

The cardinal features of Beckwith-Wiedemann syndrome are exomphalos, macroglossia, and gigantism in the neonate. It is mentioned here because hypertrophy of the pancreas is an imaging feature and severe hypoglycemia of affected neonates is the most threatening early clinical complication of Beckwith-Wiedemann syndrome. The symptom triad was the origin of the acronym EMG syndrome (*e*xomphalos-*m*acroglossia-*g*igantism syndrome), used earlier as the preferred designation. Beckwith-Wiedemann syndrome patients are at increased risk of developing specific tumors. Beckwith-Wiedemann syndrome is caused by alterations of imprinted genes in the chromosome 11p15.5 region. Duplication or paternal uniparental disomy in this region seems to be involved in the pathogenesis, which is still incompletely understood. Most cases are sporadic. The mode of inheritance is complex. Possible patterns include autosomal-dominant inheritance with variable expressivity, de novo contiguous gene duplication at 11p15, and genomic imprinting defects of the maternally derived allele. The enlarged tongue, together with the omphalocele or other umbilical abnormalities, permits recognition of the disorder at birth. Because many of the affected infants have hypoglycemia in the first days of life, anticipation of this complication can prevent serious neurologic sequelae. Visceromegaly, adrenocortical cytomegaly, and dysplasia of the renal medulla are conspicuous features later in life. Adrenal carcinoma, nephroblastoma, hepatoblastoma, and rhabdomyosarcoma occur with increased frequency. The variable degree of visceromegaly can affect the kidneys, liver, pancreas, and adrenals. The long-term prognosis varies with the development of the intra-abdominal tumors and their degree of malignancy [8,9]. The short-term prognosis depends on the severity of neonatal hypoglycemia, and macroglossia, which can affect swallowing and may cause respiratory problems.

Shwachman-Diamond syndrome (OMIM 260400)

Shwachman-Diamond syndrome is an autosomal-recessive disorder with clinical features that include pancreatic exocrine insufficiency, hematologic dysfunction, and skeletal abnormalities. Shwachman-Diamond syndrome is the second-most common cause of exocrine pancreatic insufficiency in children and imaging features with replacement of pancreatic tissue by fat or diffuse fatty infiltration are rather characteristic [10,11]. Manifestations outside the pancreas sometimes concern the skeletal features (eg, metaphyseal dysplasia) but most often involve hematologic abnormalities including intermittent neutropenia. Affected patients are short in stature and most commonly suffer from diarrhea and failure to thrive. In contrast to cystic fibrosis sweat chloride concentration is normal. Although most of the pancreatic tissue is replaced by fat resulting in a variable degree of steatorrhea, which can even somewhat improve when the children get older, the islet cells of Langerhans and the ductal architecture remain largely intact. Neither diabetes nor pancreatitis are consistent features of Shwachman-Diamond syndrome. The disease is caused by germline mutations in an only recently characterized gene, SBDS (for the full name Shwachman-Bodian-Diamond syndrome) on chromosome 7q11 [12]. SBDS encodes a predicted protein of 250 amino acids. A pseudogene copy (SBDSP) with 97% nucleotide sequence identity resides in a locally duplicated genomic segment of 305 kilobase (kb). Interestingly, recurring mutations often (89%) result from gene conversion with at least one of two pseudogene-like sequence changes that result in protein truncations. SDBS is a member of a highly conserved protein family of unknown function with putative orthologs in diverse species including archaea and eukaryotes. The protein is most likely involved in RNA metabolism.

Pearson marrow pancreas syndrome (OMIM 557,000)

Pearson's syndrome is characterized by refractory sideroblastic anemia with vacuolization of marrow precursors and exocrine pancreatic dysfunction. Severe, transfusion-dependent, macrocytic anemia usually starts in infancy. In contrast to the Shwachman syndrome, the pancreas shows fibrosis in Pearson's syndrome; the disorders also differ in bone marrow morphology. Pearson's syndrome was found to be a mitochondrial disorder resulting from deletions of the mitochondrial DNA [13]. The disorder may be progressive and phenotypic shift from a predominantly hematopoietic disorder (Pearson's syndrome) to a disease with overt muscle dysfunction (mitochondrial myopathy) was repeatedly observed, with the eventual evolution to a full picture of Kearns-Sayre syndrome, depending on the distribution of deleted mitochondrial DNA [14].

Cystic disorders of the pancreas

By far most cysts in the pancreas are multiple cysts; pseudocysts (no true epithelial lining); and a complication of chronic pancreatitis. True single congenital cysts of the pancreas are extremely rare. They have a female pre-dominance and typically present as an asymptomatic palpable mass, or epi-gastric pain, jaundice, and vomiting [10] related to compression of surrounding visceral structures. These cysts are most commonly located in the tail and body of the pancreas [15] and are typically unilocular cysts with thin-walled cavities ranging in size from microscopic up to 5 cm in di-ameter. Ductal communication is rare. These cysts are usually anechoic on ultrasound and are low-attenuation cystic structures on CT studies with no wall enhancement. Associated congenital anomalies include renal tubular ectasia, polydactyly, anorectal malformations, polycystic kidneys, and as-phyxiating thoracic dystrophy [15]. Most congenital cysts with these symp-toms and clinical manifestations are diagnosed in children. When they are found in adults the differential diagnosis of chronic pancreatitis-associated cysts with cystic tumors of the pancreas (cystic adenomas and carcinomas, also more common in females) becomes an important and sometimes diffi-cult differential diagnosis.

Von Hippel-Lindau disease (OMIM 193300)

One of the inherited disorders associated with single or multiple cysts in different parenchymal organs including the pancreas is von Hippel-Lindau disease. Von Hippel-Lindau disease is an autosomal-dominant familial can-cer syndrome predisposing to a variety of malignant and benign neoplasms. It is caused by mutations in the VHL tumor-suppressor gene on chromo-some 3p25 but genetic changes in the cyclin D1 gene on chromosome 11q13 may further modify the phenotype. The incidence is estimated at 3 per 100,000 and affected patients are at risk of developing cerebellar, spinal, and retinal hemangioblastoma; renal cell carcinoma; pheochromocytoma; pancreatic neuroendocrine tumors; pancreatic and renal cysts; and epididy-mal cystadenoma. Von Hippel-Lindau disease has previously been classified as type 1 (without pheochromocytoma) and type 2 (with pheochromocy-toma) [16]. Other authors have subdivided von Hippel-Lindau disease fur-ther into type 2A (with pheochromocytoma) and type 2B (with pheochromocytoma and renal cell carcinoma). A von Hippel-Lindau disease register in the northwest of England has shown in 83 affected persons that the age at onset of first symptoms is 26 years, with cerebellar hemangioblas-toma being the most common presenting manifestation. The mean age at di-agnosis of von Hippel-Lindau disease was 31 years and the mean age at death was 41 years. The most common causes of death from von Hippel-Lindau disease are metastases from renal cell carcinoma and neurologic complications from cerebellar hemangioblastomas. Pancreatic lesions in von Hippel-Lindau disease include multiple cysts, serous cystadenoma, and islet cell tumors (see the article endocrine tumors of the pancreas else-where in this issue). Pancreatic carcinoma and adenocarcinoma of the am-pulla of Vater have also been reported. Pancreatic cysts are relatively common in von Hippel-Lindau disease, and involvement can range from a single cyst to multiple cysts, virtually replacing the pancreas. Cysts are reported in up to 30% of patients on imaging studies [10], but can be found in up to 72% in patients with von Hippel-Lindau disease at autopsy. Peripheral calcifications may also be present. These cysts may be the first indication of disease during routine screening and may precede any other manifestation of von Hippel-Lindau disease by several years.

Polycystic kidney disease (OMIM 263,200 and 173900)

Multiple congenital cysts of the pancreas can be present as part of a polycystic systemic disorder including autosomal-recessive and autosomal-dominant polycystic disease. Autosomal-recessive polycystic disease is caused by mutations in the PKHD1 (polycystic kidney and hepatic disease 1) gene on chromosome 6p12, a large gene spanning 470 kb of genomic DNA [17]. Micromutations in the 66 exons encoding the longest open reading frame have been described and account for about 80% of known cases. The disease presentation of autosomal-recessive polycystic disease is highly variable. In infancy, the disease results in significantly enlarged polycystic kidneys, with pulmonary hypoplasia resulting from oligohydramnios as a major cause of morbidity and mortality. Liver involvement is detectable in approximately half of infants and is often the major feature in adults indicating that collecting-duct ectasia in affected organs is a general feature and pathogenetic principle. This also explains the frequent association with Caroli's disease, a gross cystic dilatation of the intrahepatic biliary tree. Caroli's disease is a rare cause of chronic cholestasis and hepatolithiasis in young adults. Although some overlap may exist the development of pancreatic cysts is much more a feature of autosomal-dominant polycystic kidney disease. Autosomal-dominant polycystic kidney disease is a common condition affecting 1 in 800 live births from all ethnic groups. It results in progressive loss of renal function, with more than half of affected individuals requiring renal replacement therapy by the age of 60 or above. Overall, this one condition accounts for 8% of the renal dialysis population in some studies. The cardinal clinical manifestations are renal cysts, liver cysts, intracranial aneurysm, and pancreatic cysts. Genetic heterogeneity exists but mutations in one gene (PKD1 on chromosome 16p) are responsible for the most common form [18]. A second gene termed PKD2 located on chromosome 4 has also been recognized as underlying the disease, and at least another locus PKD3 must exist where the causative gene has not been so far identified.

The more variable features of the disease include hepatic and pancreatic cysts, hypertension, cardiac valvular abnormalities, and intracranial vascular malformations. The PKD1 gene product, polycystin-1, is an evolutionarily conserved 4302–amino acid protein that is predicted to contain a large N-terminal extracellular domain of approximately 2500 residues, several multiple transmembrane domains, and a short cytoplasmic C-terminal region. Immunolocalization demonstrates that the protein is expressed widely in a variety of epithelial cell types and is located at lateral cell membranes. Pancreatic cysts are present in about 10% of the patients and pancreatic involvement is typically less severe than renal and hepatic involvement.

Duplication cysts

Gastrointestinal duplication cysts are abnormalities of the developing foregut and have, as opposed to the pseudocysts seen in chronic pancreatitis, alimentary tract epithelial lining. Most of these cysts contain gastric mucosa or pancreatic tissue, and digestive secretions can facilitate hemorrhage within the cyst. Juxtapancreatic duplication cysts typically originate from the stomach or duodenum and may compress the pancreas. Rarely, the cysts may be sequestered within the pancreas itself [10]. Communication between the cyst and the pancreatic duct is uncommon.

Metabolic disorders

Acute and chronic recurrent pancreatitis has been reported in patients with a variety of inborn errors of metabolism. Among these are hyperlipidemia, various disorders of branched-chain amino acid degradation, homocystinuria, hemolytic disorders, acute intermittent porphyria, and several amino acid transporter defects. Some of these disease entities are exceedingly rare. In most of these disorders pancreatitis is not very common and, with the exception of lipoprotein lipase and apolipoprotein C-II deficiency, is neither the leading nor the clinically most distressing manifestation of the underlying metabolic defect. Most of these syndromes are inherited, however, and often entire kindreds are carriers of well-defined germline mutations that can, to varying degrees, be associated with pancreatitis. The clinical, biochemical, and genetic characteristics of those inborn errors of metabolism differ from those of other pancreatic disorders and they need to be distinguished from other hereditary causes of pancreatic diseases.

Pancreatitis caused by hyperlipidemia

Hyperlipidemia is one of the most common inherited causes of recurrent pancreatitis. A number of familial disorders, including lipoprotein lipase deficiency, apolipoprotein C-II deficiency, and common hypertriglyceridemia, can result in massive plasma accumulations of chylomicrons or triglycerides. Triglyceride levels above 2000 mg/dL are generally considered to put patients at a significant risk of developing pancreatitis.

Hereditary lipoprotein lipase deficiency (OMIM 246650)

Lipoprotein lipase is a glycoprotein serine esterase that forms homodimers at the luminal surface of endothelial cells. The human gene has 10 exons and is located on chromosome 8p22. Lipoprotein lipase activity at the endothelial membrane together with its cofactor apolipoprotein C-II, which is contained in chylomicrons, is major components in the processing of circulating lipoproteins. Lipoprotein lipase deficiency as a cause of hyperlipidemia was first reported in 1960, and in the meantime more than 30 disease-relevant mutations have been reported. The mode of inheritance is autosomal-recessive and the disease has a low incidence of 1 per 1,000,000, but is more frequent in parts of Canada and areas of the world where consanguinity is common. The first symptoms often arise in early childhood and the most common clinical presentation includes abdominal pain caused by recurrent attacks of pancreatitis, eruptive cutaneous xanthomatosis, and hepatosplenomegaly. Almost 30% of patients with lipoprotein lipase deficiency develop pancreatitis. Another characteristic clinical finding is the presence of eruptive xanthomas. These are lipid deposits in the patient's skin that most commonly affect the buttocks, knees, and extensor surfaces of the arms. They can become generalized but disappear over a period of months under effective lipid-lowering therapy. Recurrence of xanthomas is regarded as a sign that triglyceride-lowering therapy is inadequate.

Lipoprotein lipase deficiency should be suspected in hyperlipidemic patients when chylomicrons are detectable in refrigerated fasting plasma and no significant very-low-density lipoprotein elevation is found. The diagnosis of lipoprotein lipase deficiency can be made by measuring the enzyme activity in postheparin plasma (heparin releases the enzyme into the bloodstream) with a commercially available ELISA. Heterozygous carriers of mutations in the lipoprotein lipase gene generally have a lower catalytic activity than wild-type controls. The diagnosis can be confirmed by molecular genetic techniques, which identify the mutation. The disease is not associated with atherosclerotic vascular disease and its most prominent clinical feature is recurrent pancreatitis. The variety of pancreatitis associated with lipoprotein lipase deficiency is most often recurrent; sometimes severe and necrotizing; and only rarely leads to diabetes, pancreatic calcifications, or exocrine pancreatic deficiency. Young patients learn to prevent the abdominal pain by avoiding foods with high fat contents. The laboratory diagnosis of pancreatitis can be difficult because chylomicrons may interfere directly with the measurement of amylase, hemoglobin, and bilirubin. Amylase levels in patients with pancreatitis caused by lipoprotein lipase deficiency can be lower than expected or even normal, whereas hyperbilirubinemia (as seen also in Sieve's syndrome) can appear without clinical relevance.

The association between pancreatitis and hypertriglyceridaemia has long been known, but the former was long considered to be the cause of the latter. It is now well established that the opposite is true, and hyperlipidemia is regarded as a well-established cause of pancreatitis [19–21] and can account for up to one quarter of hospital admissions for pancreatitis [22–24]. The severity of pancreatitis in patients with lipoprotein lipase deficiency can vary greatly and is not always paralleled by a proportionate chylomicronemia.

Even patients with severe necrotizing pancreatitis have been admitted with normal or only mildly elevated amylase levels, because hyperlipidemia interferes with amylase measurements, leading to false-negative results [19,20,23–26].

The treatment of pancreatitis in these patients is not different from that with other causes of the disease, but an aggressive lipid-lowering therapy by dietary restriction of fat intake is paramount to prevent recurrence. Both animal and vegetable fat intake should be lowered to 15% of calories with the goal of lowering plasma triglyceride levels to below 1000 or 2000 mg/dL. Medium-chain triglycerides can serve as a substitute because they are not incorporated into chylomicrons after absorption. Parents of affected children need to be counseled about the benefits of medium-chain triglyceride fats and their initially inferior taste, and the fact that unsaturated and saturated fat must be restricted. Other important counseling factors are the requirements for extremely aggressive fat-lowering strategies during pregnancy; the futility of fat-lowering drugs; and the avoidance of agents that increase endogenous triglyceride levels, such as alcohol, estrogens, diuretics, isoretinoin, and β-blockers [27–33].

Apolipopopoprotein C-II deficiency (207750)

Apolipoprotein C-II deficiency is caused by mutations in the APOC2 gene, was first reported in 1978, is inherited as an autosomal-recessive disorder with a worldwide distribution, and results in an impaired clearance of chylomicrons from the blood. The gene for apolipoprotein II-C (APOC2) is located on chromosome 19 and has four exons. The enzyme belongs to a family of apolipoproteins with other known members, such as apolipoproteins E and C-I on chromosome 19 and apolipoproteins A-I, C-III, and A-IV on chromosome 11. Apolipoprotein C-II deficiency is less common than lipoprotein lipase deficiency, and more than 10 disease-relevant mutations in the apolipoprotein C-II gene have been reported. All affected patients were homozygous, although compound heterozygosity could also be disease-relevant. Apolipoprotein C-II is synthesized in the liver and secreted in great abundance into the plasma. The most prominent function of apolipoprotein C-II is that as an activator for lipoprotein lipase. The enzyme recycles between high-density lipoprotein and the triglyceride-rich lipoproteins, chylomicrons, and very-low-density lipoprotein and plays a gatekeeper function for lipid metabolism and energy storage. It regulates the hydrolysis of triglycerides in the core of lipoproteins, which results in free fatty acids.

Apolipoprotein C-II deficiency is generally diagnosed later than lipoprotein lipase deficiency in older children or young adults and the most frequent clinical presentation is that of recurrent episodes of pancreatitis. The diagnosis is made by measuring lipoprotein lipase activity in postheparin plasma as described previously or on gel electrophoresis of very-low-density lipoprotein apolipoproteins. A distinction from lipoprotein lipase deficiency can be readily made because the addition of apolipoprotein C-II to the assay completely restores lipolytic activity but does not affect the plasma of patients with lipoprotein lipase deficiency.

A transfusion of normal plasma into a patient with apolipoprotein C-II deficiency results in a rapid decrease in plasma triglyceride levels and can even be used therapeutically when aggressive lipid-lowering therapy is indicated for an episode of severe pancreatitis. Clinically, apolipoprotein C-II deficiency resembles lipoprotein lipase deficiency, but generally has a milder course and later onset of symptoms (between 13 and 60 years).

Pancreatitis represents a more frequent and sometimes severe complication of apolipoprotein C-II deficiency, however, and up to 60% of patients are affected by episodes of pancreatitis [34–36]. If lipid-lowering treatment is not initiated early, pancreatitis can result in chronic exocrine and endocrine pancreatic insufficiency. As in patients with lipoprotein lipase deficiency, premature atherosclerosis is not a clinical feature of the disease.

The treatment of apolipoprotein C-II deficiency is similar to that of lipoprotein lipase deficiency and consists in restricting the dietary intake of fat. The lipid-lowering therapy can often be less aggressive than for patients with lipoprotein lipase deficiency because of the milder phenotype and the less dramatic increase in plasma triglycerides. Heterozygote carriers have an approximately 50% reduction in apolipoprotein C-II activity, but because only 10% of apolipoprotein C-II is physiologically required for the clearance of chylomicrons from the plasma, these patients have normal circulating lipid levels.

Familial hypertriglyceridemia and chylomicronemia (OMIM 145750)

Several other disorders of lipid metabolism have been reported that can lead to either chylomicronemia or hypertriglyceridaemia and are not associated with defects in the lipoprotein lipase system. As shown for lipoprotein lipase deficiency and apolipoprotein C-II deficiency, they represent a significant risk factor for the development of acute or recurrent pancreatitis when plasma triglyceride levels rise above 2000 mg/dL. The incidence of patients with lipid disorders that result in such elevated triglyceride levels is estimated to be between 10 and 20 per 100,000 and is much higher than that of disorders caused by inborn errors of the lipoprotein lipase system. Often, the high triglyceride levels are not caused by the disorder alone, but are precipitated by additional factors, such as diabetes mellitus, alcohol use, β-adrenergic blockers, glucocorticoids and estrogens, diuretics, and other drug therapies. All of these factors can greatly increase the extent of hypertriglyceridemia and raise it above the threshold level for developing pancreatitis. The most common familial disorders associated with chylomicronemia are the type I and type V hyperlipoproteinemias (according to Levy and Fredrickson [36]). They comprise a diverse group of primary and secondary disorders with moderate to severe hypertriglyceridemia.

Individuals with monogenic familial hypertriglyceridemia are rare and often have only mild hypertriglyceridemia, and the previously mentioned additional factors are often required before the risk of developing pancreatitis becomes significant. Unrelated diseases that have been found to increase plasma lipids in these predisposed patients are plasmocytoma, systemic lupus erythematosus, and lymphomatous disease. In terms of therapy, most patients require a low-fat diet. In addition, and in contrast to lipoprotein lipase or apolipoprotein C-II deficiency, lipid-lowering drugs can be effective.

Glycogen storage disorders (OMIM 240600-306000)

In Europe, the incidence of glycogen storage diseases is approximately 1 per 20,000. The first patient with "hepatonephromegalia glycogenica" was described by von Gierke in 1928 (OMIM 232,200). Since that initial description, over 10 different disease varieties involving disturbances of glycogen metabolism have been described and they can present with a wide spectrum of clinical symptoms. The liver and striated muscles store most of the body's glycogen and are most commonly affected by inborn errors of glycogen metabolism.

Acute and chronic pancreatitis have been reported in patients with type I (von Gierke) glycogen storage disease [37–39]. The underlying mechanism for the development of pancreatitis in these patients is not known, but the most common biochemical changes in this disease variety include hypoglycemia, lactic acidosis, hyperuricemia, and hyperlipidemia, any of which could contribute to the onset of pancreatitis. Although the liver is most prominently affected (hepatomegaly caused by excessive storage of glycogen and fat), other organs, including the kidneys (nephrocalcinosis and proteinuria) and the intestinal mucosa (intermittent diarrhea), can be involved in addition to the pancreas. Most patients are diagnosed in early childhood (3–5 months) and present with hypoglycemia, lactic acidosis, or hepatomegaly. Fat and glycogen deposits can be detected in some patients as skin xanthomas over the arms and legs or as yellowish lesions on the retina. Impaired platelet aggregation leads to recurrent epistaxis and frequent bruising and may also contribute to a hemorrhagic course of acute pancreatitis. Clinical symptoms often deteriorate during pregnancy in affected women but fertility seems to be normal. Glycogen storage disorder type I is caused by a deficiency of glucose-6-phosphatase. The most frequent disorder is glycogen storage disorder Ia, caused by a defect in the glucose-6-phosphatase gene, whereas a glucose-6-phosphatase translocase is deficient in glycogen storage disorder Ib. Disease-causing mutations have been identified in both of these genes. The aim of therapeutic approaches is the maintenance of normal concentrations of blood glucose, because normoglycemia leads to a normalization of nearly all disease-associated abnormalities. In general, most affected patients receive frequent meals with a high carbohydrate content and restriction of galactose and fructose during the day and nocturnal nasogastric infusions, leading to an impressive improvement in the clinical outcome.

Branched-chain ketoaciduria (maple syrup urine disease,
OMIM 248,600)

Branched-chain ketoaciduria, or maple syrup urine disease (MSUD), is an autosomal-recessive disorder with an incidence of between 0.5 and 1 per 100,000 in the Western world. MSUD can be caused by mutation in at least four genes: (1) BCKDHA, (2) BCKDHB, (3) DBT, and (4) DLD. These genes encode the catalytic components of the branched-chain α-keto acid dehydrogenase complex, which catalyzes the catabolism of the branched-chain amino acids, leucine, isoleucine, and valine. Cases of MSUD have been reported from virtually every ethnic group and the incidence is much higher than indicated previously in countries where a ban on consanguineous marriages is not legally or socially enforced (some Middle Eastern and Asian nations). The highest rate of MSUD has been reported from isolated and highly inbred societies, such as Pennsylvania Mennonites and Amish (1 per 180). The first cases of central nervous degeneration and death in early childhood caused by deficient branched-chain amino acid metabolism were reported in 1954 by Menkes and coworkers [40], and because the urine of these children had a peculiar smell that was reminiscent of maple syrup or burned sugar, the disease was called "maple syrup urine disease." The odor was later found to be caused by urinary excretion of branched-chain keto acids (2,4-dinitrophenylhydrazones) derived from greatly elevated serum levels of the branched-chain amino acids leucine, isoleucine, and valine. This observation suggested that the catabolism of branched-chain amino acids was blocked and the respective α-keto acids (1-14C) did not undergo decarboxylation (branched-chain ketoaciduria).

Between the late 1970s and the late 1980s, not only the enzyme responsible for keto acid breakdown (branched-chain α-keto acid dehydrogenase) but also its molecular structure, composed of three catalytic components and two regulatory enzymes that are encoded by six genetic loci, were identified. A variety of deletions, insertions, and frameshift mutations in these loci have been found to be associated with the MSUD phenotype. Today, sequencing of the most commonly affected catalytic subunits E1a, E1b, E2, and E3 permits prenatal and carrier detection in many cases. Five clinical and biochemical phenotypes of branched-chain aminoaciduria are distinguished: (1) classic, (2) intermediate, (3) intermittent, (4) thiamin-responsive, and (5) dihydrolipoyl dehydrogenase–deficient MSUD. Patients with classic MSUD have the most severe phenotype. Because of the accumulation of leucine and ketoisocaproic acid, they present with a neonatal onset of encephalopathy, seizures, coma, and rapid weight loss, which leads to death if treatment is not initiated immediately and severe neurologic damage in surviving patients. Pancreatitis has been reported in patients with several organic acidemias, including MSUD [41,42].

Patients with intermediate MSUD have residual enzyme activity of up to 30% and, as a result of their milder phenotype, are often diagnosed later in childhood because of developmental delay or seizures. Patients with intermittent MSUD have a normal childhood development, grow normally, and develop a normal intelligence. Physiologically, they have normal laboratory values including branched-chain amino acid levels, but under stressful situations, such as infection or surgery, they can suffer acute metabolic decompensation. Thiamin-responsive and dihydrolipoyl dehydrogenase (E3)–deficient MSUD are both very rare and represent more complex clinical entities. MSUD is one of the few examples of the successful implementation of population-wide newborn screening to detect inherited metabolic disease. The formerly widely used Guthrie test, which was legally required in 20 countries and also in most states of the United States, is based on the observation that the growth of *Bacillus subtilis* is inhibited by 4-azaleucine under culture conditions with nutrient-depleted medium. Tandem mass spectrometry (MS/MS)–based amino acid profiling of dried blood spots obtained between 24 and 48 hours of life has made newborn screening with the Guthrie bacterial inhibition assay obsolete. This growth inhibition is reversed by the high leucine levels in the blood spot from a newborn with MSUD. The test detects only children with classic MSUD, the intermediate form, and E3 deficiency, but generally not those with the intermittent or thiamin-responsive forms of MSUD.

The life-threatening sequelae of MSUD can be largely prevented when treatment is initiated immediately following a positive test. Therapy options include rapid removal of toxic metabolites (ie, by hemodiafiltration); reversal of the patient's catabolism (insulin replacement and high-carbohydrate diet); and nutritional support, including branched-chain amino acid–free formulas. These principals also apply to patients with pancreatitis caused by MSUD [42]. Once the acute episode of clinical deterioration in an MSUD patient has been controlled, the long-term treatment includes a diet with restricted intake of branched-chain amino acids or supplementation of thiamin at pharmacologic doses. It needs to be remembered that diagnostic branched-chain amino acid levels in patients with intermittent MSUD are detected only during acute episodes and that these acute attacks are often exacerbated by infections, operations, or trauma. Although not applicable in most patients, orthotopic liver transplantation is a new treatment option with which this metabolic disorder can be fully corrected.

Homocystinuria caused by cystathionine β-synthase deficiency (OMIM 236200)

Cystathionine β-synthase (CBS) deficiency is a disorder of methionine degradation inherited in an autosomal-recessive manner that has been reported from all regions of the world with an estimated prevalence of between 1 per 20,000 and 1 per 1,000,000 The disease entity was initially reported in the early 1960s as homocystinuria and the enzymatic defect was later found to affect CBS. In terms of the underlying genetic alterations, a considerable heterogeneity seems to be present in different CBS-deficient families. The CBS gene was identified on chromosome 21q22.3 and more than 100 different disease-causing mutations have been identified so far. CBS is the key enzyme in the metabolism of methionine. Because of insufficient activity of CBS, there is an accumulation of homocysteine (an intermediate metabolite in the degradation of methionine) in the plasma of affected individuals (20- to 50-fold increase). Affected patients reveal a depletion of cysteine resulting in various biochemical abnormalities including the metabolism of glutathione.

A variety of clinical signs and symptoms have been reported to affect patients with homocystinuria caused by CBS deficiency. They predominantly involve the patients' eyes (eg, luxation or subluxation of the lens, myopia, retinal abnormalities); skeletal bones (osteoporosis, scoliosis, marfanoid stature); vascular system (recurrent and often severe thromboembolism, livedo reticularis); and central nervous system (mental retardation, psychiatric abnormalities, seizures). Other less frequently found signs are thin and brittle skin, endocrine abnormalities, and myopathy.

The major cause of morbidity and mortality in patients with CBS deficiency remains the thromboembolic events that can affect the vessels of any organ system including the brain, the coronary arteries, and pulmonary and peripheral arteries. On postmortem histology of CBS-deficient patients, almost every large- or medium-sized artery may be affected by marked fibrous thickening of the intima and frayed and split muscle and elastic fibers of the media. Lipid deposition is usually absent. The pancreatitis of patients with CBS deficiency [43–45] could correspond to the known vascularly induced varieties of the disease. Disturbance of glutathione metabolism might be another explanation, however, for the increased risk of pancreatitis. About 50% of patients with CBS deficiency respond to treatment with pharmacologic doses of pyridoxine, the cofactor of CBS, in combination with folic acid with a decrease or complete normalization of homocysteine, methionine, and cysteine plasma levels. B6-nonresponders have to be treated with a strict diet reduced in methionine and supplemented with cystine and betaine, the latter supporting remethylation of homocysteine.

3-Hydroxy-3-methylglutaryl–coenzyme A lyase deficiency
(OMIM 246450)

Pancreatitis has been repeatedly seen in organic acidurias caused by impaired degradation of leucine. One of these rare disorders is 3-hydroxy-3-methylglutaric aciduria, which is most commonly found in patients of Arabic parentage. It is inherited in an autosomal-recessive manner and thought to represent a monogenic disease. It was first reported in 1976 and its symptom onset typically begins either in the first days of life or later in infancy and childhood. Some patients remain asymptomatic throughout their lifetime. Patients present with metabolic acidosis and hypoglycemia, which can be characteristically associated with vomiting, hypotonia, and lethargy progressing to coma. The biochemical parameters may resemble Reye's syndrome. In metabolic acidosis, children typically do not develop ketosis because 3-hydroxy-3-methylglutaryl–coenzyme A lyase activity is deficient and is required for ketone formation. Half of the patients have hepatomegaly and elevated transaminases. The cause of pancreatitis in patients with 3-hydroxy-3-methylglutaryl–coenzyme A lyase deficiency is not known [46,47], but its onset may be related to either acidosis or hypoglycemia. Psychomotor retardation is common and probably secondary to severe or recurrent hypoglycemia. Diagnosis is confirmed by detecting a characteristic profile of organic acids of leucine catabolism in the urine (increase in urinary 3-hydroxy-3-methylglutaric acid, 3-methylglutaconic acid, 3-hydroxyisovaleric acid, or 3-methylglutaric acid).

Treatment during acute episodes of hypoglycemia consists of glucose infusions and the correction of acidosis. Patients are then fed a diet low in fat and leucine together with a high-carbohydrate diet. Patients should avoid extended fasting because of the associated hypoglycemia and fatty acid oxidation. During infection or following immunization, however, an increased protein catabolism results in elevated leucine metabolism. Under both conditions, a catabolic state must be avoided or aggressively treated. It should be mentioned that 3-hydroxy-3-methylglutaryl–coenzyme A lyase deficiency is but one example of inborn errors of branched-chain amino acid metabolism (examples of other organoacidiurias are methylmalonaciduria and propionaciduria) that can be associated with pancreatitis.

Acute intermittent porphyria (OMIM 176000)

Porphyrias are inherited or acquired disorders that affect specific enzymes required for the biosynthesis of heme, the critical component of hemoglobin, and lead to accumulation of porphyrin and porphyrin precursors. Acute intermittent porphyria is an autosomal-dominant disorder caused by a relative deficiency of the enzyme porphobilinogen deaminase (porphobilinogen ammonia-lyase [polymerizing] [EC 4.3.1.8]). Affected patients have only 50% of porphobilinogen deaminase activity compared with wild-type relatives. Most affected carriers of porphobilinogen deaminase mutations never develop the disease phenotype throughout their lives, and acute episodes of porphyria are usually triggered exogenously by fasting, stress, steroid hormones, and a multitude of pharmaceutical agents and drugs that induce hepatic microsomal cytochrome P-450 and δ-aminolevulinic acid synthase. The incidence varies between different parts of the world (5–10 per 100,000 for the mutation, 1–2 per 100,000 for the disease phenotype) but is highest among northern Europeans. If symptoms develop, they usually begin after puberty and more frequently affect women than men. The most prominent clinical symptoms involve the peripheral, autonomic, or central nervous system and result in neuropathy with a plethora of symptoms.

The great clinical variety of porphyria-associated neurologic and central nervous system symptoms is, unfortunately, still responsible for the fact that the prevalence among psychiatric patients remains higher than in the general population. Another leading clinical symptom during acute episodes of intermittent porphyria is severe abdominal pain, which can involve nausea and vomiting, diarrhea and constipation, ileus, back pain, and renal and hepatic dysfunction. Although episodes of acute pancreatitis associated with acute intermittent porphyria have been reported [48–52], they represent less a pathophysiologic dilemma than an important differential diagnosis. The symptoms of both diseases can overlap to a significant extent and distinguishing between them is important because it has therapeutic consequences. The diagnosis of acute intermittent porphyria is commonly made by demonstrating increased porphobilinogen, porphyrin, and δ-aminolevulinic acid levels in the patient's urine, which in 50% of cases has a red or brownish color. Therapy for an acute episode is initially symptomatic, with glucose or fructose infusions; induced diuresis; and, failing that, infusion of hemearginate, which suppresses δ-aminolevulinic acid synthase in the liver.

The human gene for porphobilinogen deaminase is located on chromosome 11q23 and contains 15 exons spread over 10 kb of DNA. Ten different mutations have so far been reported and have been grouped into four subclasses of structural changes. Two different enzyme isoforms are expressed, respectively, in erythrocytes and the liver. Molecular diagnosis is not usually required unless predictive testing for at-risk relatives is specifically asked for and should generally be discouraged for asymptomatic subjects. The critical advice for affected patients is to avoid stress, alcohol, and catabolic situations. Patients are regularly given a booklet of pharmaceutical agents with known porphyria-inducing potential, as can be found in almost every national drug formulary.

Pyruvate kinase deficiency (OMIM 266200)

Because erythrocytes have no mitochondria, they rely entirely on anaerobic glycolysis for energy generation. One of the critical enzymes involved in anaerobic glycolysis is pyruvate kinase. Pyruvate kinase deficiency is the most common erythrocyte enzymopathy and an autosomal-recessive disorder. Only homozygous and compound heterozygous carriers are clinically affected. Mutant alleles have been found at a frequency of between 0.1% and 6% in different populations. The disease has a worldwide distribution but is most common in northern Europeans and particularly prevalent among Pennsylvania Amish. Deficiency of pyruvate kinase results in impaired glycolysis and in a hereditary form of lifelong chronic hemolysis of variable severity. The characteristic symptoms are recurrent chronic jaundice, mild to moderate splenomegaly, and an increased incidence of gallstone disease. Symptoms usually begin in early infancy or childhood but some rare patients are diagnosed as adults. The diagnosis is made by demonstrating decreased erythrocyte pyruvate kinase activity, but an increase in the ratio of 2,3-diphosphoglycerate to ATP is already indicative of this specific enzymopathy. Pyruvate kinase has a broad range of molecular heterogeneity; most affected patients are compound heterozygotes because, most likely, homozygosity is potentially lethal. Pancreatitis can occur in patients with pyruvate kinase deficiency [53] and is most frequently caused by gallstones. Gallstone disease is very common in this group of patients and can develop as early as infancy.

Cystinuria OMIM (220100)

Cystinuria type I is caused by mutation in the SLC3A1 amino acid transporter gene located on chromosome 2p16.3. Cystinuria type III seems to be caused by mutation at a separate locus. Cystinuria is a rare inborn error of metabolism, and renal stones composed of cystine crystals were recognized as a disease entity in the nineteenth century. Cystinuria has a worldwide distribution with an incidence of between 1 and 10 per 100,000 but is found more frequently among North African Jews. Cystinuria is transmitted as an autosomal-recessive trait. The underlying mechanism is defective amino acid transport for the dibasic amino acids cystine, lysine, arginine, and ornithine, which mainly involves the epithelial cells of the kidneys and the gastrointestinal tract. The gene for the human sodium-independent transporter of cystine and dibasic amino acids (SLC3A1, or previously rBAT) encodes a protein of 680 amino acids and is located on chromosome 2q16-q21. More than 10 mutations and polymorphisms in different portions of the protein have been reported from unrelated kindreds. The predominant clinical feature of patients with cystinuria is the formation of radiopaque cystine stones in the urinary tract. Most patients are diagnosed with calculous kidney or urinary tract disease in their twenties or thirties, but some patients can be children or already in their eighties when they first develop symptoms. Often, the correct diagnosis in a patient with urinary calculi can be made by simple microscopy of the sediment of morning urine and the demonstration of the characteristic hexagonal cystine crystals. Acidification of the urine specimen precipitates cystine crystals and makes them easier to detect, and a cyanide-nitroprusside test has been widely applied as a chemical screening procedure. More sophisticated techniques include thin-layer chromatography, high-voltage electrophoresis, column amino acid analysis, liquid chromatography, and mass spectrometry to identify cystine and dibasic amino acids.

Urinary tract stones generally develop when the cystine excretion rate exceeds 300 mg/g of creatinine in acid urine, and therapy is directed at reducing cystine uptake and increasing cystine solubility in the urine. This is achieved by alkalinizing the patient's urine above pH 7.5 and diluting it by high oral fluid intake. If these measures are insufficient to prevent stone formation, treatment with D-penicillamine, N-acetyl-D-penicillamine, or mercaptopropionylglycine is considered, but troubling side effects including hypersensitivities, skin disorders, and epidermolysis must be anticipated. Angiotensin-converting enzyme inhibitors (ie, captopril) have therapeutic potential that needs to be further evaluated in clinical trials. Patients with cystinuria are susceptible to all complications of urinary stone disease including painful colics, recurrent infection, and chronic renal failure. They often require interventional removal of their calculi by lithotripsy or open surgery and a significant number of them become transplant recipients. Cystinuria has been associated with a variety of other disorders, including familial pancreatitis [54]. It is not clear whether this association is caused by cotransmission of one of the recently identified trypsinogen mutations that characterize hereditary pancreatitis, might indicate a de novo formation of pancreatic duct calculi in cystinuria, or is based on the known association between chronic renal failure and pancreatic disease [55,56].

Lysinuric protein intolerance (OMIM 222,700) and other cationic aminoacidurias

Lysinuric protein intolerance is a rare autosomal-recessive disorder that was first described in 1965. By far the highest incidence (1 per 60,000) is found among the Laplander population of Finland. The disease is characterized by postprandial hyperammonemia caused by a primary defect in the transport of the cationic amino acids lysine, arginine, and ornithine in the epithelial cells of the kidneys and gastrointestinal tract and secondarily by a disturbance of the urea cycle. Lysinuric protein intolerance has been found to be caused by mutations in the amino acid transporter gene SLC7A7, located on chromosome 14q.

Because of the increased urinary excretion and decreased intestinal absorption of cationic amino acids in general and of the essential amino acid lysine in particular, the bodies of patients with lysinuric protein intolerance are progressively depleted of these amino acids. Deficiency of ornithine subsequently leads to an impairment of the urea cycle. Affected patients experience periods of hyperammonemia and accordingly develop nausea and vomiting and avoid protein-rich foods. Newborns and infants after the breast-feeding period fail to thrive, and symptoms of protein malnutrition are further aggravated by lysine deficiency. Subsequently, patients develop hepatosplenomegaly; osteoporosis and bone fractures; sparse hair; muscle hypotonia; anemia and coagulopathies; and pulmonary, renal, and sometimes central nervous system disorders.

In patients with lysinuric protein intolerance, the plasma concentration of cationic amino acids in plasma is low and the concentrations of glutamine, alanine, serine, proline, citrulline, and glycine may be elevated. The urinary excretion of lysine is excessive and that of arginine and ornithine is also elevated. Serum ammonia increases after protein-containing meals but is normal under fasting conditions. Patients with lysinuric protein intolerance are treated with a protein-restricted and citrulline-supplemented diet and usually respond with an improvement of symptoms, although the aversion to dietary proteins remains. Patients with lysinuric protein intolerance–associated pulmonary disease, but not with renal complications, have been reported to respond to steroids.

Several cases of pancreatitis have been reported in patients with lysinuric protein intolerance, and the morphologic alterations in the pancreas can include inflammatory changes, necrosis, intraductal protein plugs, atrophy, and fibrosis [57,58]. The underlying defect is thought to be the severe protein deficiency, because similar pancreatic changes have been found in patients with kwashiorkor. In at least one kindred that was previously classified as having familial pancreatitis [59], the underlying cause may have been either primary lysinuric protein intolerance or coinheritance of lysinuric protein intolerance together with one of the other gene mutations that predispose to familial pancreatitis and are discussed elsewhere in this issue.

Summary

Most of the inborn errors of metabolism reviewed here are rare disorders. For a complete and extensive overview of their genetics, biochemistry, and clinical treatment, the reader is referred to the latest edition of the authoritative textbook of Scriver and coworkers [58]. In many of these diseases, pancreatitis is neither common nor is its pathogenesis well understood. Because many of these disorders "run in families" from regions of the world where consanguineous marriages are common, they should be kept in mind (and sometimes need to be ruled out) when patients with hereditary pancreatitis present with unusual clinical symptoms and signs. Particularly, the organic acidurias and inherited hyperlipidemia should be considered as a possible cause of recurrent pancreatitis. As far as the cystic and polycystic syndromes are concerned, their pathogenetic role in pancreatic disease is much more evident and straightforward. Genetic conditions and syndromes with specific relevance to the pancreas, such as hereditary pancreatitis, cystic fibrosis, von Hippel-Lindau disease, and Johanson-Blizzard syndrome are discussed in more detail elsewhere in this volume. Pancreatic changes associated with cationic trypsinogen mutations (hereditary pancreatitis) and cystic fibrosis transmembrane conductance regulator and SPINK1 mutations (idiopathic pancreatitis) are discussed in dedicated articles of this issue.

References

[1] Pictet RL, Rall LB, Phelps P, et al. The neural crest and the origin of the insulin-producing and other gastrointestinal hormone producing cells. Science 1976;191:191–2.

[2] Rizzo RJ, Szucs RA, Turner MA. Congenital abnormalities of the pancreas and biliary tree in adults. Radiographics 1995;15:49–68.

[3] Choudari CP, Imperiale TF, Sherman S, et al. Risk of pancreatitis with mutation of the cystic fibrosis Gene. Am J Gastroenterol 2004;99:1358–63.

[4] Skandalakis JE. The pancreas. In: Skandalakis J, Gray S, editors. Embryology for surgeons. Baltimore: Williams and Wilkins; 1994. p. 366–404.

[5] Prasad TR, Gupta SD, Bhatnagar V. Ectopic pancreas associated with a choledochal cyst and extrahepatic biliary atresia. Pediatr Surg Int 2001;17:552–4.

[6] Stoffers DA, Zinkin NT, Stanojevic V, et al. Pancreatic agenesis attributable to a single nucleotide deletion in the human IPF1 gene coding sequence. Nat Genet 1997;15:106–10.

[7] Sellick GS, Barker KT, Stolte-Dijkstra I, et al. Mutations in PTF1A cause pancreatic and cerebellar agenesis. Nat Genet 2004;36:1301–5.

[8] Beckwith JB. Macroglossia, omphalocele, adrenal cytomegaly, gigantism, and hyperplastic visceromegaly. Birth Defects 1969;5:188–96.

[9] Nijs E, Callahan MJ, Taylor GA. Disorders of the pediatric pancreas: imaging features. Pediatr Radiol 2005;35:358–73.

[10] Johnson PR, Spitz L. Cysts and tumors of the pancreas. Semin Pediatr Surg 2000;9: 209–15.

[11] Lacaille F, Mani TM, Brunelle F, et al. Magnetic resonance imaging for diagnosis of Schwachman's syndrome. J Pediatr Gastroenterol Nutr 1996;23:599–603.

[12] Boocock GRB, Morrison JA, Popovic M, et al. Mutations in SBDS are associated with Shwachman-Diamond syndrome. Nat Genet 2003;33:97–101.

[13] Rotig A, Colonna M, Bonnefont JP, et al. Mitochondrial DNA deletion in Pearson's marrow/pancreas syndrome. Lancet 1989;1:902–3.

[14] Krauch G, Wilichowski E, Schmidt KG, et al. Pearson marrow-pancreas syndrome with worsening cardiac function caused by pleiotropic rearrangement of mitochondrial DNA. Am J Med Genet 2002;110:57–61.

[15] Auringer ST, Ulmer JL, Sumner TE, et al. Congenital cyst of the pancreas. J Pediatr Surg 1993;28:1570–1.

[16] Neumann HPH, Wiestler OD. Clustering of features of von Hippel-Lindau syndrome: evidence for a complex genetic locus. Lancet 1991;337:1052–4.

[17] Ward CJ, Hogan MC, Rossetti S, et al. The gene mutated in autosomal recessive polycystic kidney disease encodes a large, receptor-like protein. Nat Genet 2002;30:259–69.

[18] Hughes J, Ward CJ, Peral B, et al. The polycystic kidney-disease-1 (PKD1) gene encodes a novel protein with multiple cell recognition domains. Nat Genet 1995;10:151–60.

[19] Brunzell JD, Schrott HG. The interaction of familial and secondary causes of hypertriglyceridemia: role in pancreatitis. Trans Assoc Am Physicians 1973;86:245–54.

[20] Siafakas CG, Brown MR, Miller TL. Neonatal pancreatitis associated with familial lipoprotein lipase deficiency. J Pediatr Gastroenterol Nutr 1999;29:95–8.

[21] Wilson DE, Hata A, Kwong LK, et al. Mutations in exon 3 of the lipoprotein lipase gene segregating in a family with hypertriglyceridemia, pancreatitis, and non-insulin-dependent diabetes. J Clin Invest 1993;92:203–11.

[22] Cameron JL, Capuzzi DM, Zuidema GD, et al. Acute pancreatitis with hyperlipidemia: the incidence of lipid abnormalities in acute pancreatitis. Ann Surg 1973;177:483–9.

[23] Farmer RG, Winkelman EI, Brown HB, et al. Hyperlipoproteinemia and pancreatitis. Am J Med 1973;54:161–5.

[24] Toskes PP. Hyperlipidemic pancreatitis. Gastroenterol Clin North Am 1990;19:783–91.

[25] Greenberger NJ, Hatch FT, Drummey GD, et al. Pancreatitis and hyperlipemia: a study of serum lipid alterations in 25 patients with acute pancreatitis. Medicine (Baltimore) 1966;45: 161–8.

[26] Dominguez-Munoz JE, Malfertheiner P, Ditschuneit HH, et al. Hyperlipidemia in acute pancreatitis: relationship with etiology, onset and severity of the disease. Int J Pancreatol 1991;10:261–7.

[27] Howard JM, Ehrlich E, Spitzer JJ, et al. Hyperlipemia in patients with acute pancreatitis. Ann Surg 1964;160:210–8.

[28] Fallat RW, Vestor JW, Glueck CJ. Suppression of amylase activity by hypertriglyceridemia. JAMA 1973;225:1331–4.

[29] Sharma P, Lim S, James D, et al. Pancreatitis may occur with a normal amylase concentration in hypertriglyceridaemia. BMJ 1996;313:1265.

[30] Flynn WJ, Freeman PG, Wickboldt LG. Pancreatitis associated with isotretinoin-induced hypertriglyceridemia. Ann Intern Med 1987;107:63.

[31] Lesser PB, Warshaw AL. Diagnosis of pancreatitis masked by hyperlipemia. Ann Intern Med 1975;82:795–8.

[32] Fortson MR, Freedman SN, Webster PD III. Clinical assessment of hyperlipidemic pancreatitis. Am J Gastroenterol 1995;90:2134–9.

[33] Warshaw AL, Bellini CA, Lesser PB. Inhibition of serum and urine amylase activity in pancreatitis with hyperlipemia. Ann Surg 1975;182:72–5.

[34] Breckenridge WC, Little JA, Steiner G, et al. Hypertriglyceridemia associated with deficiency of apolipoprotein C–II. N Engl J Med 1978;298:1265–73.

[35] Cox DW, Breckenridge WC, Little JA. Inheritance of apolipoprotein C–II deficiency with hypertriglyceridemia and pancreatitis. N Engl J Med 1978;299:1421–4.

[36] Levy RI, Fredrickson DS. Familial hyperlipoproteinemia. In: Stanbury JB, Wyngaarden JB, Fredrickson DS, editors. The metabolic basis of inherited disease. 3rd edition. New York: McGraw-Hill; 1972. p. 545.

[37] Michels VV, Beaudet AL. Hemorrhagic pancreatitis in a patient with glycogen storage disease type I. Clin Genet 1980;17:220–2.

[38] Kikuchi M, Hasegawa K, Handa I. Chronic pancreatitis in a child with glycogen storage disease type I. Eur J Pediatr 1991;150:852–3.

[39] Herman TE. Type IA glycogenosis with acute pancreatitis. J Radiol 1995;76:51–3.

[40] Menkes JH, Hurst PL, Craig JM. A new syndrome: progressive familial infantile cerebral dysfunction associated with an unusual urinary substance. Pediatrics 1954;14:462–7.

[41] Friedrich CA, Marble M, Maher J, et al. Successful control of branched-chain amino acids (BCAA) in maple syrup urine disease using elemental amino acids in total parenteral nutrition during acute pancreatitis. Am J Hum Genet 1992;51:A350.

[42] Kahler SG, Sherwood WG, Woolf D, et al. Pancreatitis in patients with organic acidemias. J Pediatr 1994;124:239–43.

[43] Collins JE, Brenton DP. Pancreatitis and homocystinuria. J Inherit Metab Dis 1990;13:232–3.

[44] Makins RJ, Gertner DJ, Lee PJ. Acute pancreatitis in homocystinuria. J Inherit Metab Dis 2000;23:190–1.

[45] Ilan Y, Eid A, Rivkind AI, et al. Gastrointestinal involvement in homocystinuria. J Gastroenterol Hepatol 1993;8:60–2.

[46] Muroi J, Yorifuji T, Uematsu A, et al. Cerebral infarction and pancreatitis: possible complications of patients with 3-hydroxy-3-methylglutaryl-CoA lyase deficiency. J Inherit Metab Dis 2000;23:636–7.

[47] Wilson WG, Cass MB, Sovik O, et al. A child with acute pancreatitis and recurrent hypoglycemia due to 3-hydroxy-3-methylglutaryl-CoA lyase deficiency. Eur J Pediatr 1984;142:289–91.

[48] Lam J, Loyola ME, Contreras L. High lipase level in a patient with porphyria crisis: cause of confusion with acute pancreatitis. Rev Med Chil 1996;124:1273–4.

[49] Shiraki K, Takase K, Tameda Y, et al. Acute pancreatitis associated with acute intermittent porphyria. Nippon Rinsho 1995;53:1479–83.

[50] Shiraki K, Matsumoto H, Masuda T, et al. A case of acute intermittent porphyria with acute pancreatitis. Gastroenterol Jpn 1991;26:90–4.

[51] Mustajoki P. Acute intermittent porphyria and acute pancreatitis. Gastroenterology 1977;72:1368.

[52] Kobza K, Gyr K, Neuhaus K, et al. Acute intermittent porphyria with relapsing acute pancreatitis and unconjugated hyperbilirubinemia without overt hemolysis. Gastroenterology 1976;71:494–6.

[53] Mahour GH, Lynn HB, Hill RW. Acute pancreatitis with biliary disease in erythrocyte pyruvate-kinase deficiency: case report and comments on management. Clin Pediatr (Phila) 1969;8:608–10.

[54] Gross JB, Ulrich JA, Jones JD. Urinary excretion of amino acids in a kindred with hereditary pancreatitis and aminoaciduria. Gastroenterology 1964;47:41–5.

[55] Lerch MM, Riehl J, Mann H, et al. Sonographic changes of the pancreas in chronic renal failure. Gastrointest Radiol 1989;14:311–4.

[56] Lerch MM, Hoppe-Seyler P, Gerok W. Origin and development of exocrine pancreatic insufficiency in experimental renal failure. Gut 1994;35:401–7.

[57] Gmaz-Nikulin E, Nikulin A, Plamenac P, et al. Pancreatic lesions in shock and their significance. J Pathol 1981;135:223–36.

[58] Klujber V, Klujber L. Hereditary pancreatitis. Orv Hetil 1989;130:1777–8.

[59] Scriver CR, Sly DS, Childs B, et al, editors. The metabolic and molecular bases of inherited disease. 8th edition. New York: McGraw-Hill; 2000.

**ELSEVIER
SAUNDERS**

Endocrinol Metab Clin N Am
35 (2006) 243–253

ENDOCRINOLOGY
AND METABOLISM
CLINICS
OF NORTH AMERICA

Genetic Basis and Pancreatic Biology of Johanson-Blizzard Syndrome

Martin Zenker, MD[a],*, Julia Mayerle, MD[b],
André Reis, MD[a], Markus M. Lerch, MD[b]

[a]*Institute of Human Genetics, University of Erlangen-Nuremberg, Schwabachanlage 10,
91054 Erlangen, Germany*
[b]*Department of Gastroenterology, Endocrinology and Nutrition,
Ernst-Moritz-Arndt-University, Freidrich-Löffler-Strasse 23A, 17487 Greifswald, Germany*

Johanson-Blizzard syndrome (JBS; OMIM 243,800) is a rare genetic disorder with a unique combination of congenital abnormalities. The condition is characterized by the association of congenital exocrine pancreatic insufficiency and hypoplasia or aplasia of the nasal wings (Fig. 1A). In addition, there are a number of variable abnormalities present in a high proportion of patients, including short stature ($>80\%$); tooth abnormalities (mainly oligodontia $>80\%$); sensorineural hearing loss (80%); mental retardation (77%); scalp defects (76%); hypothyroidism (40%); imperforate anus (39%); and genitourinary malformations (38%) (Fig. 1B, C) (reviewed in [1,2]). Mental retardation is moderate to severe in most JBS patients, but normal intelligence has been reported in some instances [2,3]. JBS was first described as a separate entity in 1971 [4], and more than 60 cases have been reported. Besides the predominance in populations with a high rate of consanguineous marriages, JBS cases have been reported from all over the world. The incidence of JBS has not been determined systematically. In a European population-based study on imperforate anus [5] including 4.6 million live births, however, seven JBS cases were mentioned. Considering that imperforate anus occurs in approximately 40% of JBS patients, this gives a rough estimate of the incidence of JBS at around 1 per 250,000.

Exocrine pancreatic insufficiency is a constant feature of JBS, rendering this disorder a potential model for genetic pancreatic disease. A small

This work was supported by grant No. ZE 524/2 from the German Research Foundation and a grant from the Marohn Foundation of the University Erlangen-Nuremberg to M.Z., and by grants from the DFG and the Deutsche Krebshilfe to M.M.L. and J.M.

* Corresponding author.
E-mail address: mzenker@humgenet.uni-erlangen.de (M. Zenker).

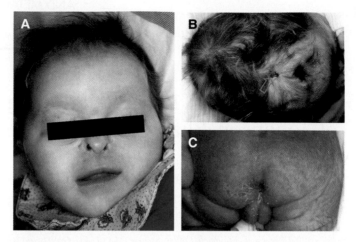

Fig. 1. Clinical phenotype of JBS. (*A*) Typical facial appearance of JBS with aplasia of the nasal wings in an 8-month-old girl. Scalp defect (*B*) and imperforate anus (*C*) in the same child as a newborn.

number of reports describing autopsy findings of children with JBS at different ages uniformly state that there is a seemingly selective defect of acinar tissue, whereas islets of Langerhans and ducts are quite well preserved [6–8]. The cause of this acinar cell loss has remained elusive. The morphologic findings correspond to an almost complete absence of zymogens from duodenal juice, whereas bicarbonate secretion was much less impaired and in contrast to patients suffering from cystic fibrosis [9]. Diabetes has been reported in several instances of JBS, mostly in older children, suggesting a somewhat progressive course of pancreatic disease [10,11].

Positional cloning of the gene underlying Johanson-Blizzard syndrome

A genome-wide linkage analysis using a panel of microsatellite markers with average distance of 10 cM (Weber panel Version 10, Research Genetics) and subsequent fine mapping identified a region of homozygosity on chromosome 15q14-q21 that was shared by all affected individuals originating from five unrelated consanguineous JBS families (Fig. 2). The maximum two-point lod score was 4.8 in a candidate region that comprised an approximately 7.5-cM interval between the flanking markers D15S1012 and D15S659. This region still contained more than 120 known genes. No obvious candidate gene was identified in the linkage interval. High throughput direct sequencing of positional candidates in JBS patients eventually detected mutations in the gene *UBR1* [12]. *UBR1* is a rather large gene that spans approximately 161 kilobases, contains 47 exons, and encodes the homonymous protein UBR1. Of the original study group comprising JBS patients from 13 families, the variations likely to be causal mutations could

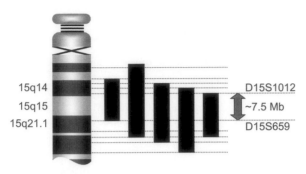

Fig. 2. Homozygosity mapping of JBS to chromosome 15. Partial ideogram of chromosome 15 and the respective regions of homozygosity (represented as black bars) in five unrelated consanguineous JBS families. The shared region of homozygosity (JBS candidate region) is flanked by the markers D15S1012 and D15S659.

be identified on both alleles of *UBR1* in 12 pedigrees. In one family (family 8, Table 1), only one mutation was found suggesting that the second mutation might be located in noncoding regions (eg, promotor) that were not sequenced. These results clearly indicate that JBS is not heterogeneous. Remarkably, most disease-associated *UBR1* mutations (12 of 14) predict premature translational stop codons (see Table 1), suggesting that a complete loss of UBR1 function is the mechanism underlying most cases of JBS. Two *UBR1* missense mutations detected in JBS patients affect conserved amino acid residues of the UBR1 protein, providing circumstantial evidence that they also perturb the activity of UBR1 [12]. None of the mutations was detected in a large number of controls.

In accordance with the mutational spectrum, investigations with specific antibodies against human UBR1 proved the complete lack of UBR1 protein expression in different tissues (fibroblasts, lymphocytes, pancreas) derived from patients with JBS [12].

Known function of the *UBR1* gene product

The UBR1 protein encoded by *UBR1* acts as an ubiquitin (Ub) ligase. Ubiquitylation and subsequent degradation of proteins at the proteasome is the universal mechanism for regulated protein degradation and control of the levels of many intracellular proteins [13,14]. A ubiquitylated protein bears a covalently linked poly-Ub chain, and is degraded by the 26S proteasome [13]. Substrates of the Ub system are conjugated to Ub through the action of three enzymes: (1) E1 (Ub activating enzyme); (2) E2 (Ub conjugating enzyme); and (3) E3 (Ub ligase). The latter represent an exceptionally large and heterogeneous group of proteins [13,14]. The ubiquitin ligases (E3) specifically recognize a substrate's degradation signal (degron) [13,15], conferring the selectivity of ubiquitylation. Of the large number of Ub ligases, some have already been implicated in the pathogenesis of various human

Table 1
UBR1 mutations observed in JBS patients from 13 families

Family	Nucleotide alterations	Exon	Predicted consequences on protein	Status
1	c.1648C→T	14	Premature stop codon: Q550X	Homozygous
2	c.1759C→T	15	Premature stop codon: Q587X	Homozygous
3	c.1537C→T	13	Premature stop codon: Q513X	Homozygous
4	c.1537C→T	13	Premature stop codon: Q513X	Homozygous
5	c.407A→G	3	Substitution of conserved residue: H136R	Compound
	IVS20+2T→C	20	Abnormal splicing	Heterozygous
6	IVS21+1G→C	2	Abnormal splicing	Homozygous
7	IVS5-2delAG	6	Abnormal splicing	Compound
	c.3835G→A	35	Substitution of conserved residue: G1279S	Heterozygous
8	c.2547insA	27	Frameshift and premature stop: M849fsX861	Heterozygous[a]
9	c.4927	45	Premature stop codon: E1643X	Homozygous
10	c.477delT	4	Frameshift and premature stop: T159fsX164	Homozygous
11	c.753-754delTG	6	Premature stop codon: C251X	Homozygous
12	IVS9-12A→G	10	Abnormal splicing	Homozygous
13	c.2598delA	28	Frameshift and premature stop: P866fsX878	Homozygous

[a] Mutation on the second allele was not identified in this family.

genetic diseases. These include Angelman's syndrome (OMIM 105,830), a nonprogressive mental retardation syndrome (UBE3A); autosomal-recessive juvenile parkinsonism (OMIM 600,116) (parkin); von Hippel-Lindau disease (OMIM 193,300) (VHL protein); and others (reviewed in [13,14,16]).

UBR1 belongs to one important branch of the Ub-proteasome system called the N-end rule pathway [15,17–22]. This highly conserved pathway is aimed at the recognition and ubiquitylation of target proteins with specific (destabilizing) amino acids at their N-terminus, relating the in vivo half-life of a protein to the identity of its N-terminal residue [15,17,18,21]. It has a hierarchic structure, where some N-terminal residues are enzymatically modified before their recognition by the pathway's Ub ligases, including UBR1. Previously known functions of the N-end rule pathway include the control of peptide import (through conditional degradation of import's repressor); the regulation of apoptosis (through degradation of a caspase-processed inhibitor of apoptosis); the fidelity of chromosome segregation (through degradation of a conditionally produced fragment of cohesion); and regulation of meiosis and cardiovascular development [17–21]. The N-end rule pathway is probably responsible for the bulk of constitutive and conditional protein degradation in cells. It is present in all cells and species, even in prokaryotes.

Mammalian UBR1 contains distinct binding sites for basic (type 1) and bulky hydrophobic (type 2) N-terminal residues of substrates, and a third binding site for substrates bearing internal (non–N-terminal) degrons [15,17,18,20,21]. The family of mouse (and human) UBR proteins, which contain a common substrate-binding domain termed the "UBR box," was found to consist of at least four E3s, including UBR1 and UBR2 [21].

It is evident that the latter have very similar substrate-binding properties, hence providing functional redundancy of the system [18,20]. Considering the functional properties of the N-end rule pathway, it can be assumed that almost every protein of which the original (stabilizing) N-terminal Met-residue has been removed by either nonspecific degradation steps or specific cleavage may become a target of the N-end rule pathway.

UBR1 is expressed in many tissues with the most prominent expression in skeletal muscle in mice. It has now been shown that in humans pancreatic expression is almost as high as in muscle. In the pancreas, UBR1 is mainly found in the cytoplasm of acinar cells [12].

Consequences of UBR1-deficiency on human pancreas

Because the exocrine pancreas is the most consistently affected organ in JBS, UBR1 has to be considered to play a critical role in either development or maintenance of acinar cells. New insights in the probable pathogenesis of the pancreatic defect in JBS have emerged from morphologic and cell biologic studies on pancreas derived from fetuses affected by JBS. It could be demonstrated that the primary development is apparently normal. Later in prenatal life (presumably coinciding with the appearance of mature zymogen granules) massive acinar cell loss, hyperemia, and leukocyte infiltration occurred. Still, at the age of 34 weeks of gestation, some apparently intact acini could be found, whereas in newborns and young infants exocrine cells had almost vanished and the inflammatory reaction had resolved, leaving a pancreas that contains some ducts and islets, whereas acinar parts are largely replaced by adipose and connective tissue (Fig. 3). To study the nature of acinar cell loss in JBS, pancreas from patients and controls was examined by 3OH-knick-end-labeling, a widely used marker for apoptosis. Surprisingly, almost no apoptotic cells were seen in remaining acinar cells and connective tissue of the pancreas from a premature JBS patient. In contrast, apoptosis was seen occasionally in acinar cells and abundantly in interspersed mesenchymal cells in pancreas from non-JBS control premature newborns (Fig. 4A–C). Apoptosis is assumed to be the leading mechanism to replace the connective tissue by exocrine cells. The replacement of mesenchymal tissue has been reported before to follow a linear increase in the ratio of acinar cells to connective tissue during gestation and postnatal life [23]. In contrast to the absence of apoptotic changes, remaining acinar cells in pancreas from a premature newborn with JBS showed ultrastructural signs of necrosis (Fig. 4D). Together these findings suggest that the destruction of the pancreas in JBS is caused by necrotic acinar cell loss resembling a severe destructive pancreatitis of intrauterine onset. This may implicate UBR1 in the defense of acinar cells against noxious stimuli. The apparent predisposition of JBS patients for the development of diabetes during adolescence may reflect an ongoing destructive process, eventually also affecting the islets.

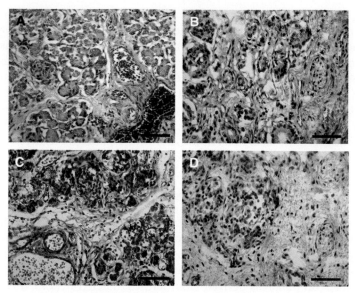

Fig. 3. Characterization of human pancreas in JBS. Hematoxylin-eosin (H & E)–stained paraf-
fin sections of the fetal pancreas of a control (*A*, 34 weeks of gestation) and of JBS fetuses and
newborns at different gestational ages (21 weeks, 34 weeks, and term newborn) (*B–D*). (*B*) H & E
staining in the JBS patient at 21 weeks of gestation shows normal development of pancreatic
acinar cells and the lack of eosin staining is indicative for the absence of proteases at this stage
of organ development. (*C*) At 34 weeks of gestation large areas of loss of the acinar tissue, hy-
pervascularization, depositions of connective tissue, and prominent inflammatory infiltrates
can be seen. Note that remaining pancreatic acini display an apparently normal architecture.
The age-matched control is shown in *A*. (*D*) In contrast, the pancreas of a term newborn has
few areas of remaining acini, and the parenchyma is largely replaced by connective tissue. Size
bars indicate 250 μm (original magnification 200-fold).

Phenotype of *ubr1* knockout mice

An *ubr1* knockout mouse model had already been published in 2001 [18].
Notably, despite the normally ubiquitous expression of UBR1, these mice
were viable, fertile, and did not display congenital malformations reminiscent of JBS or morphologic abnormalities of internal organs, including
the pancreas. The only physical differences compared with wild-type mice
were confined to a 10% to 20% reduction in weight (with disproportionate
decreases of skeletal muscle and adipose tissue) and some behavioral abnormalities. Some more detailed investigations done in these mice might suggest
metabolic abnormalities that are compatible with a nutritional deficit, but
this could not be substantiated [18]. After the identification of *UBR1* as
the gene responsible for JBS, pancreatic morphology and function were
re-evaluated in *ubr1* knockout mice. Although it was confirmed that these
animals have a reduced weight (Fig. 5A) and normal histomorphologic
and ultrastructural appearance of the pancreas under control conditions,

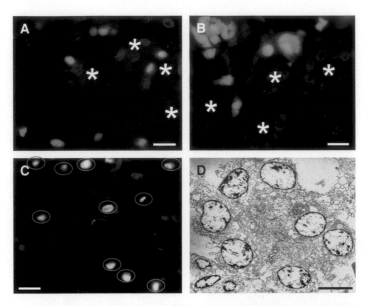

Fig. 4. Apoptosis versus necrosis in human JBS pancreas. To discriminate whether organ de-struction was caused by apoptosis, labeling of free 3-OH-DNA termini was performed using the terminal deoxynucleotidyl transferase method with fluorescein-labeled digoxigenin nucleo-tides staining apoptotic nuclei in yellow. DAPI counterstain of nuclei (blue). Autofluorescence of erythrocytes is displayed in green. In control sections from a fetus at 34 weeks of gestation apoptosis rate was around 1% in pancreatic acinar cells (*A*). In contrast, in pancreatic tissue from a JBS patient of the same gestational age no apoptotic cells were present in both remaining pancreatic acini (*asterisks*) and mesenchymal cells (*B*). Remarkably, nearly 30% of mesenchymal cells of the control display free 3-OH-DNA termini, consistent with the fact that turnover in mesenchymal cells in a normally developing fetal pancreas is driven by apoptosis (*C*). Electron microscopy of acinar cells in the premature JBS newborn (34. week gestational age) show ultra-structural characteristics of necrosis. Those are progressive cellular hydration, which results in membrane discontinuities, and disruption of the intracellular organelles. In comparison with apoptosis where nuclei show chromatin margination and the plasma membrane and organelles remain intact, the nuclei in necrosis represent the only stable cellular structure and the mem-branes of organelles become disrupted rapidly, as seen in *D*.

specific testing for fecal chymotrypsin and elastase activity indicated a signif-icantly reduced zymogen excretion suggesting that the obvious nutritional deficit might stem at least in part from exocrine pancreatic insufficiency [12]. By measuring protein content and pancreatic tissue activities of trypsin-ogen and proelastase in $UBR1^{-/-}$ mice versus wild-type mice it can be ex-cluded that the observed defects are caused by a strongly reduced synthesis of these enzymes or caused by significant defects in their activation (Fig. 5B).

Most remarkably, in vitro exposure of isolated pancreatic acini from $ubr1^{-/-}$ and wild-type mice to increasing concentrations of the physiologic se-cretagogue cholecystokinin [24] revealed a considerably (approximately 100-fold) lower responsiveness of mouse $ubr1^{-/-}$ pancreas to stimulation (Fig. 5C).

Moreover, studying the ultrastructure of pancreatic acini after cerulein stimulation in electron microscopy, the authors surprisingly detected the rare phenomenon of secretory granule fusion, which is most likely the morphologic
correlate to impaired secretion (Fig. 5D). This difference may explain the observed secretory defect of the pancreas in $ubr1^{-/-}$ mice, and suggests that sig-
nal-secretion coupling in exocrine pancreas cells is controlled by the N-end
rule pathway. In addition, it can be demonstrated that $ubr1^{-/-}$ mice, compared
with wild-type, display an increased susceptibility to cerulein-induced pancreatitis as shown by both histologic evidence and serum amylase and lipase
levels, and other parameters of local pancreatic injury like elastase activity
or systemic inflammatory response (Fig. 5E, F) [25]. These results emphasize
that the intact (as distinguished from UBR1-deficient) N-end rule pathway

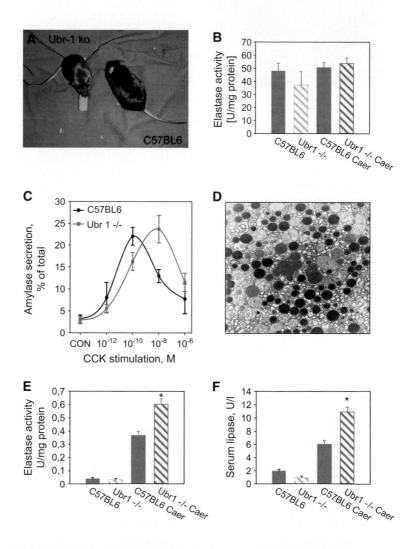

contributes to pancreatic homeostasis and defense against noxious stimuli in pancreatic acinar cells.

Despite the large phenotypic differences between UBR1-deficiency in man and mouse, common pathogenetic mechanisms seem to exist, including a block of zymogen excretion and eventually a liability to irreversible acinar cell damage. Given the almost ubiquitous expression of the N-end rule pathway and the known functional overlaps among Ub ligases of the N-end rule pathway, it may be speculated that the observed difference in phenotypic severity of UBR1 deficiency between human JBS and its mouse $ubr1^{-/-}$ counterpart [18,20,21] reflects species-specific differences in the ability of UBR2 or other UBRs to compensate for the lack of UBR1.

Perspectives

The gene responsible for JBS being an Ub ligase implicates that the basic pathogenetic event leading to all the features of that syndrome is a metabolic stabilization or increased half-life of certain proteins that are specific UBR1 targets. It is challenging to identify these targets, the excess of which is capable of driving such a deleterious process. Regarding the exocrine pancreas one might consider molecules that are involved in the intracellular processing or export of zymogens. Future research has to address these issues. The lessons learned from this rare disorder may point at a relevance of disturbances of the N-end rule pathway or its substrates also for other pancreatic disorders. Given the strong predominance of null alleles of *UBR1* associated with the JBS phenotype, it is an intriguing question whether hypomorphic

◀───

Fig. 5. Characterization of pancreatic abnormalities in $ubr1^{-/-}$ mice. (*A*) Physical appearance of *ubr1* knockout mice: reduction in weight in the $ubr1^{-/-}$ animal on the left side compared with an age-matched wild-type littermate. (*B*) To rule out that the decreased fecal elastase levels of *ubr1* knockout animals is caused by decreased zymogen synthesis elastase activity after enterokinase activation was measured in pancreatic homogenate. No significant difference between wild-type and knockout littermates was detected. (*C*) Amylase release was determined in freshly isolated pancreatic acini incubated with increasing concentrations of the secretagogue cholecystokinin (CCK; 10^{-12} M–10^{-6} M). Wild-type acini responded with maximal secretion to 10^{-10} M CCK, whereas the maximum shifted two logs upward (10^{-8} M CCK) in $ubr1^{-/-}$ acini, indicating an impaired stimulus-secretion coupling in *Ubr1*-deficient pancreas. Asterisks indicate $P < .005$. (*D*) Ultrastructural analysis of pancreatic tissue from *ubr1* knockout animals after supramaximal cerulein stimulation shows here the rarely seen phenomenon of zymogen granule fusion at the apex indicative for an impaired stimulus secretion coupling. In vivo induction of pancreatitis by supramaximal concentrations of cerulein in $ubr1^{-/-}$ animals. This treatment is known to lead to a block of pancreatic secretion and intracellular zymogen activation, eventually resulting in acinar cell necrosis and local and systemic inflammatory response. Pancreatic homogenates from $ubr1^{-/-}$ mice treated with cerulein contained significantly higher elastase activity than wild-type homogenates (*E*). There was no increased spontaneous elastase activity in untreated $ubr1^{-/-}$ mice *versus* wild-type mice. Consistent with these findings, serum lipase levels were significantly higher in $ubr1^{-/-}$ mice (*F*). For each group, N = 6, error bars represent SEM.

UBR1 alleles may be relevant for partial phenotypes out of the JBS spectrum. The authors' findings may implicate UBR1 and its unknown pancreatic targets in the pathogenesis of idiopathic chronic pancreatitis.

Moreover, the phenotypic defects in JBS involve, in a consistently recurring pattern, several organ systems in addition to pancreas [1–4,6–8]. This suggests that UBR1-mediated protein degradation plays a critical role at certain stages of human development, and in specific cell types. Moreover, it implies that in those settings the role of UBR1 cannot be effectively taken over by other E3s of the N-end rule pathway. The protein targets that are of pathogenetic relevance at these different sites are probably not the same as in the pancreas. Some pathomechanisms, however, like those responsible for the various endocrine disorders that may be associated with JBS (hypothyroidism, growth hormone deficiency) might turn out to be quite similar. Further advances in understanding JBS require identification of specific UBR1 substrates whose levels or functions are perturbed in the absence of UBR1, and in ways that underlie the pathogenesis of JBS.

References

[1] Hurst JA, Baraitser M. Johanson-Blizzard syndrome. J Med Genet 1989;26:45–8.
[2] Rudnik-Schoneborn S, Keller B, Beemer FA, et al. Johanson-Blizzard syndrome. Klin Padiatr 1991;203:33–8.
[3] Moeschler JB, Lubinsky MS. Johanson-Blizzard syndrome with normal intelligence. Am J Med Genet 1985;22:69–73.
[4] Johanson A, Blizzard R. A syndrome of congenital aplasia of the alae nasi, deafness, hypothyroidism, dwarfism, absent permanent teeth, and malabsorption. J Pediatr 1971;79:982–7.
[5] Cuschieri A. Anorectal anomalies associated with or as part of other anomalies. Am J Med Genet 2002;110:122–30.
[6] Daentl DL, Frias JL, Gilbert EF, et al. The Johanson-Blizzard syndrome: case report and autopsy findings. Am J Med Genet 1979;3:129–35.
[7] Moeschler JB, Polak MJ, Jenkins JJ III, et al. The Johanson-Blizzard syndrome: a second report of full autopsy findings. Am J Med Genet 1987;26:133–8.
[8] Vanlieferinghen PH, Borderon C, Francannet CH, et al. Johanson-Blizzard syndrome: a new case with autopsy findings. Genet Couns 2001;12:245–50.
[9] Jones NL, Hofley PM, Durie PR. Pathophysiology of the pancreatic defect in Johanson-Blizzard syndrome: a disorder of acinar development. J Pediatr 1994;125:406–8.
[10] Steinbach WJ, Hintz RL. Diabetes mellitus and profound insulin resistance in Johanson-Blizzard syndrome. J Pediatr Endocrinol Metab 2000;13:1633–6.
[11] Trellis DR, Clouse RE. Johanson-Blizzard syndrome: progression of pancreatic involvement in adulthood. Dig Dis Sci 1991;36:365–9.
[12] Zenker M, Mayerle J, Lerch MM, et al. Deficiency of UBR1, a ubiquitin ligase of the N-end rule pathway, causes pancreatic dysfunction, malformations and mental retardation (Johanson-Blizzard syndrome). Nat Genet 2005;37:1345–50.
[13] Pickart CM. Back to the future with ubiquitin. Cell 2004;116:181–90.
[14] Hershko A, Ciechanover A, Varshavsky A. The ubiquitin system. Nat Med 2000;6:1073–81.
[15] Varshavsky A. The N-end rule: functions, mysteries, uses. Proc Natl Acad Sci U S A 1996;93: 12142–9.
[16] Ciechanover A, Schwartz AL. The ubiquitin system: pathogenesis of human diseases and drug targeting. Biochim Biophys Acta 2004;1695:3–17.

[17] Turner GC, Du F, Varshavsky A. Peptides accelerate their uptake by activating a ubiquitin-dependent proteolytic pathway. Nature 2000;405:579–83.

[18] Kwon YT, Xia Z, Davydov IV, et al. Construction and analysis of mouse strains lacking the ubiquitin ligase UBR1 (E3alpha) of the N-end rule pathway. Mol Cell Biol 2001;21:8007–21.

[19] Kwon YT, Kashina AS, Davydov IV, et al. An essential role of N-terminal arginylation in cardiovascular development. Science 2002;297:96–9.

[20] Kwon YT, Xia Z, An JY, et al. Female lethality and apoptosis of spermatocytes in mice lacking the UBR2 ubiquitin ligase of the N-end rule pathway. Mol Cell Biol 2003;23:8255–71.

[21] Tasaki T, Mulder LCF, Iwamatsu A, et al. A family of mammalian E3 ubiquitin ligases that contain the UBR box motif and recognize N-degrons. Mol Cell Biol 2005;25:7120–36.

[22] Bachmair A, Finley D, Varshavsky A. In vivo half-life of a protein is a function of its amino-terminal residue. Science 1986;234:179–86.

[23] Lee PCLE. Prenatal and postnatal development of the human exocrine pancreas. 2nd edition. New York: Raven Press; 1993.

[24] Halangk W, Kruger B, Ruthenburger M, et al. Trypsin activity is not involved in premature, intrapancreatic trypsinogen activation. Am J Physiol Gastrointest Liver Physiol 2002;282: G367–74.

[25] Halangk W, Lerch MM, Brandt-Nedelev B, et al. Role of cathepsin B in intracellular trypsinogen activation and the onset of acute pancreatitis. J Clin Invest 2000;106:773–81.

ELSEVIER
SAUNDERS

Endocrinol Metab Clin N Am
35 (2006) 255–269

ENDOCRINOLOGY
AND METABOLISM
CLINICS
OF NORTH AMERICA

Polygenetic Traits in Pancreatic Disorders

David C. Whitcomb, MD, PhD

*Departments of Medicine, Cell Biology and Physiology, and Human Genetics,
University of Pittsburgh, GI Administration, UPMC Presbyterian,
Mezzanine Level 2, C Wing, 200 Lothrop Street, Pittsburgh, PA 15213, USA*

Chronic pancreatitis is a compound complex disorder, meaning that in each case there are multiple contributing and interacting causes, and that different people within a population have different sets of causal factors [1]. Acute pancreatitis is equally complex, as reflected by the current inability to predict accurately the clinical course of a patient who sustains an insult to the pancreas. Human genetics has provided revolutionary insights into uncommon disorders of the pancreas, including hereditary pancreatitis [2,3], childhood and familial pancreatitis [4,5], and tropical pancreatitis [6,7], and to a lesser extent alcoholic and idiopathic pancreatitis in adults [8–10]. On careful analysis, however, the genes associated with chronic pancreatitis actually cause recurrent acute pancreatitis [11,12], and most of the genes associated with pancreatic disorders only occur in a minority of subjects. These observations suggest the causes of pancreatic diseases are more complex than earlier imagined, and that the interaction of multiple genes and environmental factors is likely [13].

Genetics is the study of inheritance patterns of specific traits. The best understood type of genetics is Mendelian genetics, which focuses on major variations in expressed genes that confer identifiable traits that are inherited in an autosomal dominant, autosomal recessive, or sex-linked pattern. Complex trait genetics focuses on traits that require gene–environment interactions, gene–gene interactions, or multiple gene–environment interactions before the phenotype is seen. Epigenetics, which is not discussed here,

This work was supported in part by NIH DK61451, DK054709, and the Wayne Fusaro Pancreatic Cancer Research Fund. This article is based on the presentation of Dr. Whitcomb at the 5th International Symposium on Inherited Diseases of the Pancreas, Graz, Austria, July 7, 2005, and on a major review by Whitcomb et al [1].

E-mail address: whitcomb@pitt.edu

focuses on altered gene expression that is caused by factors other than changes in DNA sequence, such as gene methylation.

Further study of genetic factors in pancreatic diseases is critical because many of the clinical observations cannot be explained by normal responses to pancreatic stressors. For example, why do some people develop acute pancreatitis whereas most people are highly resistant? Why do 20% of individuals with acute pancreatitis develop a severe clinical course? Why is there no obvious link between recurrent acute pancreatitis and chronic pancreatitis? Why does only a subset of people with chronic pancreatitis develop severe pain, diabetes, malabsorption, or cancer? Our research group and others have been testing the hypothesis that the reasons reflect genetic variability and that the underlying pathophysiologic mechanism can be understood and used to predict clinical courses, outcomes, and targets for intervention.

If the above hypothesis is true, then the multiple factors determining susceptibility and clinical course fall under the category of complex genetic disorders. Fortunately, the widespread availability of high throughput genotyping techniques makes possible the exploration of the role of genetic variations in various diseases, including pancreatitis. Unfortunately, the early availability of genetic testing was followed by an explosion of articles reporting statistically significant associations between DNA sequence variants and various common disorders with a suspected genetic component, but without clear autosomal dominant or recessive disease inheritance patterns. It soon became apparent that many of these reports, often published in prestigious journals, could not be replicated in subsequent studies [14–16]. The challenge has been to determine why.

The irreproducibility factor in the study of complex genetic disorders

The basis of the scientific method is that the results of experiments conducted by one scientist will be reproduced by other scientists. The observation that some reported genetic associations could not be reproduced by others suggests that there is a major problem in the study design, study methods, study execution, or study interpretation. Postmortem analysis of these studies has not yet diagnosed the cause of this apparent system failure, or what steps should be taken to prevent this in the future.

Currently, the strongest arguments for the genetic basis of specific diseases come from epidemiologists who have used meta-analysis to compare hundreds of studies [15–17]. Based on this approach, the general consensus among many leaders in the field is that (1) most genetic susceptibility factors have only a small effect on common diseases, and (2) studies generally are unreliable unless they have greater than 1000 subjects per study arm. Other leaders suspect that there is something wrong with these conclusions, however. Furthermore, accepting these conclusions means that the genetic basis of uncommon diseases (in which greater than 1000 well-characterized cases cannot be ascertained easily) cannot be determined, nor genetic associations proven. Finally, the conclusions of studies that require greater than 1000 subjects to demonstrate a small but statistically significant conclusion likely are medically trivial.

The author recently addressed the issues of study size and study design in simple and complex genetic traits and suggested that the problem of nonreproducibility is not study size, but study design [1]. From our perspective, the use of meta-analysis in evaluating multiple studies on complex disorders with possible systematic design flaws may have generated erroneous inferences regarding the mechanism of common diseases [1]. If the goal of investigating complex traits is to provide insight into the disease mechanism for individual patients, then complex genetics should be approached from a systems-based case series approach, in which multiple genetic effects are considered in independent and properly powered mechanistically based association studies before the independent effects are integrated into a complex disease model. The outcomes of these studies should be a mathematically based tool that has outstanding performance characteristics on a patient-by-patient basis.

Strengths and limitations of case-control studies

Scientific investigation into human medical genetics has required many approaches and methods. Pure genetics focuses on the inheritance of specific traits in related subjects. Genetic epidemiology seeks to understand the interaction of genes and environmental factors and to identify genes determining susceptibility to disorders. Medical genetics considers the contribution of genetic variability, plus epigenetics factors, environmental and metabolic factors, disease susceptibility, pathogenesis, natural history, and complications. Other academic disciplines, such as population genetics, are also relevant, especially in considering targets for pharmaceutic agents and public health policy. Because of the broad spectrum of human diseases and disorders with differing degrees of complexity and incidence within populations a single approach cannot be used.

Many lines of evidence (eg, the lack of strong environmental factors) suggest that sporadic cases of chronic pancreatitis, severe acute pancreatitis, and pancreatic cancer have a strong genetic or epigenetic basis. The general paucity of a family history of pancreatic disease in most clinical cases, however, means that the disease pathogenesis is complex. The relative rarity of either large families or multiple small families means that standard methods of genetic linkage analysis cannot be used. Those who study chronic pancreatitis and other disorders of the exocrine pancreas are faced with investigations of a limited group of subjects with a complex syndrome and a complex genetic contribution to the pathogenesis. The options are to approach the questions with either a case-control study design with a limited number of patients, or to invent new approaches that are not dependent totally on single statistical tests. The theory and application of case-control studies to human genetics has been reviewed recently (eg, genetic association studies) [18]. Here the author focuses on the factors that determine study power and study design, and considers how to reorganize experimental approaches to complex genetic disorders that maximize insight with limited numbers of complex and inhomogeneous patients.

Design and analysis of genetic association studies

Statistics involves the gathering and interpretation of data from a sample taken from a population. The concern using statistical methods is that the inferences are wrong, either because a true inference is rejected as false, or because a false inference is accepted as true. Investigations into the genetic contribution to a medical condition is especially challenging because most of the fully penetrant discrete genetic disorders that are common have been discovered. The design for most genetic studies depends on the available patient population and some idea about the nature of the disorder. Examples include case–control, cohort, cross-sectional, extreme values, case–parent triads, case–parent–grandparent septets, general pedigrees, DNA pooling, and case-only study design [18]. Each approach has its strengths and weaknesses, but issues of study power, multiple testing, and false positive results have driven many epidemiologists to conclude that larger and larger studies are needed.

The importance of study size in genetic association studies recently has been highlighted in a series of papers by Ioannidis and colleagues [15–17] and others [19]. The thrust of the Ioannidis's argument is that many of the smaller studies that were reported in major journals could not be reproduced in subsequent studies, primarily because the sample size was too small (ie, underpowered). Based on extensive meta-analysis of many published reports, Ioannidis [14] suggests that the studies that were adequately powered to detect single genetic associations typically included one thousand subjects or more, depending on the prevalence of the polymorphism and the effect size on the outcome. These types of evaluations appear to contribute to the general premise that most genuine genetic associations represent modest effects with odds ratios of 1.1 to 1.5 [14]. To obtain a significant P value and to avoid inappropriately reporting a false association as true, a large sample size is required.

Although bigger is better for well-designed epidemiologic studies, setting an arbitrary threshold of greater than 1000 subjects for publishing genetic association studies has several inherent downsides. First, it eliminates the chance to report early and important results for common and uncommon disorders. Second, it precludes the ability to compare differences in study results of the same phenotype from multiple populations, an exercise that can provide tremendous insight into disease mechanism. Third, it makes most studies cost-prohibitive. Finally, it facilitates the reporting of statistically significant but medically insignificant results.

Before accepting the 1000-subject threshold suggested by meta-analysis, it is important to consider the factors that influence study size for a given study power, study design, and some concerns about using meta-analysis to gain insight into the cause of complex disorders.

Study power

Although study size clearly is an important consideration, it is only one of four factors that determine study power, which is the likelihood of identifying a true positive association (or effect) in a population, if there is one. The key variable in linking study power to study size (assuming the variance and significance level are constant) is the effect size, commonly expressed in population studies as the odds ratio (OR) or relative risk (RR). Studies with higher OR (eg, OR > 2) thus require fewer subjects than studies with lower OR (eg, OR < 1.5). Furthermore, genetic variables with stronger effect are more likely to be medically relevant, suggesting that smaller studies of major effects can be valid and important. The real question is: How many patients are required to demonstrate with confidence that a genetic variant is associated with a measured effect?

Pretest probability

Most basic laboratory experiments are designed to answer specific question about the interactions or effects of a known agent on a defined parameter in a controlled environment when significant information about the mechanism is known. In these cases it is highly likely that any differences in outcome between experimental and control conditions are attributable to the effects of the agent being tested. The problem is more complex in biologic systems in which the mechanism is not well understood and the agent causing an effect is uncertain. For cases in which the mechanism is unknown and multiple variables are being compared with a clinically defined outcome, the likelihood that a statistical association between a random variable and the outcome define the mechanism is small [1]. The second situation is one commonly faced in human and medical genetics.

In controlled basic laboratory studies the prior probability that a statistically significant finding reflects a true effect is high. If little is known about the disease mechanism, however, as in a genome-wide association study involving thousands of markers, then the prior probability that a specific DNA variation that is found to be statistically associated with an outcome is a true disease-associated factor is small. Because the foundation of science is that a logical deduction from well-defined experiments is true, there may be serious consequences for the credibility of scientists reporting that a conclusion to an experiment is true when in fact it is false.

What are the chances that a report describes a biologically false association? Recently Wacholder and colleagues [20] published an approach to assessing the probability that a statistically positive genetic association is actually false. They demonstrated that the false positive report probability (FPRP) was influenced strongly by the prior probability that the genetic variation contributed to the measured effect (ie, the hypothesis being tested was both plausible and likely). This approach differs from classic frequentist statistical theory in which the truth of the null hypothesis and alternate hypothesis are unknown, and the support for the null hypothesis is considered [20]. The P value thus is the probability of a statistically significant finding given that the null hypothesis is true, whereas FPRP, as defined by Wacholder and coworkers [20], is the probability that the null hypothesis is true given that the test of association is statistically significant.

These issues have significant implications for study design in human genetics. If one is searching for an unknown genetic variation that is hypothesized to be associated with a human disease, then the prior probability that a given DNA sequence variation is the one is low. To compensate for the lower FPRP one can increase the threshold for significance (eg, $P < .0001$), which in turn requires many patients (eg, $n >> 1000$) [20]. In addition, complementary and compelling lines of additional evidence that the DNA variant has a biologic effect also are required by most journals for publication of findings. These are the types of issues that challenge the discovery of genetic risk factors for major diseases using linkage analysis. This challenge is of special concern for rare diseases in which study size is the limiting factor.

Uncommon diseases, such as chronic pancreatitis, present some major challenges because most cases appear to be sporadic. We do know a significant amount about the disorder from other perspectives, however, including pathology studies, the central role of trypsin (based on the autosomal dominant hereditary pancreatitis) [2,21], animal models [22], mathematical models [23], and epidemiology studies [24]. This information can be used to develop detailed models [25] and influence diagrams [1] (Fig. 1) that point the investigators to a limited number of specific, mechanism-associated candidate genes. Having a structured, mechanistic understanding of underlying pathology markedly improves the prior probability that a statistically significant association is true. If the hypothesis is specific and the outcome measures precisely it follows that the study size need not be large (eg, ~ 100 cases and controls may be adequate) when the pretest probability is high (~ 1) and the effect size high (eg, $OR > 5$). Of course, this assumes that we truly understand the pathologic mechanisms causing the disorder, that the phenotyping is highly accurate and discriminating, and that the question is simple. (An example of a simple study would be to measure the effect of a candidate gene promoter polymorphism on protein expression rather than on eventual disease outcome). The successful analysis of various complex disorders requires consideration of all of these factors with appropriate adjustments in study design based in part on the opportunity to improve the prior probability [1].

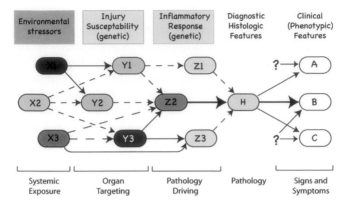

Fig. 1. Hypothetic model of a chronic inflammatory disorder. This model illustrates a condition with nine different risk factors organized according to general categories (red = environmental factors, blue = weakened protective mechanism, green = inflammatory response elements) and effect strength (darker = stronger effect). Solid arrows indicate that presence of the factor has a strong effect on the linked factor, whereas dashed arrows indicate a weak effect that requires either a double dose (eg, recessive trait) or complementary factors (eg, Y1/Y1 or Y1/Y2). For the disease to occur (defined by histology, H), there must be risk in all three categories of risk factors, but the disease is not pathway dependent. Note also that the presence or absence of H in a subject is inferred. (*From* Whitcomb DC, Aoun E, Vodovotz Y, et al. Evaluating disorders with a complex genetics basis: the future role of meta-analysis and systems biology. Dig Dis Sci 2005;50(12):2195–202.)

Study population

The success and reproducibility of genetic association studies highly depends on the populations in which the associations are being tested. In the basic science laboratory most animal experiments are conducted within a highly homogeneous group of inbred, age- and sex-matched animals raised under diet- and environment-controlled conditions. In most cases the study size is small (eg, <10 animals per group) and the effect size is unknown. These studies are powered adequately, because the variability is low and the required significance level is typically and appropriately set at $P<.05$. Under these conditions we know from experience that scientists in other laboratories from around the world can reproduce these results on the premise that identical animals and conditions are used. Meeting these stipulations in human studies, however, is impossible.

The reason that laboratory studies are powered adequately to detect a true effect with a small study size is that the variability (one of the factors that determine study power) is low. In most cases, six animals per group is sufficient. If one is interested in determining if a genetic variant has an effect on a disorder then choosing a study population with minimal variance can be used either to strengthen the study power or reduce study size. Populations with small variance are said to be homogenous. The challenge is finding large populations that are homogenous and include many subjects with the disorder. It is unlikely that geographically (and ethnically) different populations are homogenous (ie, have the same variance) and exhibit the same effects in equivalent proportions. Variations in populations become increasingly important for complex disorders in which multiple pathologic variables from multiple domains (eg, environmental factors, injury protection mechanisms, immunologic responses, disease modifiers) are required. Reproducibility of small genetic association studies may depend more on population variances than study size. Furthermore, observing different effect sizes of a single variable within a multivariant disorder in different populations does not invalidate either study.

Defining phenotypes

The ultimate goal of genetic association studies should be to determine if specific genetic variations contribute to the pathologic mechanism of a disorder. A major problem is that clinically defined disorders often are assumed to be or are approached as if they were caused through a single mechanism with a precisely determined cause-associated phenotype, and that most patients develop characteristic pathology through the same pathway. For example, chronic inflammatory disorders, such as chronic pancreatitis, are defined by the presence of scar tissue (ie, fibrosis) rather then features of the causal defect. Furthermore, and unlike laboratory animal studies, physicians recognize that homogenous groups of patients do not exist; not even two patients are homogenous. These considerations are but a few of the issues that compound the complexity of phenotyping a disorder.

There are two approaches to solving the phenotyping problem [1]. One is to use a genetic factor that is associated with a subset of patients and work backward to better define the phenotypic features [26]. The other is to break a disease process down into progressive steps, each with phenotypic features, and focus on each step in a highly mechanistic way (see Fig. 1) [11,13]. In this model, the phenotype represents the normal function of a single defined protein (eg, Y2 of Fig. 1), with the effect of a genetic variation being measured in terms of alterations in the gene-associated protein expression and function rather than the presence or absence of end-stage disease. These approaches require a systems biology framework (see later discussion).

Statistical approaches to complex disorders

Statistical genetics is an academic discipline that focuses on determining the probability that a genetic polymorphism contributes to a phenotypic trait. The most common methods include linear and logistic regression, χ^2, transmission/disequilibrium tests, log-linear models, pedigree disequilibrium tests, quantitative transmission/disequilibrium tests, and others [18]. The approaches generally are based in classic statistic theory and epidemiologic methods and are useful for determining the risk for a factor with respect to a phenotype within a population. These approaches tend to require large amounts of data to make small inferences and are best suited for making predictions within a training set, with little insight into mechanisms and biologic principles. They often are incorrect in predicting outside of the data set. Standard statistical methods triangulate on single factors or determine the independent contribution of several additive factors. These approaches fail in more complex, multivariant, multiple pathway, non-linear, time-dependent, feedback-controlled processes, especially when physicians are intervening actively in some of the steps.

Meta-analysis of multiple genetic association studies raised major concerns about study size. Meta-analysis is a systematic method that uses statistical techniques for combining results from different studies to obtain a quantitative estimate of the overall effect of a particular intervention or variable on a defined outcome. The author has discussed the limitations of meta-analysis in complex traits elsewhere [1]. Here the study designs of some of the association studies considered in major systematic reviews using meta-analysis are examined.

In 2003 Ioannidis and colleagues [16] published a report of 55 meta-analyses based on 579 association studies to test whether the magnitude of the genetic effect differs in large versus smaller studies. All but one reported example had small effects with OR < 2. The exception was a poor clozapine response associated with the serotonin receptor gene subtype 2A (*HTR2A*) H452Y mutation. In this case the combined studies had an OR 5.55 (CI 1.15–26.8) or OR 3.37 (CI 0.97–11.6), depending on method. Note that the clozapine studies focused on a more specific mechanistic step, the effect of specific receptor mutations on antagonist effect. But even in this case, the phenotype and mechanisms are complex.

Clozapine is an atypical antipsychotic drug and antagonist of the post-synaptic HTR2A G-coupled receptor, the neuronal receptor that mediates the effects of LSD. Because it is know that a major target of clozapine is HTR2A, the pretest probability that a mutation in this receptor could alter the interaction of agonists or antagonist is high. The primary challenge in this case is determining the phenotype accurately. Because schizophrenia and other mental illnesses are complex and multidimensional disorders, treatment usually is reserved for patients who fail typical antipsychotic drugs, the effects often take months to develop, and measurement of the response can be subjective. Furthermore, the molecular mechanism of clozapine's effect is complex compared with the enzyme-specific metabolism of a compound, for example. Clozapine, as a receptor antagonist, requires a functional receptor that recognizes serotonin and possesses otherwise normal second messenger signaling properties. This means that any mutation could have multiple effects, and multiple polymorphisms must be considered in diverse human populations. Furthermore, the pharmacology of clozapine is complex, with high (~50%) first-pass clearance in the liver and other factors that influence bioavailability so that there is no clear dose-response curve for this compound [27,28]. Another confounding effect is that clozapine is a multireceptor antagonist and response to treatment also varies with polymorphisms in the dopamine 2 receptor and ethnicity [29]. A strong effect is associated with the polymorphism in the HTR2A gene, however, suggesting that the interaction of clozapine with HTR2A is a major determinant in biologic responses in a subset of subjects with psychiatric disorders.

In the meta-analysis of other genetic association studies considered by Ioannidis and colleagues [16] most studies tested associations between specific gene mutations and complex effects that often were remote, indirect, and delayed, with multiple additional links and risk factors intervening. Examples include the *ACE* (insertion/deletion), DD versus DI + II polymorphism (which increases function), myocardial infarction, ischemic heart disease, ischemic cerebrovascular disease, ischemic stroke, diabetic neuropathy, and IGA nephropathy [16]. For the *ACE* DD genotype to be linked to stroke, for example, there must be a link between the polymorphism and the end-stage disorder. ACE is only one of many relevant factors in the highly regulated rennin-angiotensin system, however. If all other factors were equal, an ACE polymorphism could lead to increased blood pressure (only in patients who have ineffective counter-regulatory mechanism and who were not treated effectively by their physicians). Hypertension is only one of many factors contributing to cardiovascular disease, and cerebrovascular disease is only one of many possible cardiovascular diseases. Finally, only a subset of patients who have cerebrovascular disease will have a stroke. From a mechanistic and systems biology perspective it is amazing that any effects of *ACE* gene polymorphisms were seen in stroke without consideration of the many other risk factors that are known to be important (eg, tobacco smoking, hypertension, obesity, diabetes, age, and so forth) [30]. Large studies are needed to demonstrate an association between a single DNA variant and an uncommon downstream effect. Furthermore, because of all of the other important variables, the relative contribution of a single factor would be expected to be small. Another interpretation of the meta-analysis of these reports is that large studies are needed to show an effect of a single factor in a poorly designed study of complex disorders.

Systems biology

Systems biology is a holistic approach to the mechanisms underlying complex biologic processes, in which these processes are viewed as integrated systems of many diverse interacting components [1]. Systems biology combines multiple perspectives in an organized way, and uses powerful computational approaches to understand the interactions among many factors and systems that are relevant to a disease process. Systems biology is becoming highly mathematical with intentional inclusion of prior knowledge embodied in multi-scale models of disease. Although systems biology previously shared many of the limitations of classic statistics, being a data-rich, knowledge-poor conceptual framework, it is evolving into a data-rich, knowledge-rich environment, making full use of reductionist science [1].

An example of the importance of adding structure to understand rich data sets is the analysis of a photograph in Fig. 2. All of the colors of a picture are accurately collected and depicted in the format of a histogram. Furthermore, the intensity of the color tones across the photograph (top panel) can be resolved into primary colors, shown in the bottom three panels. With this information in hand one could ask what type of statistical analysis should be done to understand the content of the photograph.

The importance of structure is illustrated in Fig. 3. The top panel provides general outlines of the major features of the picture. The bottom panel integrates the information from Fig. 2 into the structure of the top panel in

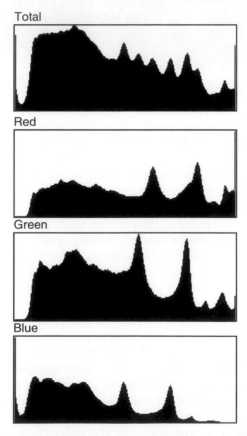

Fig. 2. Histograms of color intensity across a photograph. The top panel illustrates tone, which is the sum of the three primary colors in the lower panels. The data are highly accurate, dense, and helpful in understanding the photograph. The picture cannot be understood, however, from this perspective alone (created in Adobe Photoshop CS).

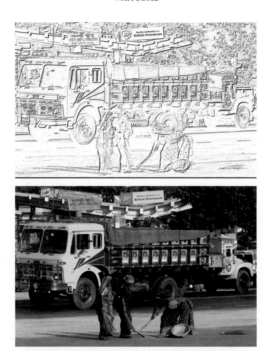

Fig. 3. Photograph of a street in Bangladesh. The top panel outlines the structures in the photograph. When the colors and tones from Fig. 2 are combined properly with the structure the details of the photograph can be understood (photograph by the author).

Fig. 3 to provide an enriched understanding of the picture (bottom panel). In a similar way, the structure provided by systems biology allows for integrates of anatomic, histologic, physiologic, and regulatory information to complement genetic or genomic data so that a full understanding of the disease in specific patients can be reached. A comparison of statistical methods and mathematical methods (used in systems biology) is given in Box 1.

Systems biology has not been used fully in the study of human genetics, but the author suggests that it should become the foundation for a proper understanding of complex genetic diseases in the future [1]. This systems biology framework allows multiple scientific questions to be answered about the elements and interactions of multiple variables in a complex disease with a high degree of accuracy and with small study sizes. This approach should allow multiple pathway-specific disease mechanisms to be teased out of a complex syndrome. Furthermore, the results of such a study should be useful in developing accurate risk models that can be applied to individual patients rather than being limited to populations.

A systems biology approach should also differ from traditional human genetic studies by focusing sequentially on all of the haplotypes that alter the function of relevant proteins, rather than exploring the effect of a single nucleotide polymorphism in a complex syndrome [1]. Finally, such an

---

Box 1. Comparison of statistical and mathematical methods

Statistics
- Association based (e.g. case control)
- Limited use of prior knowledge
- Requires large amounts of data
- Prediction within training data yet often used incorrectly to predict outside such data

Mathematics
- Highly causal
- Extensive use of prior knowledge
- Allows explanation of emergent phenomena
- More difficult
- Predictions outside of training data

---

approach should allow scientists to evaluate complex syndromes that may be a combination of several complex disorders with a similar phenotype. Understanding complex trait genetics from a systems biology perspective also helps understand the limits of meta-analysis in complex trait genetics. Such approaches have been used in many biologic disciplines.

A simple model of a chronic inflammatory disease was presented in Fig. 1. This figure could be used to illustrate multiple possible pathways through all of the major domains leading to end-stage pathology as is seen in end-stage chronic pancreatitis, inflammatory bowel disease, chronic liver disease, and so forth. This model is an extension of the domain model of Whitcomb [13] in which the necessity of having contributing factors in all three domains of environmental stressors, impaired protective factors, and altered immune responses is illustrated in a Venn diagram. Fig. 1 represents a plausible model that helps divide and organize relevant risk factors for further consideration as a systems biology model is developed [1]. It also suggests that to develop an end-stage disease there must be some pathologic factors in each domain to provide a continuous link from start to finish.

Summary

Genetic variations underlie much of the susceptibility to and characteristics of human diseases [1]. It is becoming evident that most chronic digestive diseases in which the cause is unclear or undefined are complex genetic traits. The goal of genetic linkage and association studies is to determine the role of specific DNA variations in human disease, but discovery of interacting or redundant genetic covariants in complex syndromes is difficult with traditional linkage and association studies. Meta-analysis of many previous studies suggested that the reproducibility of small studies was reduced.

Meta-analysis is designed to take advantage of the cumulative support for factors from multiple studies, and has limited usefulness in understanding complex genetic disorders [1]. Instead, the study of human genetics should be grounded in systems biology because it offers an approach that is more accurate and more informative, and may provide insights into complex disorders that can be translated into a comprehensive risk-assessment model for individual patients.

References

[1] Whitcomb DC, Aoun E, Vodovotz Y, et al. Evaluating disorders with a complex genetics basis: The future role of meta-analysis and systems biology. Dig Dis Sci 2005;50(12):2195–202.
[2] Whitcomb DC, Gorry MC, Preston RA, et al. Hereditary pancreatitis is caused by a mutation in the cationic trypsinogen gene. Nat Genet 1996;14(2):141–5.
[3] Gorry MC, Gabbaizedeh D, Furey W, et al. Mutations in the cationic trypsinogen gene are associated with recurrent acute and chronic pancreatitis. Gastroenterology 1997;113(4): 1063–8.
[4] Witt H, Luck W, Hennies HC, et al. Mutations in the gene encoding the serine protease inhibitor, Kazal type 1 are associated with chronic pancreatitis. Nat Genet 2000;25(2):213–6.
[5] Pfützer RH, Barmada MM, Brunskil APJ, et al. SPINK1/PSTI polymorphisms act as disease modifiers in familial and idiopathic chronic pancreatitis. Gastroenterology 2000;119: 615–23.
[6] Rossi L, Pfützer RL, Parvin S, et al. SPINK1/PSTI mutations are associated with tropical pancreatitis in Bangladesh: a preliminary report. Pancreatol 2001;1(3):242–5.
[7] Chandak GR, Idris MM, Reddy DN, et al. Mutations in the pancreatic secretory trypsin inhibitor gene (PSTI/SPINK1) rather than the cationic trypsinogen gene (PRSS1) are significantly associated with tropical calcific pancreatitis. J Med Genet 2002;39(5):347–51.
[8] Cohn JA, Friedman KJ, Noone PG, et al. Relation between mutations of the cystic fibrosis gene and idiopathic pancreatitis. N Engl J Med 1998;339(10):653–8.
[9] Sharer N, Schwarz M, Malone G, et al. Mutations of the cystic fibrosis gene in patients with chronic pancreatitis. N Engl J Med 1998;339(10):645–52.
[10] Witt H, Luck W, Becker M, et al. Mutation in the SPINK1 trypsin inhibitor gene, alcohol use, and chronic pancreatitis. JAMA 2001;285(21):2716–7.
[11] Whitcomb DC. Value of genetic testing in management of pancreatitis. Gut 2004;53(11): 1710–7.
[12] Whitcomb DC. Gene mutations as a cause of chronic pancreatitis. In: Adler G, Ammann R, Buchler M, et al, editors. Pancreatitis: advances in pathobiology, diagnosis and treatment (Falk Symposium 143). Lancaster (UK): Springer; 2005. p. 139–52.
[13] Whitcomb DC. Advances in understanding the mechanisms leading to chronic pancreatitis. Nat Clin Practice, Gastro Hepatol 2004;1(1):46–52.
[14] Ioannidis JP. Genetic associations: false or true? Trends Mol Med 2003;9(4):135–8.
[15] Ioannidis JP, Ntzani EE, Trikalinos TA, et al. Replication validity of genetic association studies. Nat Genet 2001;29(3):306–9.
[16] Ioannidis JP, Trikalinos TA, Ntzani EE, et al. Genetic associations in large versus small studies: an empirical assessment. Lancet 2003;361(9357):567–71.
[17] Trikalinos TA, Ntzani EE, Contopoulos-Ioannidis DG, et al. Establishment of genetic associations for complex diseases is independent of early study findings. Eur J Hum Genet 2004; 12(9):762–9.
[18] Cordell HJ, Clayton DG. Genetic association studies. Lancet 2005;366(9491):1121–31.
[19] Dahlman I, Eaves IA, Kosoy R, et al. Parameters for reliable results in genetic association studies in common disease. Nat Genet 2002;30:149–50.

[20] Wacholder S, Chanock S, Garcia-Closas M, et al. Assessing the probability that a positive report is false: an approach for molecular epidemiology studies. J Natl Cancer Inst 2004; 96(6):434–42.

[21] Whitcomb DC, Preston RA, Aston CE, et al. A gene for hereditary pancreatitis maps to chromosome 7q35. Gastroenterology 1996;110(6):1975–80.

[22] Deng X, Wang L, Elm MS, et al. Chronic alcohol consumption accelerates fibrosis in response to cerulein-induced pancreatitis in rats. Am J Pathol 2005;166(1):93–106.

[23] Whitcomb DC, Ermentrout GB. A mathematical model of the pancreatic duct cell generating high bicarbonate concentrations in pancreatic juice. Pancreas 2004;29(2):E30–40.

[24] Etemad B, Whitcomb DC. Chronic pancreatitis: Diagnosis, classification, and new genetic developments. Gastroenterology 2001;120:682–707.

[25] Schneider A, Whitcomb DC. Hereditary pancreatitis: a model for inflammatory diseases of the pancreas. Best Pract Res Clin Gastroenterol 2002;16(3):347–63.

[26] Schneider A, Barmada MM, Slivka A, et al. Clinical characterization of patients with idiopathic chronic pancreatitis and SPINK1 Mutations. Scand J Gastroenterol 2004;39(9): 903–4.

[27] Zhou S, Chan E, Duan W, et al. Drug bioactivation, covalent binding to target proteins and toxicity relevance. Drug Metab Rev 2005;37(1):41–213.

[28] Davis JM, Chen N. Dose response and dose equivalence of antipsychotics. J Clin Psychopharmacol 2004;24(2):192–208.

[29] Hwang R, Shinkai T, De Luca V, et al. Association study of 12 polymorphisms spanning the dopamine D(2) receptor gene and clozapine treatment response in two treatment refractory/ intolerant populations. Psychopharmacology (Berl) 2005;181(1):179–87.

[30] Padwal R, Straus SE, McAlister FA. Evidence based management of hypertension. Cardiovascular risk factors and their effects on the decision to treat hypertension: evidence based review. BMJ 2001;322(7292):977–80.

ELSEVIER
SAUNDERS

Endocrinol Metab Clin N Am
35 (2006) 271–287

ENDOCRINOLOGY
AND METABOLISM
CLINICS
OF NORTH AMERICA

Trypsinogen Mutations in Pancreatic Disorders

Louis J. Vitone, MB, ChB, MRCS,
William Greenhalf, PhD,
Nathan R. Howes, MB, ChB, MD, FRCS,
Michael G.T. Raraty, MB, BS, PhD, FRCS,
John P. Neoptolemos, MA, MB, BChir, MD, FRCS*

*Division of Surgery and Oncology, The University of Liverpool, 5th Floor UCD Building,
Daulby Street, Liverpool, L69 3GA, United Kingdom*

All but one of the human trypsinogen genes are intercalated between the β T-cell receptor genes on chromosome 7 [1]. Three nonfunctioning trypsinogen genes are located at the 5′ end of the β T-cell receptor locus (7q35), and five tandemly arrayed genes including the cationic and anionic trypsinogen genes are located at the 3′ end. Trypsinogen is encoded by the protease serine (PRSS) genes 1, 2, and 3, which are defined according to their respective isoelectric points. Three different isoforms of trypsinogen have been identified in human pancreatic juice: (1) cationic trypsinogen (product of PRSS1); (2) anionic trypsinogen (PRSS2); and (3) mesotrypsinogen (PRSS3). The PRSS3 gene encoding mesotrypsinogen translocated from chromosome 7 to 9p11.2(1) and was named to reflect the intermediate pI and electrophoretic mobility of the zymogen. Mesotrypsinogen was observed to have resistance to inhibitory proteins, such as SPINK1 (described later), and it may act to degrade these inhibitors in foodstuffs, which are otherwise resistant to digestion [2]. Cationic trypsinogen accounts for approximately 60% of the total trypsinogen content in the pancreas, anionic trypsinogen 30%, and mesotrypsinogen less than 5% [3]. The cationic/ionic ratio is roughly 1:1.5.

In 1896, Chiari speculated that pancreatitis is a result of pancreatic autodigestion. Trypsin remains the most abundant protein produced by the pancreas. Furthermore, a key role has been attributed to the activation of trypsinogen to trypsin in the chain of events leading to and regulating

---

* Corresponding author.
E-mail address: j.p.neoptolemos@liverpool.ac.uk (J.P. Neoptolemos).

0889-8529/06/$ - see front matter © 2006 Elsevier Inc. All rights reserved.
doi:10.1016/j.ecl.2006.02.006

conversion of other proteolytic enzymes to their active forms. Intrapancreatic activation was a long-standing candidate as the initiating event in the pathogenesis of acute pancreatitis, although this has always been controversial. The discovery by Whitcomb and coworkers [4] of disease-causing mutations in a trypsinogen gene verified the significance of the pancreatic protease cascade in the cause of chronic pancreatitis; however, uncertainties about the mechanistic role of the mutations has left open the possibility that trypsinogen activation is protective rather than causative of pancreatic injury.

The mutations identified by Whitcomb and coworkers [4] were all in the cationic trypsinogen gene, PRSS1 [5]. These mutations lead to hereditary pancreatitis, an autosomal-dominant disease [6,7] with incomplete penetrance (80%) [8], accounting for approximately 1% of all cases of pancreatitis. It is characterized by the onset of recurrent attacks of acute pancreatitis in childhood and frequent progression to chronic pancreatitis. PRSS1 is about 3.6 kilobases long with five exons. The preprotein is 247 amino acids, including a 15–amino acid signal peptide and an 8–amino acid activation peptide.

Normal exocrine pancreatic enzyme function

One of the key functions of the exocrine pancreas is to produce and secrete digestive enzymes. These include the proteolytic enzymes, trypsin, chymotrypsin, carboxypeptidase, and elastase; also included are lipase, phospholipase A, amylase, ribonuclease, and deoxyribonuclease. Several protective mechanisms are in place to safeguard the functional unit of the exocrine pancreas, the acinar cell:

1. Production, packaging, and secretion of proenzymes (inactive zymogens [eg, trypsinogen]), which are only activated in the duodenum (eg, trypsinogen is activated by enterokinase). Most digestive enzymes are secreted in this way, the exceptions being lipase, amylase, ribonuclease, and deoxyribonuclease.
2. Condensed packaging of zymogens in granules with localized environments (eg, stable high calcium concentrations), reducing the risk of activation of the zymogen and protecting the acinar cell from the effects of small concentrations of activated protein.
3. Protease inhibitors within the acinar cells, such as serine protease inhibitor, Kazal type I (SPINK1).
4. Autolysis or lysis by other digestive enzymes activated in a protease cascade (eg, trypsin can be deactivated by autolytic cleavage or the action of mesotrypsin).

Models for the pathogenesis of pancreatitis

Biochemical and clinical observations can be applied in a variety of ways to produce contrasting models for the pathogenesis of pancreatitis. To take these theories from the laboratory to a point where they can be practically applied in a clinical setting they must first be tested in experimental animal models, the most common being the application of supraphysiologic doses of CCK-8 or its analogue cerulein to rodents. This leads to a rapid breakdown of intracellular trafficking with destruction of acinar cells. According to one model of the pathogenesis of pancreatitis, fusion of zymogen granules with lysosomes enables the lysosomal enzyme cathepsin B to activate trypsinogen. Blocking of intracellular trafficking by cerulein has this effect. Treating mice unable to express cathepsin B with cerulein is expected to lead to a decrease in induction of pancreatitis. Indeed, when this was done the level of intracellular trypsinogen activation declined dramatically in comparison with the wild-type mouse [9]. There was still some trypsinogen activation (albeit at a level of only 10%), however, and surprisingly the level of pancreatitis (pancreatic necrosis and systemic inflammatory response) did not alter dramatically in the knockout mouse. This raises the issue not only of the importance of cathepsin in the pathogenesis of pancreatitis but also the role of trypsin activation.

Identification of instigating events in human diseases is often facilitated by the existence of a genetic syndrome predisposing to the disease; an inherited predisposing mutation identifies a defect that was present (at least in the syndromic patients) before any other pathogenic event. In the case of pancreatitis the central role of trypsin is supported by patients with inherited mutations in the cationic trypsinogen gene. Intuitively, it is assumed that the mutations must increase the activity of trypsin within the acinar cell; possible scenarios consistent with this are that the mutant trypsinogen is more easily activated or alternatively less readily inhibited or digested.

Activation of the mutant trypsinogen is difficult to study in vivo because no transgenic animal model of hereditary pancreatitis exists. Also, one of the amino acid changes found in hereditary pancreatitis, a change from an arginine to a histidine at position 122 (R122H), coincides with the naturally occurring amino acid found at the equivalent position in the dominant form of trypsinogen expressed in healthy rats, suggesting that the mutation is context-dependent and is difficult to model in animals. In vitro studies with recombinant cationic trypsinogen mutants, however, could at least answer some questions that can be related back to disease pathology. The role of cathepsin B in trypsinogen activation has been investigated with recombinant cationic trypsinogen [10] and synthetic peptides [11]. The activation of hereditary pancreatitis–associated mutants by the lysosomal cysteine protease was unchanged or reduced [10,11]. Hence, increased susceptibility to cathepsin B is not the underlying cause of hereditary pancreatitis.

The crystal structure of cationic trypsinogen suggests that the commonly occurring mutations of PRSS1 could both affect the site of inactivating cleavage (discussed later). Biochemical studies suggest, however, that at least one of the mutations leads to increased autoactivation at low pH [12]. Increased autoactivation or reduced inactivation is possible and although the mutations seem to be distant to the site of SPINK1 association, the possibility of reduced inhibitor binding has not been excluded. It is likely that the activity of the mutant enzymes is qualitatively different in in vivo conditions. Gaiser and coworkers [13] addressed this recently by expression of mutated cationic trypsinogen in a pancreatic acinar cell line (AR4-2J). They found that expression of the R122H mutant trypsinogen induced intracellular trypsin activity suggesting increased autoactivation. The experiment does not exclude reduced inactivation, however, and the cell line is derived from an azaserin-induced rat pancreatic acinar tumor (not ideal because naturally expressed rat trypsinogen has a histidine at site 122). Also, the authors noted that in this model there was an increased level of caspase-3 activation, suggesting a noninflammatory apoptotic result of trypsin activation, not consistent with the inflammatory event seen in humans. This raises the issue of whether the mutations are in any case gain of function. If, as the authors speculate, acinar cells may react to intracellular trypsin activity by triggering apoptosis, then a mutation that reduces trypsin activity (loss of function) might be more likely to result in pancreatitis.

It seems incredible after so many years of study that the nature of the initiating event in hereditary pancreatitis is so poorly understood, that such diametrically opposing theories (trypsin activation or inactivation) can still coexist. It is quite possible that elastase and not trypsin is at the start of the protease cascade that leads to pancreatitis; it is even possible that the elastase need not even be expressed in the acinar cells themselves, but be provided by peripheral blood monocytes invading the pancreatic tissue [14]. If the culprit is elastase rather than trypsin, a protective role for trypsin can quite easily be envisaged. A wide range of inactivating mutations is also far easier to accept than multiple gain of function mutations. Against this must be placed, however, the evidence that trypsin activation (and not inactivation) has been observed in models of pancreatitis, such as ceruleintreated mice. Also, trypsin activation can be explained by changes in calcium levels seen in experimental models [15] and predicted to occur as a result of alcohol excess, the most frequent etiologic factor associated with acute or chronic pancreatitis [16]. A better understanding of how the different trypsinogen variants function and impact on disease progression is of great clinical and scientific importance.

Mutations in the cationic trypsinogen gene and variants

The European Registry of Hereditary Pancreatitis and Familial Pancreatic Cancer (EUROPAC) aims to identify and make provisions for those affected by hereditary pancreatitis and familial pancreatic cancer. The most common mutations in hereditary pancreatitis are R122H, N29I, and A16V but many families have been described with clinically defined hereditary pancreatitis where there is no PRSS1 mutation [8].

Since identification of PRSS1 as a disease gene, a number of different mutations have been identified. At least 19 gene variants resulting in

17 amino acid exchanges have been described (http://www.uni-leipzig.de/pancreasmutation/) (Table 1). The two most frequently occurring mutations in hereditary pancreatitis are R122H and N29I. These two mutations have been identified in families with hereditary pancreatitis from Europe, Asia, the Americas, and recently in a Thai family and a family of Aboriginal descent.

R122H

The R122H mutation is a single guanine (G) to adenine (A) transition mutation in the third exon of PRSS1 that results in an arginine (CGC) to histidine (CAC) missense substitution at amino acid residue 122. Note that originally residue 122 was referred to as "position 117" according to the consensus position with chymotrypsinogen; hence, the mutation was referred to as "R117H." The nomenclature presently used is that recommended by the Nomenclature Working Group and also used by the Human Gene Mutation Database.

The trypsin molecule contains a calcium-binding pocket near the side chain connecting the two globular domains of the molecule. This side chain (the autolysis loop) contains amino acid position 122, which is a target for attack by other trypsin molecules. Enzymatic cleavage of the side chain at arginine 122 (R122) by the second trypsin leads to rapid destruction of the first trypsin molecule (autolysis). The autolysis loop is flexible and R122 may come near to the calcium-binding pocket. As the concentration of soluble calcium rises, calcium enters the calcium-binding pocket and limits exposure of R122 to enzymatic attack by another trypsin [17]. It is widely assumed, with some biochemical support [12,18,19], that the substitution of histidine for arginine results in a reduction in the destruction of autoactivated trypsinogen in a calcium-dependent fashion.

In most cases the R122H mutation is easily identified because it created a novel recognition site for the restriction endonuclease AflIII. Howes and coworkers [20], however, demonstrated that a neutral polymorphism within this enzyme recognition site may produce a false-negative result. An alternative mutation-specific polymerase chain reaction approach was developed for detection of the mutation even in the presence of the polymorphism [20].

N29I

A second mutation in PRSS1 was subsequently discovered in two affected families without the R122H mutation [5]. A single adenine (A) to thymine (T) transversion mutation (N29I) was identified in exon 2, which results in a change from asparagine (AAC) to isoleucine (ATC) at amino acid 29. The mutation was previously known as "N21I" according to the chymotrypsinogen consensus numeration.

The mechanism accounting for how N29I causes pancreatitis is uncertain, although in light of the assumed mechanism of action of R122H and the clinical similarities between R122H and N29I phenotypes it was suggested

Table 1
Details of reported PRSS1 mutations and variants

Authors	Mutation: amino acid change[a], nucleotide change, position in genomic DNA[b]	Site	Frequency	Comments
Ferec et al, 1999	-28delTCC (3 base pair deletion at position -28 from ATG)	5'UTR3 (promoter)	Rare	One individual; may increase transcription of PRSS1
Witt et al, 1999	A16V (C > T transition, at nucleotide position 131906, GCC > GTC)	Exon 2	Third commonest	Increased autoactivation?
Chen et al, 2003	D19A (A>C transversion at codon position 56)	Exon 2	Rare	One patient with chronic pancreatitis; facilitation of autoactivation
Teich et al, 2000	D22G (A>G transition, at nucleotide 131924, GAC>GGC)	Exon 2	Rare	One family with hereditary pancreatitis; facilitation of autoactivation
Ferec et al, 1999	K23R (A>G transition, at nucleotide position 131927, AGG>AAG)	Exon 2	Rare	One family with hereditary pancreatitis; facilitation of autoactivation
Gorry et al, 1997	N29I (A>T transversion, at nucleotide position 131945, AAC>ATC)	Exon 2	Second commonest	Increased autoactivation; decreased degradation?
Pfützer et al, 2002	N29T (A>C transition, at nucleotide position 131945)	Exon 2	Rare	Increased autoactivation; decreased degradation?
Chen et al, 2001	P36R (C>G transversion, at nucleotide position 131966, CCC>CGC)	Exon 2	Rare	Found in one patient with idiopathic chronic pancreatitis
Chen et al, 2003	Y37X (C>A missense mutation at codon position 111)	Exon 2	Rare	Found in one patient with alcoholism but not chronic pancreatitis

Reference	Mutation	Exon	Frequency	Comment
Chen et al, 2003	IVS2 + 1G>A (splice mutation)	Exon 2	Rare	Found in one patient with alcoholism but not chronic pancreatitis
Chen et al, 2001; Teich et al, 2002	E79K (G>A transition, at nucleotide position 133153, GAA>AAA)	Exon 3	Rare	Found in three families with hereditary pancreatitis; one patient with idiopathic chronic pancreatitis and two controls
Chen et al, 2001	G83E (G>A transition, at nucleotide position 133166, GGG>GAG)	Exon 3	Rare	Found in one patient with idiopathic chronic pancreatitis
Chen et al, 2001	K92N (G>T transversion, at nucleotide position 133194, AAG>AAT)	Exon 3	Rare	Found in one patient with idiopathic chronic pancreatitis
Teich et al, 2002	L104P (T>C transition at nucleotide position 133229)	Exon 3	Rare	Found in one family with hereditary pancreatitis and could possibly be linked to the disease
Le Maréchal et al, 2001; Teich et al, 2002	R116C (C>T transition at nucleotide position 133246, CGT>TGT)	Exon 3	Rare	Found in three patients with idiopathic chronic pancreatitis and not in phase with disease in one family with hereditary pancreatitis
Whitcomb et al, 1996	R122H (G>A transition, at nucleotide position 133283, CGC>CAC)	Exon 3	Most common	Elimination of the autolysis site; increased autoactivation, decreased degradation
Howes et al, 2001; Chen et al, 2001	R122H (GC>AT transition, at nucleotide positions 133283-4, CGC>CAT)	Exon 3	Rare	Found in one family with hereditary pancreatitis and in one patient with idiopathic chronic pancreatitis; neutral polymorphism that destroys the AflIII restriction site

(continued on next page)

Table 1 (*continued*)

Authors	Mutation: amino acid change[a], nucleotide change, position in genomic DNA[b]	Site	Frequency	Comments
Pfützer et al, 2002; Simon et al, 2002; Le Maréchal et al, 2001	R122C (C>T transition at nucleotide position 133282, CGC>T GC)	Exon 3	Rare	Increased autoactivation; decreased degradation
Chen et al, 2001	V123M (G>A transition, at nucleotide position 133285, GTG>ATG)	Exon 3	Rare	Found in one patient with idiopathic chronic pancreatitis; modification of the autolysis site?
Teich et al, 2002	C139F (G>T transversion, at nucleotide position 133334)	Exon 3	Rare	Found in one individual; could be linked to idiopathic chronic pancreatitis
Teich et al, 2002	D162D (G>T transversion, at nucleotide position 133807)	Exon 4	Rare	Found in one family with hereditary pancreatitis; neutral polymorphism, not disease related
Teich et al, 2002	N246N (C>T transition, at nucleotide position 134309)	Exon 5	Rare	Found in one family with hereditary pancreatitis; neutral polymorphism, not disease related

[a] Numbering of amino acids begins with ATG; [b] or codon position, named in accordance with GenBank accession number U66061.
From Howes N, Greenhalf W, Stocken DD, et al. Cationic trypsinogen mutations and pancreatitis. Gastroenterol Clin North Am 2004;33:770–1.

that the mechanism must involve increased trypsin activity [5]. This may be caused by enhanced autoactivation of trypsinogen, alteration of the binding of pancreatic secretory trypsin inhibitor (SPINK1), or impairment of trypsin inactivation by altering the accessibility of the initial hydrolysis site to trypsin. Whitcomb [21] predicted conformational changes in the crystallographic structure of trypsin, which could explain a reduced accessibility to the calcium-binding pocket. An alternative model was proposed by Nishimori and coworkers [22], who suggested that the N29I mutation alters the native structure of the PRSS1 gene to a sheet structure. It was implied that this conformational alteration might impair trypsin activation. Sahin-Toth and collaborators [12] used direct biochemical approaches to investigate the mechanism rather than structural modeling and concluded that the N29I mutation increased autoactivation under acidic conditions. This is the most widely accepted mechanism at the time of writing and contrasts with the perceived model for R122H pathology (ie, reduced inactivation following autoactivation). Despite the apparently significant difference between the pathologic mechanisms of N29I and R122H, initial reports from the EUROPAC registry indicate a remarkably similar pathophysiology of the disease in patients with the two mutations [8].

A16V

A third mutation where there is a cytosine (C) to thymine (T) missense mutation has been identified in exon 2 that leads to an alanine (GCC) to valine (GTC) substitution at codon 16 (A16V) [23]. This mutation affects the first amino acid of the trypsinogen molecule and directly the cleavage site for the signal peptide. The mechanism by which pancreatitis is initiated remains speculative, but given the position of the mutation at the edge of the signal peptide it is widely believed to involve defects in secretion.

The A16V mutation was originally identified during a study to determine the spectrum and frequency of mutations in the PRSS1 gene in 44 children and adolescents with chronic pancreatitis. Thirty of these individuals were found to have idiopathic pancreatitis and 14 were found to have hereditary pancreatitis. R122H was identified in one individual; A16V was found in three individuals with presumed idiopathic pancreatitis and in one said to have hereditary pancreatitis. The A16V mutation was also identified in seven first-degree relatives of these patients but only one had clinically apparent pancreatitis, suggesting low penetrance of this mutation.

Variants

Recently, in vitro experiments using recombinant trypsinogen preparations have provided some insight into the pathogenesis of genetically determined chronic pancreatitis. The main mutations (N29I and R122H) have exclusively been found in patients with hereditary pancreatitis and, although A16V mutations were originally identified in patients with no clear family history, this mutation has not yet been identified in individuals with ethanol-induced or tropical pancreatitis [8,24–27]. In addition to these three principle mutations, there are multiple variants of the PRSS1 gene as detailed in a recent review by Howes and coworkers [8]. These include -28delTCC (a three–base pair deletion 28 base pairs upstream from the start codon) [28]; D19A [29]; D22G [30]; K23R [28]; N29T [31]; P36R [25]; Y37X [32]; G83E [25]; K92N [25]; L104P [24]; R116C [24]; V123M [25]; C139F [24]; and most recently V39A [33]. All these variants are rare and in some cases the link with inherited pancreatitis is only suggestive. Two neutral polymorphisms (D162D and N246N [24]) have also been described (see Table 1). Clearly, the actions of all of these mutant trypsinogens could upset the balance of pancreatic protease-antiprotease equilibrium resulting in supraprotease activity in the functional acinar unit.

Anionic trypsinogen and mesotrypsinogen

Because mutations in the cationic trypsinogen gene cause pancreatitis, it is reasonable to state that genetic alterations in the other two trypsinogen genes expressed in pancreatic tissue may also cause pancreatitis. The involvement of anionic trypsinogen and mesotrypsinogen in chronic pancreatitis has been excluded in one study of six symptomatic families with no PRSS1 mutation [34]. More recently, the E79K mutation of cationic trypsin leads to an enhanced transactivation of anionic trypsinogen [35]. The presumption is that the ensuing imbalance may initiate a further activation of trypsinogen and other pancreatic zymogens with sequential pancreatic autodigestion. A recent report from India excludes the association of mutations in the anionic trypsinogen gene in tropical calcific chronic pancreatitis, suggesting a role for other genetic or nongenetic factors in the disease pathogenesis [36].

Chen and coworkers [32] recently identified a stop codon mutation in exon 2 of an alcoholic patient without pancreatitis, suggesting that a loss of function mutation in PRSS1 may act as a protective factor against pancreatitis.

Sahin-Toth [37] recently found that mesotrypsin rapidly hydrolyzed the reactive-site peptide bond of the Kunitz-type soybean trypsin inhibitor and completely degraded the Kazal-type pancreatic secretory trypsin inhibitor, suggesting that mesotrypsin has a purpose in protease inhibitor degradation and may, in a prematurely activated form, degrade protease pancreatic secretory trypsin inhibitor, predisposing to pancreatitis. This is consistent with the notion that mesotrypsinogen is strongly activated by the pathologic trypsinogen activator cathepsin B [37]. In vitro, mesotrypsinogen is robustly activated by the lysosomal cysteine protease cathepsin B [2], which is responsible for trypsinogen activation in experimental pancreatitis [9]. Hence, if mesotrypsinogen is converted to mesotrypsin prematurely in the pancreas, then resultant degradation of SPINK1 may represent an immediate risk factor for an acute attack of pancreatitis [38]. To explore this model, Nemoda and coworkers [38] tested the hypothesis that the E32del genetic variant of mesotrypsin may represent a risk factor for chronic pancreatitis, as a result of enhanced degradation of SPINK1. They screened almost equal numbers (N approximately 100 in each group) of healthy controls and individuals with alcohol-induced chronic pancreatitis for the E32del variant and characterized the biochemical properties of E32del mesotrypsinogen. They found that E32del mesotrypsinogen is a frequent polymorphic variant not associated with chronic alcoholic pancreatitis.

Other disease genes

SPINK1 plays a crucial role in the regulation of intra-acinar trypsin activity and is a good candidate for a hereditary pancreatitis disease gene. A mutation in SPINK1 (N34S) has been shown to be associated with pancreatitis; however, it is common in the general population and it is unlikely that in isolation it results in the initiation of pancreatitis. It may be that the N34S mutation acts in conjunction with another susceptibility mutation, such as mutations in the cystic fibrosis transmembrane conductance regulator (CFTR). Cystic fibrosis is one of the most common inherited diseases of the exocrine pancreas. The main pathology of cystic fibrosis results from obstruction of ducts in several organs, including the pancreas, by mucous secretions. Although cystic fibrosis is associated with pancreatic insufficiency rather than pancreatitis, heterozygous mutations in CFTR [39] gene may result in chronic pancreatitis in cystic fibrosis carriers.

Although mutations in the SPINK1 and CFTR genes have been associated with cases of pancreatitis of various etiology, no other gene apart from PRSS1 has been shown to have mutations that cause hereditary pancreatitis. Many families, however, have been described with clinically defined hereditary pancreatitis where there is no PRSS1 mutation [8]. This indicates that there is at least one more disease gene left to be identified.

Genotype-phenotype correlation

Hereditary pancreatitis has an extremely variable clinical course with some patients suffering early onset debilitating acute attacks, followed by rapid progression to chronic disease and exocrine-endocrine failure, whereas others (even within the same family) may have late onset with mild attacks and little or no long-term pancreatic failure. Some mutation carriers (approximately 20%) do not develop the disease at all. An understanding of the mechanism of disease pathology would be greatly assisted by accurate correlation between the features of disease and the genotype of the patient. This requires a mechanism for description of disease severity and an understanding of nongenetic factors that influence the disease. Chronic pancreatitis has been defined as a progressive inflammatory disease characterized by irreversible histologic transformation that clinically presents with pain or loss of function [40]. Any causative factor resulting in an acute episode of pancreatitis may incite further, recurrent attacks. Alcohol consumption and choledocholithiasis account for approximately 70% of all acute cases of pancreatitis.

All forms of pancreatitis seem to be associated with cancer to some degree [41], although the exact mechanism linking various forms of pancreatitis to pancreatic cancer remains to be elucidated. The risk of pancreatic cancer in alcoholic chronic pancreatitis seems to rise only after several decades with chronic pancreatitis [42]. Lowenfels and coworkers [42] found a cumulative risk of pancreatic cancer in individuals with alcoholic chronic pancreatitis of 1.8% after 10 years and 4% after 20 years. Augustine and coworkers [43] reported pancreatic adenocarcinoma in 22 (8.3%) of 266 individuals with tropical pancreatitis presenting over an 8-year period. Chari and coworkers [44] followed 185 individuals with tropical pancreatitis for an average of 4.5 years and found 24 individuals died from all causes, with six deaths from pancreatic cancer. The average age of onset of pancreatic cancer was 45.6 ± 7.3 years, which is younger than for Western populations. When compared with the background pancreatic cancer rate, individuals with tropical pancreatitis had a significantly increased risk of pancreatic cancer (relative risk = 100; 95% confidence interval [CI], 37–218). All forms of pancreatitis may be modified by genetic components, such as CFTR gene and the SPINK1 gene, which have been found to be associated with chronic pancreatitis as modifier genes.

Lowenfels and coworkers [45] on behalf of the International Hereditary Pancreatitis Study Group estimated the cumulative lifetime risk (to the age of 70 years) of cancer of the pancreas to be 40% in patients with hereditary pancreatitis. This was supported by Howes and coworkers [8] in a larger study. Tobacco smoking seems further to increase this risk [8,45,46]. Lowenfels and coworkers [45] also reported that paternal transmission of hereditary pancreatitis was associated with a much greater lifetime risk of developing pancreatic cancer, but it was subsequently shown that there was no significant difference between paternal and maternal transmission [47].

Clinical progress of hereditary pancreatitis patients with different mutations

Conceptually, it is assumed that different mechanisms of action of the two main PRSS1 mutations lead to variation in pathologies. Analysis of clinical data from patients with different PRSS1 mutations was performed by EUROPAC using multilevel proportional hazards modeling and was published in 2004 [8]. This study looked at 112 families in 14 countries (418 affected individuals): 58 (52%) families carried the R122H; 24 (21%) carried the N29I; 5 (4%) carried the A16V mutation; 2 had rare mutations;

and 21(19%) had no PRSS1 mutation. The median (95% CI) time to first symptoms for R122H was 10 (8,12) years of age and 14 (11,18) years for N29I. The cumulative risk (95% CI) at 50 years of age was 37.2% (28.5%–45.8%) for exocrine failure and 47.6% (37.1%–58.1%) for endocrine failure. The cumulative risk (95% CI) of pancreatic cancer was 44% (8%–80%) at 70 years from symptom onset with a standardized incidence ratio of 67% (50%–82%). Curves for age of onset of pancreatitis in EURO-PAC patients are shown in Fig. 1. Although R122H patients did have a statistically significant earlier age of onset, the difference was marginal and certainly did not give grounds for different clinical management of the two groups. In addition to endocrine failure, exocrine failure and development of pancreas cancer all appeared equivalent in the two groups of patients. This suggests, regardless of the biochemical controversy, that the mutations function similarly in causing disease.

Gene conversion

An argument for the loss-of-function model of hereditary pancreatitis mutations is the relatively large number of mutations or variants associated with the disease; there are many ways to break something, but only specific changes result in a gain of function [48]. Similarly, it is easy to explain why the principal mutations have similar pathologies if both mutations cause function to be lost, but if they result in gain of different functions then different pathologies are assumed. Alternatively, the gains of function can be programmed into the

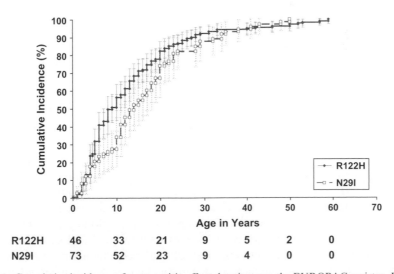

R122H	46	33	21	9	5	2	0
N29I	73	52	23	9	4	0	0

Fig. 1. Cumulative incidence of pancreatitis-affected patients on the EUROPAC registry. Data for R122H and N29I patients are given with the number of at-risk individuals for each group given under the graph.

cell by evolution; this is not too far fetched given that there are multiple forms of trypsinogen all contributing to an exquisite balance of pancreatic proteases and antiproteases. The source of genetic material for the observed mutations in PRSS1 might be one of the other trypsinogen genes. Gene conversion relates to the nonreciprocal transfer of genetic information between homologous chromosomes. Trypsinogen genes are tandemly repeated within the T-cell receptor β locus (TCR β), which is a hotspot for gene conversion events to generate a broad variety of TCR β genes. It has been speculated that conversion mutations within the interpolated trypsinogen gene family are likely [49]. This was first suggested by Chen and Ferec [50] for the N29I mutation but is also a possible explanation for the occurrence of R122H. Gene conversion normally involves the transfer of multiple bases; if conversion rather than spontaneous mutation is responsible for the base changes at codon 122 or 29, then base changes in the near vicinity are expected. In the case of gene conversion of codon 122 from the pseudogene TRY6, a minimum of a dinucleotide substitution (c.365_366GC > AT) is expected. This dinucleotide substitution has been observed [50]; however, single nucleotide substitutions causing R122H (c.365 > A), N29I (c.86A > T), and A16V (c.47 > T) are more common [51].

Recently, Teich and coworkers [49] reported a unique gene conversion that leads to complete replacement of exon 2 of the PRSS1 gene (acceptor gene) by the corresponding PRSS2 sequence (donor gene), confirming the original notion that gene conversion is a relevant mechanism for pancreatitis-associated trypsinogen mutations. The conversion event observed by Teich and coworkers [49] resulted in a second amino acid change on exon 2 (N54S and N29I), but they found no difference in the biochemical characterization of the N29I-N54S double mutant compared with the previously investigated N29I mutant, suggesting that the N54S mutation has no additional deleterious effect.

Summary

Acute pancreatitis is a common debilitating and frequently fatal disease. The major etiologic factors are alcohol consumption and choledocholithiasis, but much debate remains on the mechanism by which these factors lead to the disease state. There is an autosomal-dominant inherited form of pancreatitis with several known disease mutations in the cationic trypsinogen gene, PRSS1. Because these mutations are clearly causative, they offer clues to the initiating event of pancreatitis in the sporadic form of the disease. Conflicting hypotheses exist as to whether the mutations represent a gain of function (eg, inappropriate activation of trypsinogen) or loss of function. This article discusses the possible pathologic mechanisms of the different PRSS1 mutations; biochemical and genetic factors are considered in the context of clinical observations. It is speculated that gene conversion of PRSS1 by transfer of information from other trypsinogen genes and pseudogenes may explain frequent founder events, allowing for exchange of function from the other proteins, disturbing the protease-inhibitor equilibrium.

References

[1] Rowen L, Koop BF, Hood L. The complete 685-kilobase DNA sequence of the human beta T cell receptor locus. Science 1996;272:1755–62.

[2] Szmola R, Kukor Z, Sahin-Toth M. Human mesotrypsin is a unique digestive protease specialized for the degradation of trypsin inhibitors. J Biol Chem 2003;278:48580–9.

[3] Kukor Z, Toth M, Sahin-Toth M. Human anionic trypsinogen: properties of autocatalytic activation and degradation and implications in pancreatic diseases. Eur J Biochem 2003;270: 2047–58.

[4] Whitcomb DC, Gorry MC, Preston RA, et al. Hereditary pancreatitis is caused by a mutation in the cationic trypsinogen gene. Nat Genet 1996;14:141–5.

[5] Gorry MC, Gabbaizedeh D, Furey W, et al. Mutations in the cationic trypsinogen gene are associated with recurrent acute and chronic pancreatitis. Gastroenterology 1997;113: 1063–8.

[6] Keim V, Bauer N, Teich N, et al. Clinical characterization of patients with hereditary pancreatitis and mutations in the cationic trypsinogen gene. Am J Med 2001;111:622–6.

[7] Amann ST, Gates LK, Aston CE, et al. Expression and penetrance of the hereditary pancreatitis phenotype in monozygotic twins. Gut 2001;48:542–7.

[8] Howes N, Lerch MM, Greenhalf W, et al. Clinical and genetic characteristics of hereditary pancreatitis in Europe. Clin Gastroenterol Hepatol 2004;2:252–61.

[9] Halangk W, Lerch MM, Brandt-Nedelev B, et al. Role of cathepsin B in intracellular trypsinogen activation and the onset of acute pancreatitis. J Clin Invest 2000;106:773–81.

[10] Kukor Z, Mayerle J, Kruger B, et al. Presence of cathepsin B in the human pancreatic secretory pathway and its role in trypsinogen activation during hereditary pancreatitis. J Biol Chem 2002;277:21389–96.

[11] Teich N, Bodeker H, Keim V. Cathepsin B cleavage of the trypsinogen activation peptide. BMC Gastroenterol 2002;2:16.

[12] Sahin-Toth M. Human cationic trypsinogen: role of Asn-21 in zymogen activation and implications in hereditary pancreatitis. J Biol Chem 2000;275:22750–5.

[13] Gaiser S, Ahler A, Gundling F, et al. Expression of mutated cationic trypsinogen reduces cellular viability in AR4–2J cells. Biochem Biophys Res Commun 2005;334:721–8.

[14] Mayerle J, Schnekenburger J, Kruger B, et al. Extracellular cleavage of E-cadherin by leukocyte elastase during acute experimental pancreatitis in rats. Gastroenterology 2005;129: 1251–67.

[15] Raraty M, Ward J, Erdemli G, et al. Calcium-dependent enzyme activation and vacuole formation in the apical granular region of pancreatic acinar cells. Proc Natl Acad Sci U S A 2000;97:13126–31.

[16] Criddle DN, Raraty MG, Neoptolemos JP, et al. Ethanol toxicity in pancreatic acinar cells: mediation by nonoxidative fatty acid metabolites. Proc Natl Acad Sci U S A 2004;101: 10738–43.

[17] Simon P, Weiss FU, Sahin-Toth M, et al. Hereditary pancreatitis caused by a novel PRSS1 mutation (Arg-122 right-arrow Cys) that alters autoactivation and autodegradation of cationic trypsinogen. J Biol Chem 2002;277:5404–10.

[18] Sahin-Toth M. The pathobiochemistry of hereditary pancreatitis: studies on recombinant human cationic trypsinogen. Pancreatology 2001;1:461–5.

[19] Sahin-Toth M, Toth M. Gain-of-function mutations associated with hereditary pancreatitis enhance autoactivation of human cationic trypsinogen. Biochem Biophys Res Commun 2000;278:286–9.

[20] Howes N, Greenhalf W, Rutherford S, et al. A new polymorphism for the R122H mutation in hereditary pancreatitis. Gut 2001;48:247–50.
[21] Whitcomb DC. Hereditary pancreatitis: new insights into acute and chronic pancreatitis. Gut 1999;45:317–22.
[22] Nishimori I, Kamakura M, Fujikawa-Adachi K, et al. Mutations in exons 2 and 3 of the cationic trypsinogen gene in Japanese families with hereditary pancreatitis. Gut 1999;44: 259–63.
[23] Witt H, Luck W, Becker M. A signal peptide cleavage site mutation in the cationic trypsinogen gene is strongly associated with chronic pancreatitis. Gastroenterology 1999;117:7–10.
[24] Teich N, Bauer N, Mossner J, et al. Mutational screening of patients with nonalcoholic chronic pancreatitis: identification of further trypsinogen variants. Am J Gastroenterol 2002;97:341–6.
[25] Chen JM, Piepoli Bis A, Le Bodic L, et al. Mutational screening of the cationic trypsinogen gene in a large cohort of subjects with idiopathic chronic pancreatitis. Clin Genet 2001;59: 189–93.
[26] Rossi L, Whitcomb DC, Ehrlich GD, et al. Lack of R117H mutation in the cationic trypsinogen gene in patients with tropical pancreatitis from Bangladesh. Pancreas 1998;17:278–80.
[27] Simon P, Weiss FU, Zimmer KP, et al. Spontaneous and sporadic trypsinogen mutations in idiopathic pancreatitis. JAMA 2002;288:2122.
[28] Ferec C, Raguenes O, Salomon R, et al. Mutations in the cationic trypsinogen gene and evidence for genetic heterogeneity in hereditary pancreatitis. J Med Genet 1999;36:228–32.
[29] Chen JM, Kukor Z, Le Marechal C, et al. Evolution of trypsinogen activation peptides. Mol Biol Evol 2003;20:1767–77.
[30] Teich N, Ockenga J, Hoffmeister A, et al. Chronic pancreatitis associated with an activation peptide mutation that facilitates trypsin activation. Gastroenterology 2000;119:461–5.
[31] Pfutzer R, Myers E, Applebaum-Shapiro S, et al. Novel cationic trypsinogen (PRSS1) N29T and R122C mutations cause autosomal dominant hereditary pancreatitis. Gut 2002;50: 271–2.
[32] Chen JM, Le Marechal C, Lucas D, et al. Loss of function mutations in the cationic trypsinogen gene (PRSS1) may act as a protective factor against pancreatitis. Mol Genet Metab 2003;79:67–70.
[33] Arduino C, Salacone P, Pasini B, et al. Association of a new cationic trypsinogen gene mutation (V39A) with chronic pancreatitis in an Italian family. Gut 2005;54:1663–4.
[34] Chen JM, Audrezet MP, Mercier B, et al. Exclusion of anionic trypsinogen and mesotrypsinogen involvement in hereditary pancreatitis without cationic trypsinogen gene mutations. Scand J Gastroenterol 1999;34:831–2.
[35] Teich N, Le Marechal C, Kukor Z, et al. Interaction between trypsinogen isoforms in genetically determined pancreatitis: mutation E79K in cationic trypsin (PRSS1) causes increased transactivation of anionic trypsinogen (PRSS2). Hum Mutat 2004;23:22–31.
[36] Idris MM, Bhaskar S, Reddy DN, et al. Mutations in anionic trypsinogen gene are not associated with tropical calcific pancreatitis. Gut 2005;54:728–9.
[37] Sahin-Toth M. Human mesotrypsin defies natural trypsin inhibitors: from passive resistance to active destruction. Protein Pept Lett 2005;12:457–64.
[38] Nemoda Z, Teich N, Hugenberg C, et al. Genetic and biochemical characterization of the E32del polymorphism in human mesotrypsinogen. Pancreatol 2005;5:273–8.
[39] Cohn JA, Noone PG, Jowell PS. Idiopathic pancreatitis related to CFTR: complex inheritance and identification of a modifier gene. J Investig Med 2002;50:247S–55S.
[40] Etemad B, Whitcomb DC. Chronic pancreatitis: diagnosis, classification, and new genetic developments. Gastroenterology 2001;120:682–707.
[41] Whitcomb DC, Pogue-Geile K. Pancreatitis as a risk for pancreatic cancer. Gastroenterol Clin North Am 2002;31:663–78.
[42] Lowenfels AB, Maisonneuve P, Cavallini G, et al. Pancreatitis and the risk of pancreatic cancer. International Pancreatitis Study Group. N Engl J Med 1993;328:1433–7.

[43] Augustine P, Ramesh H. Is tropical pancreatitis premalignant? Am J Gastroenterol 1992;87: 1005–8.

[44] Chari ST, Mohan V, Pitchumoni CS, et al. Risk of pancreatic carcinoma in tropical calcifying pancreatitis: an epidemiologic study. Pancreas 1994;9:62–6.

[45] Lowenfels AB, Maisonneuve P, DiMagno EP, et al. Hereditary pancreatitis and the risk of pancreatic cancer. International Hereditary Pancreatitis Study Group. J Natl Cancer Inst 1997;89:442–6.

[46] Lowenfels AB, Maisonneuve P, Whitcomb DC, et al. Cigarette smoking as a risk factor for pancreatic cancer in patients with hereditary pancreatitis. JAMA 2001;286:169–70.

[47] Lerch MM, Ellis I, Whitcomb DC, et al. Maternal inheritance pattern of hereditary pancreatitis in patients with pancreatic carcinoma. J Natl Cancer Inst 1999;91:723–4.

[48] Halangk W, Lerch MM. Early events in acute pancreatitis. Gastroenterol Clin North Am 2004;33:717–31.

[49] Teich N, Nemoda Z, Kohler H, et al. Gene conversion between functional trypsinogen genes PRSS1 and PRSS2 associated with chronic pancreatitis in a six-year-old girl. Hum Mutat 2005;25:343–7.

[50] Chen JM, Ferec C. Origin and implication of the hereditary pancreatitis-associated N21I mutation in the cationic trypsinogen gene. Hum Genet 2000;106:125–6.

[51] Chen JM, Raguenes O, Ferec C, et al. CGC > CAT gene conversion-like event resulting in the R122H mutation in the cationic trypsinogen gene and its implication in the genotyping of pancreatitis. J Med Genet 2000;37:E36.

ELSEVIER
SAUNDERS

Endocrinol Metab Clin N Am
35 (2006) 289–302

ENDOCRINOLOGY
AND METABOLISM
CLINICS
OF NORTH AMERICA

Germline Mutations and Gene Polymorphism Associated With Human Pancreatitis

F. Ulrich Weiss, PhD, Peter Simon, MD,
Julia Mayerle, MD, Matthias Kraft, MD,
Markus M. Lerch, MD*

Department of Gastroenterology, Endocrinology, and Nutrition, Ernst-Moritz-Arndt Universität Greifswald, Friedrich-Loeffler-Strasse 23A, 17485 Greifswald, Germany

A wide range of mutations and polymorphisms in genes that relate to pancreatic function seem to be involved in the development of pancreatitis. They have been found either to determine an individual's susceptibility to develop pancreatitis or to determine the severity of the disease and the disease progression. Some of these genetic alterations lead to disease phenotypes with unequivocal mendelian inheritance patterns, whereas others seem to act as modifier genes in conjunction with environmental or, as yet unidentified, genetic cofactors. This article reviews germline changes in the genes for trypsin, pancreatic secretory trypsin inhibitor, the cystic fibrosis conductance regulator, lipid metabolism proteins, inflammatory mediators for cytokines, and cathepsin B (CTSB). International guidelines recommend genetic testing only for the former and only when chronic pancreatitis develops or two or more episodes of acute pancreatitis occur in patients with no known risk factor for pancreatitis (particularly alcohol) and specifically when the patient is under 25 years of age, and when one or more relatives of a patient also suffer from pancreatitis in the absence of known risk factors.

Chronic pancreatitis

Pancreatitis is an inflammatory disease initiated by events that cause acinar cell injury, the release of prematurely activated digestive enzymes,

---

* Corresponding author.
E-mail address: lerch@uni-greifswald.de (M.M. Lerch).

0889-8529/06/$ - see front matter © 2006 Elsevier Inc. All rights reserved.
doi:10.1016/j.ecl.2006.02.001

subsequent tissue and endothelial damage, and the development of a potentially lethal inflammatory response [1].

Chronic pancreatitis is clinically characterized by acinar cell degeneration and fibrosis that may lead to a destruction of exocrine and endocrine organ function and results in maldigestion and diabetes mellitus. Several underlying conditions seem to play a role in the pathogenesis of chronic pancreatitis. Recent progress in molecular techniques has intensified the search for genetic changes that cause or participate in the onset and progression of pancreatitis, and various germline changes and polymorphisms have been found to be associated with the disease.

Hereditary pancreatitis

In 1952, a hereditary predisposition to chronic pancreatitis that is independent of additional environmental factors was reported in a number of families by Comfort and Steinberg [2]. Hereditary pancreatitis is an autosomal-dominant disorder with a clinical manifestation that is indistinguishable from other etiologic varieties of pancreatitis. In affected patients, hereditary pancreatitis begins with recurrent attacks of acute pancreatitis that usually start in childhood or young adulthood, but in occasional patients symptom onset can begin in the seventh decade of life [3]. The severity of disease at onset ranges from mild to a complicated course with progression to pancreatic necrosis and, rarely, organ failure. Recurrent attacks of pancreatitis frequently progress to chronic disease at an early age and are associated with a significant lifetime risk for the development of pancreatic cancer [3,4]. This 60- to 70-fold increased pancreatic cancer risk is greatly increased when the patient smokes [5,6]. Although the incidence of hereditary pancreatitis is low and to date only several hundred families have been identified worldwide, the studies addressing the onset of hereditary pancreatitis have permitted several breakthroughs in the general understanding of the pathophysiology of acute and chronic pancreatitis.

Cationic trypsinogen

Whitcomb and coworkers [7] reported 10 years ago that a point mutation in the cationic trypsinogen gene on chromosome 7 is associated with hereditary pancreatitis. This finding represented a major success in the effort to understand the pathophysiology of acute and chronic pancreatitis on a molecular level. The mutation leads to a substitution of the amino acid arginine (R) to histidine (H) at position 122 and is now established as the most common mutation in the cationic trypsinogen in patients with hereditary pancreatitis. The pathophysiologic mechanisms through which carriers of the R122H mutation develop pancreatitis are unknown. It has, however, been proposed that the amino acid substitution leads to a gain of trypsin function by either a more rapid or efficient intracellular trypsinogen activation or by an impaired inactivation and autolysis, once the trypsin is enzymatically activated. In either event this results in extended trypsinogen activity that may initiate an autodigestive process within the acinar cell. The trypsin crystal structure [8] and recent biochemical data [9] are consistent with the hypothesis that R122 represents the trypsin autolysis site, which may become disrupted by the R122H mutation and impairs an important failsafe mechanism against premature or overactivation of trypsin. Recently, three groups independently reported families with an arginine-cystein exchange mutation within this same codon 122 (R122C) [10–12]. Interestingly, R122C-trypsinogen seems to differ from the R122H mutant by a greatly reduced autoactivation and an increased resistance to autolysis. Activation of recombinantly expressed R122C mutant human trypsinogen by CTSB was also greatly reduced, which is presumably a result of misfolding caused by disulfide mismatches. If this protein misfolding reflects the in vivo situation, a dramatic loss of cellular trypsin activity should be observed that raises the fundamental question whether a gain or a loss of trypsin function is crucial for the triggering mechanism in hereditary pancreatitis. A very similar loss of trypsin function mutation (E79K) was recently reported from another hereditary pancreatitis family and extensively characterized in vitro [13]. Taken together the data obtained from recombinant human trypsin variants with disease-relevant mutations are inconsistent as to whether a gain or loss of trypsin function causes hereditary pancreatitis.

Despite the remaining uncertainty about the molecular events that precede the induction of pancreatitis it is remarkable that two different mutations, and a silent polymorphism, have been found at the same codon 122 of cationic trypsinogen. This arginine 122 not only seems to represent a critical site for the biochemical properties of trypsin and the events that determine the onset of pancreatitis but also a "hot spot" for frequent genetic alterations, as recently shown with the discovery of a spontaneous de novo R122H mutation at this site [14]. Without knowing the frequency of such spontaneous mutations this finding suggests that the diagnosis of hereditary pancreatitis (as defined by a genetic predisposition) cannot entirely be ruled out even in the absence of a familial history for pancreatitis.

Another disease-relevant trypsinogen mutation leading to a substitution of asparagine by isoleucine at position 29 (N29I) has been suggested to result in a conformational change of the trypsin molecule that prevents proteolytic accession of its autolysis site and renders trypsin more resistant to inactivation. Crystallographic data confirm that N29 is in short proximity to R122H on the protein surface and the main support for this hypothesis comes from in vitro studies of recombinant rat cationic trypsinogen [15]. Enhanced autoactivation at pH 5.0 has also been reported [9], however, suggesting an alternative explanation for an increased trypsin function. A comparison of clinical data from R122H and N29I hereditary pancreatitis patients suggests that both have a fairly similar clinical course with most patients having developed exocrine and endocrine pancreatic insufficiency by the age of 70 years [3,16].

Furthermore, a mutation in the signal peptide cleavage site has been found to be associated with chronic pancreatitis [17]. A substitution of valine by alanine at position 16 (A16V) is presumed to interfere with the intracellular processing of trypsinogen but the pathophysiologic mechanisms remains unclear. It has been speculated that A16V may disturb the activation of trypsinogen by lysosomal CTSB. The colocalized hydrolase CTSB might activate A16V mutated trypsinogen more readily. A16V seems to be a relatively frequent mutation, whose penetrance is much lower than that of the mutations described previously and it was most frequently found in children with seemingly idiopathic pancreatitis (ie, without a family history).

Other rare mutations have been identified within the trypsinogen activation peptide (D22G, K23R) [18], which is cleaved from the N-terminus of trypsinogen during its proteolytic activation to trypsin. The pathophysiologic mechanism suggested here is an increased autoactivation of trypsinogen leading to elevated intracellular trypsin-levels.

Further trypsinogen variants L104P, R116C, and C139F [19] have been described in a mutational screening of patients with nonalcoholic chronic pancreatitis. To date, however, these mutations have been reported only in single individuals and their relevance to the pathogenesis of pancreatitis remains questionable. In the absence of functional data, that may represent phenotypically silent polymorphisms.

The discovery of not only one single mutation, but of at least 20 different germline alterations in the cationic trypsinogen gene, is evidence for the genetic heterogeneity in hereditary pancreatitis.

Pancreatic secretory trypsin inhibitor (SPINK-1)

The pancreatic secretory trypsin inhibitor (PSTI), a 59–amino acid Kazal type 1 serine protease inhibitor (the gene is named SPINK-1), is synthesized in acinar cells as a 79–amino acid single-chain polypeptide precursor that is subsequently processed to the mature peptide and secreted into the pancreatic ducts together with digestive proteases. It is regarded as a first-line defense system capable of inhibiting up to 20% of the total intracellular trypsin activity that could result from accidental premature trypsinogen activation within acinar cells. First studies on the role of PSTI mutations in chronic pancreatitis patients reported that some of these patients had a point mutation in exon 3 of the PSTI gene that leads to the substitution of an asparagine by serine at position 34 (N34S) [20]. Analysis of intronic sequences showed that the N34S mutation is in complete linkage disequilibrium with four additional sequence variants: (1) IVS1-37TC, (2) IVS2 + 268AG, (3) IVS3-604GA, and (4) IVS3-69insTTTT. In a number of studies further mutations and polymorphisms have been detected in PSTI, which also include a methionine to threonine exchange that destroys the start codon of PSTI. These are a leucine to proline exchange in codon 14 (L14P); an aspartate to glutamine exchange in codon 50 (D50E); and a proline to serine exchange in codon 55 (P55). Few studies have reported the frequencies of these mutations and they seem to be fairly low in comparison with the clearly disease-relevant N34S variant. Most subsequent studies have apparently restricted their analysis to the most frequent N34S mutation. N34S is found at a low abundance (0.4%–2.5%) in the normal healthy population but seems to be accumulated in selected groups of chronic pancreatitis patients. Because of inconsistent selection criteria different groups reported N34S mutations in 6%, 19%, 26%, or even 86% of alcoholic, hereditary, or familial idiopathic pancreatitis patient groups [20–24]. Although the prevalence of the N34S mutation seems to be increased in pancreatitis it does not follow a clear mendelian inheritance pattern. In hereditary pancreatitis associated with mutations in the cationic trypsinogen gene, studies have demonstrated that the additional presence of a SPINK1 mutation affects neither the penetrance nor the disease severity or the onset of a secondary diabetes mellitus in affected patients [25]. Although this does not rule out that SPINK1 is a weak risk factor for the onset of pancreatitis in general, it makes a role in the onset of hereditary pancreatitis associated with strong PRSS1 mutations very unlikely.

In studies that analyzed the association of PSTI with tropical pancreatitis, an endemic variety of pancreatitis in Africa and Asia, several groups reported a strong association of N34S in populations from India and Bangladesh. Tropical pancreatitis is a type of idiopathic chronic pancreatitis of so far unknown etiology that is sometimes categorized according to its predominant clinical manifestations into either tropical calcific pancreatitis or fibrocalculous pancreatic diabetes. Although frequencies of the N34S mutation in the normal control population are comparable with previous reports from Europe and North America (1.3%), the mutation was found in 55% and 29% of tropical calcific pancreatitis patients and in 20% and 36% of tropical calcific pancreatitis patients in Bangladesh and South India, respectively [26,27]. Mutations in the PSTI gene may define a genetic predisposition for pancreatitis or could lower the threshold for pancreatitis caused by other factors with the exception of cationic trypsinogen mutations [25].

Why SPINK1 mutations cause pancreatitis remains unclear. Because one of the known functions of PSTI is that of a serine protease (specifically trypsin) inhibitor it is tempting to speculate that a defective PSTI lowers the cellular defenses against premature and intracellular trypsinogen activation and that is a risk factor for tropical pancreatitis. An animal model in which PSTI was overexpressed in the pancreas and that in an experimental disease model of pancreatitis was found to become more resistant to acinar injury would support this notion [28]. Recombinant PSTI into which the most disease-relevant SPINK1 mutation (N34S) was introduced has a completely unimpaired trypsin-inhibiting capacity compared with the wild-type protein [29]. This suggests that the risk for developing pancreatitis conveyed by the human SPINK1 mutations may involve the perturbation of a function of PSTI that is unrelated to the inhibition of trypsin and as yet unidentified. Clear support for this assumption comes from studies involving SPINK-1–PSTI knockout mice [30]. Although the congenital absence of SPINK1 leads to severe developmental abnormalities of the pancreas it leaves the premature intracellular activation of trypsinogen (for some authors the key event to explain hereditary and SPINK1 mutation-associated pancreatitis) completely unaffected. The inconsistency of available experimental data involving cationic trypsin and SPINK1 suggests that the pathophysiologic mechanism underlying the onset of pancreatitis is more complex than a mere proteolytic degradation by a digestive protease as innocuous as trypsin.

Cystic fibrosis transmembrane conductance regulator gene

Two groups [31,32] reported independently in 1998 a strong association of cystic fibrosis transmembrane conductance regulator gene (CFTR) mutations with idiopathic chronic pancreatitis. CFTR mutations were then well known to cause cystic fibrosis, the most frequent autosomal-recessive inherited disease in whites. Typical features of cystic fibrosis include progressive obstructive pulmonary disease, pancreatic insufficiency, abnormal sweat secretion, and male infertility, but only rarely pancreatitis. Children with CFTR mutations are often born with a severely damaged, fibrotic pancreas and pancreatic insufficiency. CFTR, an adenosine 3′, 5′-cAMP and phosphorylation-regulated chloride channel, plays a critical role in the regulation of epithelial ion transport. The degree of impaired CFTR protein function for the gene variations registered so far (www.genet.sickkids.on.ca/cftr/) seems to determine the type and severity of epithelial disease phenotypes.

In the pancreas, CFTR is expressed in centroacinar and proximal intralobular duct cells and also in the apical cell membranes [33] of acinar cells. In a recent study [34] , insight into the pathomechanisms of cystic fibrosis–related pancreatic disease, expanding the theory of inspissated pancreatic secretions as a main factor for pancreatic injury, was provided. The study revealed that a proinflammatory, antiapoptotic pathway is responsible for the susceptibility to acute experimental pancreatitis in mice with defective CFTR expression.

To date more than 1000 CFTR mutations have been reported. Widely used commercial tests, however, including those used in the studies that established an association between CFTR mutations and idiopathic chronic pancreatitis [31,32], can detect only a few (approximately 30) CFTR mutations and only those that are known to cause classical cystic fibrosis. Although individuals with two identified CFTR mutations identified by standard screening tests suffer from at least mild cystic fibrosis, it was until recently unknown whether the risk for developing pancreatitis conveyed by CFTR mutations regarded homozygote, compound heterozygote, or even healthy heterozygote carriers of such mutations. In a recent publication it was shown that even cystic fibrosis carrier status for different types of

CFTR mutations, including uncommon-mild mutations, significantly increases the risk of developing pancreatitis [35]. This study also indicates that a coinheritance of SPINK1 mutations in idiopathic chronic pancreatitis is not required for CFTR mutations to confer their risk for developing pancreatitis. The degree of CFTR functional impairment is important for the increased susceptibility to pancreatitis but even uncommon-mild mutations must be considered as potential risk factors for the disease. The increase in risk that the latter confer should, however, not be overestimated because it does not exceed twofold to threefold over background.

Genetic predisposition in chronic alcoholic pancreatitis

Alcohol remains one of the most important risk factors associated with chronic pancreatitis. In industrialized countries, long-term alcohol abuse accounts for approximately 70% of chronic pancreatitis cases, whereas in 25% the cause remains unknown. Although acute pancreatitis is caused by events unrelated to alcohol in approximately 50%, alcohol-related pancreatitis is diagnosed most commonly as a chronic disease state. Recurrent episodes of acute inflammation may lead in the long-term to chronic inflammation and fibrosis. The correlation between alcohol abuse and chronic pancreatitis is not linear because it seems that less than 5% of severe alcoholics develop pancreatitis as a consequence of their excessive ethanol consumption. Why the pancreas of one individual is more susceptible to damage caused by alcohol than that of others and why the development of pancreatitis seems to follow such different routes in individual alcoholics has prompted many investigators to study the genetic predisposition. The discovery of specific gene mutations in hereditary pancreatitis was taken as an opportunity to search for the potential genetic factors determining the association between alcohol intake and chronic pancreatitis.

A number of studies screened for hereditary pancreatitis–associated cationic trypsinogen mutations in alcoholic pancreatitis patients [36,37] but the results indicated that neither R122H nor N29I mutations represent a major risk factor for alcoholic pancreatitis. The frequency of the SPINK N34S mutation in alcoholics was also analyzed by several groups and determined to be slightly elevated over the control population [22,23].

Even if this low, but statistically significant frequency rules out a major role of the N34S mutations it allows for some possible relevance of SPINK1 in certain individuals with alcoholic pancreatitis. So far, however, detailed reports about the clinical characteristics of patients with SPINK1 N34S mutations and alcoholic pancreatitis are sparse and it remains unclear whether SPINK1 mutations convey a real impact on the clinical course of alcoholic chronic pancreatitis.

Further studies have analyzed mutations in other genes, such as CFTR gene or the gene for alcohol dehydrogenase [38–40], but revealed no conclusive evidence for the association with alcoholic chronic pancreatitis. Although the SPINK1 N34S mutation may represent a minor genetic risk factor for the development of alcoholic pancreatitis, it does not seem to be the triggering event.

Inherited hyperlipidemia

A number of inherited hereditary metabolic disorders have been reported to be associated with chronic pancreatitis. Although in most of these diseases pancreatitis is not the most serious clinical manifestation of the underlying metabolic defect, it may become the dominant phenotype in the disorder known to cause dramatically increased plasma concentrations of chylomicrons and triglycerides. Hyperlipidemia, as a consequence of familial disorders of lipid metabolism, is generally considered to put patients at a significant risk of developing pancreatitis [41–43]. An extensive plasma accumulation of chylomicrons and triglycerides is found in patients with lipoprotein lipase deficiency or apolipoprotein C-II deficiency. Both proteins confer an important metabolic function in the hydrolysis of triglycerides and the production of free fatty acids. Genetic disorders in either of these genes can lead to a genetic predisposition for pancreatitis. Carriers of currently more than 30 disease-relevant lipoprotein lipase gene mutations can be identified by reduced catalytic activity in postheparin plasma or by genetic testing. The mode of inheritance is autosomal-recessive and the disease has a low incidence of 1 in 1,000,000. The first symptoms arise in early childhood and nearly 30% of patients with lipoprotein lipase deficiency develop recurrent episodes of pancreatitis. Apolipoprotein C-II deficiency is usually diagnosed at a later age during adolescence or in young adults, often with a similar clinical presentation of recurrent episodes of pancreatitis. More than 10 disease-relevant mutations have been so far identified in the apolipoprotein C-II gene, which apparently interfere with the biologic function of apolipoprotein C-II as an activator of lipoprotein lipase. Up to 60% of affected patients develop pancreatitis as a frequent and severe complication, which can result in chronic exocrine and endocrine pancreatic insufficiency [44,45].

Several other disorders of lipid metabolism have been reported, which can lead to chylomicronemia or hypertriglyceridemia and which are independent of the lipoprotein lipase system. They represent a significant risk factor for the development of pancreatitis when plasma triglyceride levels rise above 2000 mg/dL. The most common familial disorders associated with chylomicronemia are type I and type V hyperlipoproteinemias (according to Levy and Fredrickson [46]), which comprise a diverse family of disorders with moderate to severe hypertriglyceridemia.

Polymorphisms in genes of the inflammatory response system

Proinflammatory and regulatory cytokines, such as tumor necrosis factor (TNF)-α and interleukin (IL)-10, play an important role in the initial stages of the disease and in the development of severe pancreatitis. In addition to mutations that act with environmental risk factors in affecting disease susceptibility, some genetic polymorphism have been shown to influence severity of diseases by their control of the inflammatory response. Although polymorphic alleles can have a high frequency in the healthy population and may be considered physiologically normal, they may also convey a modulating effect of the function of a gene product. Their disease-relevant mechanism may involve the transcription efficiency, the stability of mRNA or protein products or an impaired protein-protein interaction that leads to a modulation in biologic function. Recently, a study investigated cytokine genotypes in 190 pancreatitis patients and found no differences in polymorphism frequencies of TNF-α, IL-10, and IL-1 receptor antagonist gene loci between pancreatitis patients and control individuals [47]. In a similar study [48] it was concluded that TNF-α and IL-10 play no role in the determination of disease severity or susceptibility to acute pancreatitis. The same group, however, found that allele 1 of IL-RN polymorphism was significantly increased in patients with acute pancreatitis and seems to affect the disease phenotype [49]. Also, polymorphisms in α_1-antitrypsin and α_2-macroglobulin have been suggested to play a modifying but not a dominant role in the course of alcoholic pancreatitis [50]. Sequence variations in the TNF-α promoter region have been analyzed and the variant TNF-238A has been suggested to be a relevant risk factor for disease manifestation in families with hereditary pancreatitis [51]. Overall, the search for cytokine and chemokine variants as risk factors, if not for pancreatitis onset but for disease severity once pancreatitis has developed, has yielded rather inconsistent results and remained mostly disappointing [52,53].

Changes affecting cathepsin B

One of the hypotheses that have addressed the question of why and how pancreatic digestive proteases become activated prematurely and within acinar cells predicts that CTSB, a lysosomal cysteine proteinase, is critically involved in the initial activation of trypsinogen [54]. This CTSB hypothesis is based on the observations that CTSB can activate trypsinogen in vitro [55], CTSB is redistributed to a zymogen-granule enriched subcellular compartment [56], and lysosomal enzymes colocalize with digestive zymogens during the early course of experimental pancreatitis [57]. Although this cathepsin hypothesis seems attractive from a cell biology point of view a number of experimental observations seem to be incompatible with its assumptions: (1) a colocalization of cathepsins with digestive zymogens has not only been observed in the initial phase of acute pancreatitis but also under physiologic control conditions and in secretory vesicles that are destined for regulated secretion from healthy pancreatic acinar cells [58]; (2) a redistribution of CTSB into a zymogen-enriched subcellular compartment can be induced in vivo by experimental conditions that interfere with lysosomal sorting and are neither associated with nor followed by the development of acute pancreatitis [59]; (3) the administration of potent lysosomal enzyme inhibitors in vivo does not prevent the onset of acute experimental pancreatitis [60] ; and (4) in experiments that used lysosomal enzyme inhibitors in vitro an increase in the rate of intracellular trypsinogen activation and a decrease in the rate of intracellular trypsinogen activation have been reported [61,62], and even a protective role against premature zymogen activation has been considered for CTSB [63].

In view of the limited specificity and bioavailability of the existing inhibitors for lysosomal hydrolases the only remaining option to address the cathepsin hypothesis conclusively was to use CTSB-deficient animals and to study them in an experimental model of acute pancreatitis. When that was done in a recent investigation the answer was very straightforward: 90% of the activation of trypsinogen during experimental pancreatitis is accounted for by the presence of CTSB and it disappears when the *ctsb*-gene is deleted [64].

The relevance for human disease, however, remained another matter. First attempts to establish the relevance of the CTSB-pancreatitis hypothesis in humans focused on the capacity of the lysosomal enzyme to activate human trypsinogen, and specifically varieties of human trypsinogen, into which disease-relevant mutations had been introduced that were identified in the context of hereditary pancreatitis studies (see previously). When recombinant trypsinogen with hereditary pancreatitis mutations was subjected to activation by CTSB in vitro it was, indeed, found that some trypsins behaved differently from their wild-type counterpart [11,65], an observation that clearly supported the CTSB hypothesis of pancreatitis. The most common PRSS1 mutations like R122H and N29I, however, did not convincingly vary from wild-type trypsin in their activation kinetics by CTSB [66]. The same study demonstrated further that CTSB is abundantly secreted from the human exocrine pancreas; plentiful contained in pancreatic secretory zymogen granules (rather than in lysosomes); and active within the secretory pathway [66]. All cellular conditions for the CTSB pancreatitis hypothesis to be operative in humans were met. Moreover, the proposed requirement for a subcellular redistribution of CTSB into the secretory compartment [56] could finally be put to test because most CTSB in the pancreas was found already to reside in the secretory compartment under physiologic conditions [58,66] rather than having to be redistributed there from lysosomes. Nevertheless, no direct evidence for an active involvement of CTSB in the onset of human pancreatitis (at least not in hereditary pancreatitis caused by the most common mutations) could be produced from these studies. That has changed with a recent study, in which a total of 306 patients with tropical pancreatitis, a disease variety in which SPINK1 mutations are the predominant risk factor in about 50% of patients, were recruited from two separate areas in Southern India and investigated for changes in *ctsb* gene. Compared with 330 controls a C76G polymorphism that results in a leucine to valine mutation at amino acid 26 was twice as common [67]. The CTSB mutation also doubled the risk for tropical pancreatitis irrespective of whether patients were positive or negative for the N34S mutation in SPINK1. Until functional data on recombinant CTSB become available it remains unclear whether this mutation in the propeptide region of CTSB affects the substrate specificity or intracellular trafficking of the lysosomal enzyme, of which the former just as the latter may be sufficient to be disease-relevant because it matters very much whether CTSB ends up in a lysosome or in a zymogen granule where dangerous substrates, such as trypsinogens, reside. What the study from India indicates is that the 30-year-old CTSB hypothesis of pancreatitis has entered the phase in which evidence from human studies is finally being presented, and that candidate gene sequencing based on pathophysiologic information is still a valid and successful research strategy, particularly when well-characterized patient cohorts are available for genotyping.

References

[1] Lerch MM, Saluja AK, Runzi M, et al. Acute necrotizing pancreatitis in the opossum: earliest morphological changes involve acinar cells. Gastroenterology 1992;103:205–13.

[2] Comfort MW, Steinberg AG. Pedigree of a family with hereditary chronic relapsing pancreatitis. Gastroenterology 1952;21:54–63.

[3] Howes N, Lerch MM, Greenhalf W, et al. Clinical and genetic characteristics of hereditary pancreatitis in Europe. Clin Gastroenterol Hepatol 2004;2:252–61.

[4] Perrault J. Hereditary pancreatitis: historical perspectives. Med Clin North Am 2000;84: 519–29.

[5] Lowenfels AB, Maisonneuve P, DiMagno EP, et al. Hereditary pancreatitis and the risk of pancreatic cancer: International Hereditary Pancreatitis Study Group. J Natl Cancer Inst 1997;89:442–6.

[6] Lowenfels AB, Maisonneuve P, Whitcomb DC, et al. Cigarette smoking as a risk factor for pancreatic cancer in patients with hereditary pancreatitis. JAMA 2001;286:169–70.

[7] Whitcomb DC, Gorry MC, Preston RA, et al. Hereditary pancreatitis is caused by a mutation in the cationic trypsinogen gene. Nat Genet 1996;14:141–5.

[8] Gaboriaud C, Serre L, Guy-Crotte O, et al. Crystal structure of human trypsin 1: unexpected phosphorylation of Tyr151. J Mol Biol 1996;259:995–1010.

[9] Sahin-Toth M. Human cationic trypsinogen: role of Asn-21 in zymogen activation and implications in hereditary pancreatitis. J Biol Chem 2000;275:22750–5.

[10] LeMarechal C, Chen JM, Quere I, et al. Discrimination of three mutational events that result in a disruption of the R122 primary autolysis site of the human cationic trypsinogen (PRSS1) by denaturing high performance liquid chromatography. BMC Genet 2001;2:19.

[11] Simon P, Weiss FU, Sahin-Toth M, et al. Hereditary pancreatitis caused by a novel PRSS1 mutation (Arg-122 → Cys) that alters autoactivation and autodegradation of cationic trypsinogen. J Biol Chem 2002;277:5404–10.

[12] Pfutzer R, Myers E, Applebaum-Shapiro S, et al. Novel cationic trypsinogen (PRSS1) N29T and R122C mutations cause autosomal dominant hereditary pancreatitis. Gut 2002;50: 271–2.

[13] Teich N, Le Marechal C, Kukor Z, et al. Interaction between trypsinogen isoforms in genetically determined pancreatitis: mutation E79K in cationic trypsin (PRSS1) causes increased transactivation of anionic trypsinogen (PRSS2). Hum Mutat 2004;23:22–31.

[14] Simon P, Weiss FU, Zimmer KP, et al. Spontaneous and sporadic trypsinogen mutations in idiopathic pancreatitis. JAMA 2002;288:2122.

[15] Sahin-Toth M. Hereditary pancreatitis-associated mutation asn(21) → ile stabilizes rat trypsinogen in vitro. J Biol Chem 1999;274:29699–704.

[16] Keim V, Bauer N, Teich N, et al. Clinical characterization of patients with hereditary pancreatitis and mutations in the cationic trypsinogen gene. Am J Med 2001;111:622–6.

[17] Witt H, Luck W, Becker M. A signal peptide cleavage site mutation in the cationic trypsinogen gene is strongly associated with chronic pancreatitis. Gastroenterology 1999;117:7–10.

[18] Teich N, Ockenga J, Hoffmeister A, et al. Chronic pancreatitis associated with an activation-peptide mutation that facilitates trypsin activation. Gastroenterology 2000;119:461–5.

[19] Ferec C, Raguenes O, Salomon R, et al. Mutations in the cationic trypsinolgen gene and evidence for genetic heterogeneity in hereditary pancreatitis. J Med Genet 1999;36:228–32.

[20] Witt H, Luck W, Hennies HC, et al. Mutations in the gene encoding the serine protease inhibitor, Kazal type 1 are associated with chronic pancreatitis. Nat Genet 2000;25:213–6.

[21] Pfutzer RH, Barmada MM, Brunskill AP, et al. SPINK1/PSTI polymorphisms act as disease modifiers in familial and idiopathic chronic pancreatitis. Gastroenterology 2000;119:615–23.

[22] Threadgold J, Greenhalf W, Ellis I, et al. The N34S mutation of SPINK1 (PSTI) is associated with a familial pattern of idiopathic chronic pancreatitis but does not cause the disease. Gut 2002;50:675–81.

[23] Drenth JP, te Morsche R, Jansen JB. Mutations in serine protease inhibitor Kazal type 1 are strongly associated with chronic pancreatitis. Gut 2002;50:687–92.

[24] Truninger K, Witt H, Kock J, et al. Mutations of the serine protease inhibitor, Kazal type 1 gene, in patients with idiopathic chronic pancreatitis. Am J Gastroenterol 2002;97:1133–7.

[25] Weiss FU, Simon P, Witt H, et al. SPINK1 mutations and phenotypic expression in patients with pancreatitis associated with trypsinogen mutations. J Med Genet 2003;40:e40.

[26] Schneider A, Suman A, Rossi L, et al. SPINK1/PSTI mutations are associated with tropical pancreatitis and type II diabetes mellitus in Bangladesh. Gastroenterology 2002;123:1026–30.

[27] Chandak GR, Idris MM, Reddy DN, et al. Mutations in the pancreatic secretory trypsin inhibitor gene (PSTI/SPINK1) rather than the cationic trypsinogen gene (PRSS1) are significantly associated with tropical calcific pancreatitis. J Med Genet 2002;39:347–51.

[28] Nathan JD, Romac J, Peng RY, et al. Transgenic expression of pancreatic secretory trypsin inhibitor-I ameliorates secretagogue-induced pancreatitis in mice. Gastroenterology 2005;128:717–27.

[29] Kuwata K, Hirota M, Shimizu H, et al. Functional analysis of recombinant pancreatic secretory trypsin inhibitor protein with amino-acid substitution. J Gastroenterol 2002;37:928–34.

[30] Ohmuraya M, Hirota M, Araki M, et al. Autophagic cell death of pancreatic acinar cells in serine protease inhibitor Kazal type 3-deficient mice. Gastroenterology 2005;129:696–705.

[31] Cohn JA, Friedman KJ, Noone PG, et al. Relation between mutations of the cystic fibrosis gene and idiopathic pancreatitis. N Engl J Med 1998;339:653–8.

[32] Sharer N, Schwarz M, Malone G, et al. Mutations of the cystic fibrosis gene in patients with chronic pancreatitis. N Engl J Med 1998;339:645–52.

[33] Zeng W, Lee MG, Muallem S. Membrane-specific regulation of Cl- channels by purinergic receptors in rat submandibular gland acinar and duct cells. J Biol Chem 1997;272:32956–65.

[34] DiMagno MJ, Lee SH, Hao Y, et al. A proinflammatory, antiapoptotic phenotype underlies the susceptibility to acute pancreatitis in cystic fibrosis transmembrane regulator (−/−) mice. Gastroenterology 2005;129:665–81.

[35] Weiss FU, Simon P, Bogdanova N, et al. Complete cystic fibrosis transmembrane conductance regulator gene sequencing in patients with idiopathic chronic pancreatitis and controls. Gut 2005;54:1456–60.

[36] Creighton J, Lyall R, Wilson DI, et al. Mutations of the cationic trypsinogen gene in patients with chronic pancreatitis. Lancet 1999;354:42–3.

[37] Monaghan KG, Jackson CE, KuKuruga DL, et al. Mutation analysis of the cystic fibrosis and cationic trypsinogen genes in patients with alcohol-related pancreatitis. Am J Med Genet 2000;94:120–4.

[38] Norton ID, Apte MV, Dixson H, et al. Cystic fibrosis genotypes and alcoholic pancreatitis. J Gastroenterol Hepatol 1998;13:496–9.

[39] Haber PS, Norris MD, Apte MV, et al. Alcoholic pancreatitis and polymorphisms of the variable length polythymidine tract in the cystic fibrosis gene. Alcohol Clin Exp Res 1999;23:509–12.

[40] Haber PS, Apte MV, Applegate TL, et al. Metabolism of ethanol by rat pancreatic acinar cells. J Lab Clin Med 1998;132:294–302.

[41] Hata A, Ridinger DN, Sutherland S, et al. Binding of lipoprotein lipase to heparin: identification of five critical residues in two distinct segments of the amino-terminal domain. J Biol Chem 1993;268:8447–57.

[42] Brunzell JD, Schrott HG. The interaction of familial and secondary causes of hypertriglyceridemia: role in pancreatitis. Trans Assoc Am Physicians 1973;86:245–54.

[43] Siafakas CG, Brown MR, Miller TL. Neonatal pancreatitis associated with familial lipoprotein lipase deficiency. J Pediatr Gastroenterol Nutr 1999;29:95–8.

[44] Breckenridge WC, Little JA, Steiner G, et al. Hypertriglyceridemia associated with deficiency of apolipoprotein C–II. N Engl J Med 1978;298:1265–73.

[45] Cox DW, Breckenridge WC, Little JA. Inheritance of apolipoprotein C–II deficiency with hypertriglyceridemia and pancreatitis. N Engl J Med 1978;299:1421–4.

[46] Levy RI, Fredrickson DS. Familial hyperlipoproteinemia. In: Stanbury JB, Wyngaarden JB, Fredrickson DS, editors. The metabolic basis of inherited disease. 3rd edition. New York: Mac Graw-Hill; 1972. p. 545.

[47] Powell JJ, Fearon KC, Siriwardena AK, et al. Evidence against a role for polymorphisms at tumor necrosis factor, interleukin-1, and interleukin-1 receptor antagonist gene loci in the regulation of disease severity in acute pancreatitis. Surgery 2001;129:633–40.

[48] Sargen K, Demaine AG, Kingsnoth AN. Cytokine gene polymorphism in acute pancreatitis. JOP 2000;1:24–35.

[49] Smithies AM, Sargen K, Demaine AG, et al. Investigations of the interleukin 1 gene cluster and its association with acute pancreatitis. Pancreas 2000;20:234–40.

[50] Teich N, Mossner J, Keim V. Screening for mutations of the cationic trypsinogen gene: are they of relevance in chronic alcoholic pancreatitis? Gut 1999;44:413–6.

[51] Beranek H, Teich N, Witt H, et al. Analysis of tumour necrosis factor alpha and interleukin 10 promoter variants in patients with chronic pancreatitis. Eur J Gastroenterol Hepatol 2003;15:1223–7.

[52] Schneider A, Barmada MM, Slivka A, et al. Transforming growth factor-beta1, interleukin-10 and interferon-gamma cytokine polymorphisms in patients with hereditary, familial and sporadic chronic pancreatitis. Pancreatology 2004;4:490–4.

[53] Schneider A, Barmada MM, Slivka A, et al. Analysis of tumor necrosis factor-alpha, transforming growth factor-beta 1, interleukin-10, and interferon-gamma polymorphisms in patients with alcoholic chronic pancreatitis. Alcohol 2004;32:19–24.

[54] Steer ML, Meldolesi J. The cell biology of experimental pancreatitis. N Engl J Med 1987;316:144–50.

[55] Figarella C, Miszczuk-Jamska B, Barrett A. Possible lysosomal activation of pancreatic zymogens: activation of both human trypsinogens by cathepsin B and spontaneous acid activation of human trypsinogen-1. Biol Chem 1988;369:293–8.

[56] Saluja A, Sadamitsu H, Saluja M, et al. Subcellular redistribution of lysosomal enzymes during caerulein-induced pancreatitis. Am J Physiol 1987;253:G508–16.

[57] Watanabe O, Baccino FM, Steer ML, et al. Supramaximal caerulein stimulation and ultra-structure of rat pancreatic acinar cell: early morphological changes during development of experimental pancreatitis. Am J Physiol 1984;246:G457–67.

[58] Tooze J, Hollinshead M, Hensel G, et al. Regulated secretion of mature cathepsin B from rat exocrine pancreatic cells. Eur J Cell Biol 1991;56:187–200.

[59] Lerch MM, Saluja AK, Dawra R, et al. The effect of chloroquine administration on two experimental models of acute pancreatitis. Gastroenterology 1993;104:1768–79.

[60] Steer ML, Saluja AK. Experimental acute pancreatitis: studies of the early events that lead to cell injury. In: Go VLW, DiMagno EP, Gardner JD, et al, editors. The pancreas: biology, pathobiology, and disease. New York: Raven Press; 1993. p. 489–500.

[61] Leach SD, Modlin IM, Scheele GA, et al. Intracellular activation of digestive zymogens in rat pancreatic acini: stimulation by high does of cholecystokinin. J Clin Invest 1991;87: 362–6.

[62] Saluja AK, Donovan EA, Yamanaka K, et al. Cerulein-induced in vitro activation of trypsinogen in rat pancreatic acini is mediated by cathepsin B. Gastroenterology 1997;113: 304–10.

[63] Gorelick FS, Modlin IM, Leach SD, et al. Intracellular proteolysis of pancreatic zymogens. Yale J Biol Med 1992;65:407–20.

[64] Halangk W, Lerch MM, Brandt-Nedelev B, et al. Role of cathepsin B in intracellular trypsinogen activation and the onset of acute pancreatitis. J Clin Invest 2000;106:773–81.

[65] Szilagyi L, Kenesi E, Katona G, et al. Comparative in vitro studies on native and recombinant human cationic trypsins: cathepsin B is a possible pathological activator of trypsinogen in pancreatitis. J Biol Chem 2001;276:24574–80.

[66] Kukor Z, Mayerle J, Kruger B, et al. Presence of cathepsin B in the human pancreatic secretory pathway and its role in trypsinogen activation during hereditary pancreatitis. J Biol Chem 2002;277:21389–96.

[67] Mahurkar S, Idris MM, Reddy DN, et al. Association of cathepsin B gene polymorphisms with tropical calcific pancreatitis. Gut, in press.

ELSEVIER
SAUNDERS

Endocrinol Metab Clin N Am
35 (2006) 303–312

ENDOCRINOLOGY
AND METABOLISM
CLINICS
OF NORTH AMERICA

Biochemical Models of Hereditary Pancreatitis

Miklós Sahin-Tóth, MD, PhD

*Department of Molecular and Cell Biology, Goldman School of Dental Medicine,
Boston University, 715 Albany Street, Evans-4, Boston, MA 02118, USA*

The past decade has witnessed remarkable progress in the genetics of chronic pancreatitis. Mutations of the *PRSS1* gene encoding cationic trypsinogen and the *SPINK1* gene encoding pancreatic secretory trypsin inhibitor were found in association with hereditary, familial, or sporadic chronic pancreatitis; and the genotype-phenotype correlations have been characterized at the clinical level. Despite these accomplishments, the understanding of the molecular mechanisms through which PRSS1 and SPINK1 mutations cause chronic pancreatitis has remained sketchy. Pancreatitis-associated gene mutations are believed to result in uncontrolled trypsin activity in the pancreas. PRSS1 mutations would cause a gain of (trypsin) function, whereas SPINK1 mutations would result in the loss of a (trypsin inhibitor) function. Experimental identification of the disease-relevant functional alterations caused by PRSS1 or SPINK1 mutations proved to be challenging, however, because results of biochemical analyses lent themselves to different interpretations. This article focuses on PRSS1 mutations and summarizes the salient biochemical findings in the context of the mechanistic models that explain the connection between mutations and hereditary pancreatitis.

Human trypsinogens and pancreatitis-associated trypsinogen mutations

The human pancreas produces the digestive proenzyme trypsinogen in three isoforms. On the basis of their relative isoelectric points and electrophoretic mobility, these are commonly referred to as "cationic trypsinogen," "anionic trypsinogen," and "mesotrypsinogen." The isoenzymes are encoded by separate genes: the *PRSS1* (protease, serine, 1); *PRSS2*; and *PRSS3* genes [1]. Cationic trypsinogen (PRSS1) and anionic trypsinogen (PRSS2) make up the

---

This work was supported by NIH grant DK58088.
E-mail address: miklos@bu.edu

bulk of secreted trypsinogens in the pancreatic juice, whereas mesotrypsinogen (PRSS3) accounts for 2% to 10% [2–6]. Typically, there is approximately twice as much cationic trypsinogen as anionic trypsinogen, but this ratio is reversed in chronic alcoholism or chronic pancreatitis [3,5]. The significance of the "isoform reversal" is unknown [7]. Human trypsinogens are synthesized as pre-pro enzymes with a signal peptide of 15 amino acids, followed by the 8–amino acid long propeptide, the trypsinogen activation peptide. The signal-peptide is removed on entry into the endoplasmic reticulum lumen and the proenzymes are packaged into zymogen granules and eventually secreted into the pancreatic juice. Physiologic activation of trypsinogen to trypsin takes place in the duodenum by enteropeptidase (enterokinase), a highly specialized serine protease in the brush-border membrane of enterocytes. Trypsin can also activate trypsinogen, a process termed "autoactivation," which in the duodenum may have a physiologic role in facilitating zymogen activation, whereas inappropriate autoactivation in the pancreas might cause pancreatitis. Mutations in the *PRSS1* gene have been identified in patients with hereditary pancreatitis or familial or sporadic chronic pancreatitis (Table 1). In contrast, genetic variants of anionic trypsinogen (PRSS2) or mesotrypsinogen (PRSS3) have not been found in association with chronic pancreatitis [8–10]. To date, 22 *PRSS1* gene variants have been described, which affect 18 different amino acid positions in trypsinogen, and result in 20 different amino acid substitutions. When classified according to frequency of occurrence, R122H (approximately 70%), N29I (approximately 25%), and A16V (approximately 4%) are the three most prevalent mutations [11–14], whereas most genetic variants have been identified in very few patients or families (see Table 1). Interestingly, the mutations are located in the N-terminal half of trypsinogen, and are clustered in the activation peptide (between Ala16 and Lys23), in the very N-terminal part of trypsin (between Asn29 and Val39) or in the longest peptide segment not stabilized by disulfide bonds (between Glu79 and Cys139).

Use of recombinant trypsinogen to study pancreatitis-associated mutations

To elucidate how mutations in cationic trypsinogen cause pancreatitis, biochemical analysis of the mutant proteins is essential. Pancreatic tissue or juice is not readily available in significant amounts from patients carrying PRSS1 mutations. In addition to limited availability, isolation of the heterozygously expressed mutant trypsinogen from the complex protein mixture poses another technical challenge. Therefore, heterologous recombinant expression has been the method of choice to generate wild-type and mutant trypsinogen proteins for biochemical analysis. The biochemical data discussed in this article were obtained on recombinant trypsinogen preparations expressed in *Escherichia coli* as denatured inclusion bodies, which were subsequently renatured through an in vitro refolding procedure [15–17]. Refolded trypsinogen was purified to homogeneity by affinity chromatography using immobilized

Table 1
Pancretitis-associated genetic variants of human cationic trypsinogen

Mutation	Frequency
-28delTCC	1 affected carrier
A16V	> 25 affected carriers
D19A	1 affected carrier
D22G	2 affected carriers
K23R	2 affected carriers
N29I	> 160 affected carriers
N29I + N54S	1 affected carrier
N29T	3 affected carriers
P36R	1 affected carrier
V39A	7 affected carriers
E79K	8 affected carriers
G83E	1 affected carrier
K92N	1 affected carrier
D100H	1 affected carrier
L104P	1 affected carrier
R116C	8 affected carriers
A121T	1 affected carrier
R122H (CAC)	> 500 affected carriers
R122H (CAT)	3 affected carriers
R122C	5 affected carriers
V123M	1 affected carrier
C139F	1 affected carrier

Only the documented affected carriers are listed; consult the appropriate references for more detailed pedigrees. For references see the Database of trypsinogen and SPINK1 variants at the Universität Leipzig. Available at: http://www.uni-leipzig.de/pancreasmutation/.

ecotin [18]. Ecotin is a protease inhibitor with broad specificity isolated from the periplasm of *E coli*. Cationic trypsin preparations produced recombinantly or isolated from pancreatic juice exhibit essentially identical catalytic activity [17], indicating that recombinant trypsinogen is a suitable experimental alternative to its native counterpart. Subtle structural differences do exist between recombinant and native preparations, however, because of different posttranslational processing in *E coli* and pancreatic acinar cells. In *E coli* cytoplasmic aminopeptidases can trim the N terminus of recombinant trypsinogens, whereas in human acinar cells trypsinogens get posttranslationally modified on Tyr154. This modification was originally described as phosphorylation [19], but more recent data suggest that the modifying group is a sulfate (M. Sahin-Tóth, unpublished data). Posttranslational sulfation is absent in *E coli*. Whether or not these structural differences between native and recombinant trypsinogen influence the effect of pancreatitis-associated mutations remains to be determined.

Phenotypic alterations caused by pancreatitis-associated mutations

The biochemical investigations reviewed here examined the following aspects of trypsinogen function: (1) trypsin activity, typically measured on the small peptide substrate N-CBZ-Gly-Pro-Arg-p-nitroanilide; (2) trypsinogen activation by trypsin (autoactivation); (3) trypsinogen activation by cathepsin B; (4) autocatalytic degradation of trypsin (autolysis); and (5) trypsin inhibition by SPINK1 (pancreatic secretory trypsin inhibitor). As listed in Table 2, trypsin activity or inhibitor binding was not affected by the mutations and the most frequently and consistently found phenotypic change was an increased propensity for autoactivation. Increased trypsin stability (ie, decreased autolysis) was also observed with three mutations. Interestingly, cathepsin B–mediated activation was either unaltered or decreased, indicating that increased susceptibility to cathepsin B does not play a role in hereditary pancreatitis. The interpretation of the biochemical data on the R122C mutant remains controversial, as discussed later.

From biochemical analysis of mutant proteins to disease mechanisms

There are three assumptions that guide the interpretation of experimental data on pancreatitis-associated mutations.

Mutations in the PRSS1 gene are the causative agents or risk factors of chronic pancreatitis

This assumption is widely accepted today as fact and the association of the studied mutations with chronic pancreatitis is well documented by a decade of genetic investigation. In the strict sense, however, this notion only holds true for the relatively frequent mutations, where disease association could be convincingly established. For most of the reported mutations, the limited sample size did not allow a conclusive genetic analysis and the authors use inference to posit that these mutations have a causative relationship with chronic pancreatitis.

Table 2
Functional properties of pancreatitis-associated cationic trypsinogen mutants

	Trypsin activity	Autoactivation of trypsinogen	Activation by cathepsin B	Trypsin autolysis	SPINK1 binding	References
D19A	Normal	Increased	Normal	Normal	Normal	[32,41]
D22G	Normal	Increased	Decreased	Normal	Normal	[31,32,37]
K23R	Normal	Increased	Decreased	Normal	Normal	[31,32,37]
N29I	Normal	Increased	Normal	Normal	Normal	[15–17,24,30,35]
N29I + N54S	Normal	Increased	Normal	Normal	Normal	[30]
N29T	Normal	Increased	Normal	Decreased	ND	[15,35]
E79K	Normal	Decreased	Normal	Normal	Normal	[33]
R122H	Normal	Increased	Normal	Decreased	ND	[16,23,25,26,35]
R122C	Decreased	Decreased	Decreased	Decreased	ND	[36]
R122C	Normal	Increased	Normal	Decreased	ND	[36]

ND, not determined; SPINK1, pancreatic secretory trypsin inhibitor.
The R122C mutant exhibited different phenotypes depending on how trypsinogen concentrations were determined in the recombinant preparations. See text and references for experimental details.

The biochemical alterations discovered through analyzing recombinant
trypsinogen mutants are relevant to the disease mechanism

Trypsinogen is highly amenable to in vitro biochemical investigations in which catalytic activity, activation, and degradation can be studied on pure, homogenous preparations either from recombinant or native source. To date, these studies are the only source of functional information regarding the effect of the PRSS1 mutations and the investigators rely on these data to formulate pathomechanistic models. It is important to remember, however, that the mutations can potentially cause defects in the synthesis, intracellular transport, or secretion of trypsinogen, and these cell-biologic aspects have not yet been studied.

There is a common mechanism through which the various mutations
cause chronic pancreatitis

Consolidation of the sometimes conflicting biochemical data into a unifying model requires value judgments, which are based on the premise that a common pathogenic pathway exists. Although it remains formally possible that a number of different, mutation-specific mechanisms are responsible for hereditary pancreatitis, such a scenario seems unlikely. A logical and wishful extension of this assumption is that biochemical models developed through analysis of hereditary pancreatitis are widely applicable to all forms of chronic pancreatitis in humans. Nonetheless, some of the models reviewed next do not conform to this notion and imply multiple mechanisms in hereditary pancreatitis.

Model 1: increased trypsin stability causes hereditary pancreatitis

The R122H mutation was the first cationic trypsinogen variant identified by Whitcomb and coworkers [20] in 1996 and still remains the most frequently found genetic alteration associated with hereditary pancreatitis. To explain why the R122H mutation might cause pancreatitis, Whitcomb proposed that the Arg122-Val123 autolytic peptide bond in trypsin plays an important role in the degradation of prematurely activated trypsin in the pancreas. Destruction of this failsafe mechanism by the R122H mutation would increase intrapancreatic trypsin activity and eventually precipitate pancreatitis. Halangk and coworkers [21] demonstrated that autodegradation of trypsin mitigates cathepsin B–mediated trypsinogen activation during cerulein-induced zymogen activation in isolated rat acini, suggesting that an autolytic failsafe mechanism might be operational in the mammalian pancreas. Biochemical evidence supports the notion that Arg122 is important for autolysis of trypsin [15,16,22–26] and mutations of this amino acid result in increased trypsin stability [16,23,6]. Because of its increased autolytic stability, R122H-trypsin was sometimes referred to as "supertrypsin." More detailed biochemical analysis indicated, however, that the R122H mutation results not only in increased trypsin stability [16] but also in increased zymogen stability [25,26] and increased autoactivation [16]. A weak trypsin-inhibitory activity associated with the Arg122 site is also lost in the R122H mutant [26]. The pleiotropic biochemical effect of R122H raises the possibility that the pathogenic alteration is unrelated to trypsin stability. More importantly, the model fails to explain how the other pancreatitis-associated PRSS1 mutations might work, because most of these do not affect trypsin stability (see Table 2).

Model 2: enhanced trypsinogen autoactivation is a common pathomechanism in hereditary pancreatitis

Indubitably, the most obvious limitation of the supertrypsin model was that it failed to offer a plausible and experimentally supported explanation for the mechanism of action of the N29I mutation. The N29I mutation is the second most frequent PRSS1 variant that causes autosomal-dominant hereditary pancreatitis with clinical and genetic features that are practically indistinguishable from those of the R122H-associated cases [11–14,27–29]. It is very likely that the underlying pathomechanisms are identical. Biochemical characterization of the N29I mutation using recombinant trypsinogen found no effect whatsoever on trypsin or trypsinogen stability [15–17,24]. Moderately increased autoactivation was observed, however, by two independent laboratories in a handful of published studies [15–17,30]. Because increased autoactivation was observed with the R122H, N29I, and N29T mutations, whereas N29I had no effect on trypsin stability, the logical conclusion was put forth that enhanced autoactivation is the common pathogenic mechanism of hereditary pancreatitis–associated PRSS1 mutations [16]. This conclusion received very strong support from the analysis of a subset of mutations that alter the activation peptide [31,32]. Conceptually, these activation peptide mutations are very important, because they do not affect trypsin structure or function, indicating that pancreatitis-associated mutations exert their effect through altering the properties of the proenzyme trypsinogen and not the active enzyme trypsin. In this context, properties of the characterized mutants D19A, D22G, and K23R confirmed that increased autoactivation of cationic trypsinogen is a relevant pathomechanism in hereditary pancreatitis [31,32]. To date, only mutation E79K seems to contradict this model, which was shown to decrease autoactivation significantly [33]. This mutant, however, exhibited enhanced transactivation of anionic trypsinogen.

Model 3: cathepsin B is a pathologic trypsinogen activator in hereditary pancreatitis

A large body of data from various animal models of experimental pancreatitis indicates that one of the early events in pancreatitis is the intra-acinar premature activation of trypsinogen, and this process seems to be mediated by the lysosomal cysteine-protease cathepsin B [34]. Intuitively, pancreatitis-associated mutations might cause pancreatitis by rendering trypsinogen more susceptible to activation by cathepsin B. This hypothesis was first described by Szilágyi and coworkers [17], who found that the N29I mutant is activated faster by cathepsin B than wild-type trypsinogen. A subsequent study, however, did not confirm this finding and demonstrated that activation of mutants N29I, N29T, and R122H by cathepsin B is unaltered relative to wild-type trypsinogen [35]. Similarly, activation of mutants E79K, R122C, or the double mutant N29I + N54S was unchanged [30,33,36]. Finally, experiments using synthetic analogues of the trypsinogen activation peptide revealed that activation of the D22G and K23R mutants by cathepsin B was actually decreased [37]. These results were also confirmed using full-length recombinant trypsinogens (M. Sahin-Tóth, unpublished data). Taken together, the evidence is overwhelming that increased activation of mutant trypsinogens by cathepsin B does not play a role in hereditary pancreatitis.

Model 4: loss of trypsin function in hereditary pancreatitis

Mutation R122C was reported in 2001 to 2002 by three independent groups [36,38,39]. The recombinantly expressed R122C mutant preparation exhibited reduced activity, autolysis, and autoactivation. This apparent loss of trypsin function was the result of in vitro misfolding caused by the introduction of the extra unpaired cysteine. When the data were normalized to the active trypsinogen fraction, however, the biochemical phenotype became very similar to that of R122H, exhibiting increased trypsin stability and increased autoactivation [36]. The complex properties of the R122C mutant were first interpreted as an example of a loss-of-function PRSS1 mutation associated with hereditary pancreatitis, suggesting that a trypsinogen mutation could cause pancreatitis by eliminating a trypsin-dependent protective mechanism [36]. Additional support for this hypothesis came from earlier studies indicating that trypsin autodegradation might play a protective role in cerulein-induced zymogen activation [21]. Although this model is provocative, the bulk of results from in vitro experiments using recombinantly expressed trypsinogen mutants remain inconsistent with it, because a loss of function could not be demonstrated for most mutations (see Table 2).

Model 5: chronic SPINK1 depletion in hereditary pancreatitis

The SPINK1-deficit model, first presented at the Fifth International Symposium on the Inherited Diseases of the Pancreas, in Graz, Austria, is an extension of the autoactivation hypothesis stating that increased autoactivation is the common pathogenic change in mutant trypsinogens. The author proposes that because human cationic trypsinogen has an unusually high propensity for autoactivation, even at acidic pH, constant physiologic autoactivation occurs during transit in the secretory pathway [40,41]. Normally, this process is controlled by SPINK1, resulting in some degree of SPINK1 consumption. An increase in autoactivation induced by trypsinogen mutations results in chronic depletion of SPINK1 and the resulting SPINK1 deficit renders the pancreas vulnerable to acute insults. Trypsinogen mutations exert their effect indirectly, by decreasing protective SPINK1 levels. It is noteworthy that within this model, loss-of-function mutations in the *SPINK1* gene or gain-of-function mutations in the *PRSS1* gene have a similar impact on SPINK 1 levels. There is some genetic evidence in support of this notion, because rare SPINK1 mutations that clearly cause loss of expression from the diseased allele seem to be associated with hereditary pancreatitis [42]. Finally, it seems likely that SPINK1 has a so far uncharacterized protective function in the pancreas, because homozygous genetic deletion of its ortholog in mice results in autophagic destruction of acinar cells [43]. It is intriguing to speculate that impairment of this novel function could play a role in hereditary pancreatitis.

Summary

Association between mutations in cationic trypsinogen and hereditary pancreatitis has been convincingly documented. Biochemical analysis of the mutation-induced effects revealed a multifaceted picture, which resulted in the formulation of multiple pathomechanistic models. Extension of the biochemical studies to cellular and animal models is mandatory.

References

[1] Chen JM, Férec C. Trypsinogen genes: evolution. In: Cooper DN, editor. Nature encyclopedia of the human genome. London: Nature Publishing Group; 2003. p. 645–50.
[2] Guy O, Lombardo D, Bartelt DC, et al. Two human trypsinogens: purification, molecular properties, and N-terminal sequences. Biochemistry 1978;17:1669–75.
[3] Rinderknecht H, Renner IG, Carmack C. Trypsinogen variants in pancreatic juice of healthy volunteers, chronic alcoholics and patients with pancreatitis and cancer of the pancreas. Gut 1979;20:886–91.
[4] Scheele G, Bartelt D, Bieger W. Characterization of human exocrine pancreatic proteins by two-dimensional isoelectric focusing/sodium dodecyl sulfate gel electrophoresis. Gastroenterology 1981;80:461–73.
[5] Rinderknecht H, Stace NH, Renner IG. Effects of chronic alcohol abuse on exocrine pancreatic secretion in man. Dig Dis Sci 1985;30:65–71.
[6] Rinderknecht H, Renner IG, Abramson SB, et al. Mesotrypsin: a new inhibitor-resistant protease from a zymogen in human pancreatic tissue and fluid. Gastroenterology 1984;86: 681–92.
[7] Kukor Z, Tóth M, Sahin-Tóth M. Human anionic trypsinogen: properties of autocatalytic activation and degradation and implications in pancreatic diseases. Eur J Biochem 2003;270: 2047–58.

[8] Chen JM, Audrézet MP, Mercier B, et al. Exclusion of anionic trypsinogen and mesotrypsinogen involvement in hereditary pancreatitis without cationic trypsinogen gene mutations. Scand J Gastroenterol 1999;34:831–2.

[9] Idris MM, Bhaskar S, Reddy DN, et al. Mutations in anionic trypsinogen gene are not associated with tropical calcific pancreatitis. Gut 2005;54:728–9.

[10] Nemoda Z, Teich N, Hugenberg C, et al. Genetic and biochemical characterization of the E32del polymorphism in human mesotrypsinogen. Pancreatology 2005;5:273–8.

[11] Applebaum-Shapiro SE, Finch R, Pfützer RH, et al. Hereditary pancreatitis in North America: The Pittsburgh-Midwest Multi-Center Pancreatic Study Group study. Pancreatology 1991;1:439–43.

[12] Keim V, Witt H, Bauer N, et al. The course of genetically-determined chronic pancreatitis. JOP 2003;4:146–54.

[13] Howes N, Lerch MM, Greenhalf W, et al. Clinical and genetic characteristics of hereditary pancreatitis in Europe. Clin Gastroenterol Hepatol 2004;2:252–61.

[14] Otsuki M, Nishimori I, Hayakawa T, et al. Hereditary pancreatitis: clinical characteristics and diagnostic criteria in Japan. Pancreas 2004;28:200–6.

[15] Sahin-Tóth M. Human cationic trypsinogen: role of Asn-21 in zymogen activation and implications in hereditary pancreatitis. J Biol Chem 2000;275:22750–5.

[16] Sahin-Tóth M, Tóth M. Gain-of-function mutations associated with hereditary pancreatitis enhance autoactivation of human cationic trypsinogen. Biochem Biophys Res Commun 2000;278:286–9.

[17] Szilágyi L, Kénesi E, Katona G, et al. Comparative in vitro studies on native and recombinant human cationic trypsins: cathepsin B is a possible pathological activator of trypsinogen in pancreatitis. J Biol Chem 2001;276:24574–80.

[18] Lengyel Z, Pál G, Sahin-Tóth M. Affinity purification of recombinant trypsinogen using immobilized ecotin. Protein Expr Purif 1998;12:291–4.

[19] Gaboriaud C, Serre L, Guy-Crotte O, et al. Crystal structure of human trypsin 1: unexpected phosphorylation of Tyr151. J Mol Biol 1996;259:995–1010.

[20] Whitcomb DC, Gorry MC, Preston RA, et al. Hereditary pancreatitis is caused by a mutation in the cationic trypsinogen gene. Nat Genet 1996;14:141–5.

[21] Halangk W, Kruger B, Ruthenburger M, et al. Trypsin activity is not involved in premature, intrapancreatic trypsinogen activation. Am J Physiol Gastrointest Liver Physiol 2002;282: G367–74.

[22] Maroux S, Desnuelle P. On some autolyzed derivatives of bovine trypsin. Biochim Biophys Acta 1969;181:59–72.

[23] Várallyai É, Pál G, Patthy A, et al. Two mutations in rat trypsin confer resistance against autolysis. Biochem Biophys Res Commun 1998;243:56–60.

[24] Sahin-Tóth M. Hereditary pancreatitis-associated mutation Asn21 → Ile stabilizes rat trypsinogen in vitro. J Biol Chem 1999;274:29699–704.

[25] Sahin-Tóth M, Gráf L, Tóth M. Trypsinogen stabilization by mutation Arg117 → His: a unifying pathomechanism for hereditary pancreatitis? Biochem Biophys Res Commun 1999; 264:505–8.

[26] Kukor Z, Tóth M, Pál G, et al. Human cationic trypsinogen. Arg(117) is the reactive site of an inhibitory surface loop that controls spontaneous zymogen activation. J Biol Chem 2002; 277:6111–7.

[27] Gorry MC, Gabbaizedeh D, Furey W, et al. Mutations in the cationic trypsinogen gene are associated with recurrent acute and chronic pancreatitis. Gastroenterology 1997;113: 1063–8.

[28] Teich N, Mössner J, Keim V. Mutations of the cationic trypsinogen in hereditary pancreatitis. Hum Mutat 1998;12:39–43.

[29] Ferec C, Raguenes O, Salomon R, et al. Mutations in the cationic trypsinogen gene and evidence for genetic heterogeneity in hereditary pancreatitis. J Med Genet 1999;36: 228–32.

[30] Teich N, Nemoda Z, Kohler H, et al. Gene conversion between functional trypsinogen genes PRSS1 and PRSS2 associated with chronic pancreatitis in a six-year-old girl. Hum Mutat 2005;25:343–7.

[31] Teich N, Ockenga J, Hoffmeister A, et al. Chronic pancreatitis associated with an activation peptide mutation that facilitates trypsin activation. Gastroenterology 2000;119:461–5.

[32] Chen JM, Kukor Z, Le Maréchal C, et al. Evolution of trypsinogen activation peptides. Mol Biol Evol 2003;20:1767–77.

[33] Teich N, Le Marechal C, Kukor Z, et al. Interaction between trypsinogen isoforms in genetically determined pancreatitis: mutation E79K in cationic trypsin (PRSS1) causes increased transactivation of anionic trypsinogen (PRSS2). Hum Mutat 2004;23:22–31.

[34] Halangk W, Lerch MM, Brandt-Nedelev B, et al. Role of cathepsin B in intracellular trypsinogen activation and the onset of acute pancreatitis. J Clin Invest 2000;106:773–81.

[35] Kukor Z, Mayerle J, Krüger B, et al. Presence of cathepsin B in the human pancreatic secretory pathway and its role in trypsinogen activation during hereditary pancreatitis. J Biol Chem 2002;277:21389–96.

[36] Simon P, Weiss FU, Sahin-Tóth M, et al. Hereditary pancreatitis caused by a novel PRSS1 mutation (Arg-122 → Cys) that alters autoactivation and autodegradation of cationic trypsinogen. J Biol Chem 2002;277:5404–10.

[37] Teich N, Bödeker H, Keim V. Cathepsin B cleavage of the trypsinogen activation peptide. BMC Gastroenterol 2002;2:16.

[38] Le Marechal C, Chen JM, Quere I, et al. Discrimination of three mutational events that result in a disruption of the R122 primary autolysis site of the human cationic trypsinogen (PRSS1) by denaturing high performance liquid chromatography. BMC Genet 2001;2:19.

[39] Pfützer R, Myers E, Applebaum-Shapiro S, et al. Novel cationic trypsinogen (PRSS1) N29T and R122C mutations cause autosomal dominant hereditary pancreatitis. Gut 2002;50:271–2.

[40] Figarella C, Miszczuk-Jamnska B, Barrett A. Possible lysosomal activation of pancreatic zymogens: activation of both human trypsinogens by cathepsin B and spontaneous acid activation of human trypsinogen-1. Biol Chem 1998;369:293–8.

[41] Nemoda Z, Sahin-Tóth M. The tetra-aspartate motif in the activation peptide of human cationic trypsinogen is essential for autoactivation control but not for enteropeptidase recognition. J Biol Chem 2005;280:29645–52.

[42] Le Marechal C, Chen JM, Le Gall C, et al. Two novel severe mutations in the pancreatic secretory trypsin inhibitor gene (SPINK1) cause familial and/or hereditary pancreatitis. Hum Mutat 2004;23:205.

[43] Ohmuraya M, Hirota M, Araki M, et al. Autophagic cell death of pancreatic acinar cells in serine protease inhibitor Kazal type 3-deficient mice. Gastroenterology 2005;129:696–705.

ENDOCRINOLOGY
AND METABOLISM
CLINICS
OF NORTH AMERICA

Endocrinol Metab Clin N Am
35 (2006) 313–331

Cell Biology of Pancreatic Proteases

Manuel Ruthenbürger, PhD, Julia Mayerle, MD,
Markus M. Lerch, MD*

*Department of Gastroenterology, Endocrinology and Nutrition, Ernst-Moritz-Arndt
Universität Greifswald, Friedrich-Loeffler-Str 23A, 17487 Greifswald, Germany*

Cause and pathogenesis of pancreatitis

Pancreatitis is a common disease with an incidence of approximately 25 cases per 100,000 population per year. It differs from other inflammatory disorders in that infectious agents and autoimmune processes are exceedingly rare causes of the disease. The mild form of acute pancreatitis, which accounts for some 75% to 80% of cases, has virtually no mortality and patients recover more or less spontaneously, whereas the severe form is characterized by local and systemic complications, may lead to multiorgan failure, and is burdened with a mortality rate between 5% and 20%. No causal treatment of pancreatitis is known today. The most common causal factors are alcohol abuse and gallstone migration, which together account for more than 80% of patients with acute pancreatitis in most Western countries. Although the mechanisms involved in alcoholic pancreatitis still are being explored and remain poorly understood, much progress has been made in elucidating the role of gallstones in the pathophysiology of acute pancreatitis.

Cellular events during pancreatic duct obstruction

A series of studies involving experimental disease models has shown that pancreatic duct obstruction, rather than reflux of bile into the pancreas, is the crucial trigger event in gallstone-induced pancreatitis [1,2]. Systematic observations in humans confirm the importance of pancreatic outflow

The authors are supported by grants from the DFG Le 625/7-1, Le 625/8-1, Mildred Scheel Stiftung 10-2031-Le I, the Alfried Krupp von Bohlen und Halbach-Stiftung (Graduiertenkolleg Tumorbiologie), and the BMBF NBL3 Programme.

* Corresponding author.
E-mail address: lerch@uni-greifswald.de (M.M. Lerch).

obstruction for the onset of pancreatitis and refute the bile reflux hypothesis [3–5]. To investigate the cellular events involved in gallstone-induced pancreatitis further, an animal model based on pancreatic duct obstruction in rodents recently was used [6]. In addition to a morphologic and biochemical characterization of this experimental disease variety the intracellular calcium release in response to hormonal stimuli was investigated. Under physiologic resting conditions most cell types, including the acinar cells of the exocrine pancreas, maintain a Ca^{2+} gradient across the plasma membrane with low intracellular (nanomolar range) facing high extracellular (millimolar range) Ca^{2+} concentrations. A rapid Ca^{2+} release from intracellular stores in response to external and internal stimuli is used by many of these cells as a signaling mechanism that regulates such diverse biologic events as growth and proliferation, locomotion and contraction, and the regulated secretion of exportable proteins. An impaired cellular capacity to maintain the Ca^{2+} gradient across the plasma membrane previously has been identified as a common pathophysiologic characteristic of vascular hypertension, malignant tumor growth, and cell damage in response to toxins. It also has been observed in a secretagogue-induced model of acute pancreatitis [7,8]. Up to 6 hours of pancreatic duct ligation in rats and mice, a condition that mimics the situation in human gallstone-induced pancreatitis, induced leukocytosis, hyperamylasemia, pancreatic edema, and granulocyte immigration into the lungs, none of which were observed in bile duct–ligated controls [6]. It also led to significant intracellular activation of pancreatic proteases such as trypsin, an event discussed later in more detail. Although the resting $[Ca^{2+}]_i$ in isolated acini rose by 45% to 205 ± 7 nmol/L, the acetylcholine- and cholecystokinin-stimulated calcium peaks and amylase secretion declined. The $[Ca^{2+}]_i$ signaling pattern, the amylase output in response to the Ca^{2+}-ATPase inhibitor thapsigargin, and the secretin-stimulated amylase release were not impaired by pancreatic duct ligation. On the single cell level pancreatic duct ligation reduced the percentage of cells in which a physiologic secretagogue stimulation was followed by a physiologic response (ie, Ca^{2+} oscillations) and increased the percentage of cells with a pathologic response (ie, peak plateau or absent Ca^{2+} signal). Moreover, it reduced the frequency and amplitude of Ca^{2+} oscillation and the capacitive Ca^{2+} influx in response to secretagogue stimulation.

To test whether these prominent changes in intra-acinar cell calcium signaling not only parallel pancreatic duct obstruction but are directly involved in the initiation of pancreatitis, animals were treated systemically with the intracellular calcium chelator BAPTA-AM. As a consequence the parameters of pancreatitis and the intrapancreatic trypsinogen activation induced by duct ligation were found to be reduced significantly. These experiments suggest that pancreatic duct obstruction, the critical event involved in gallstone-induced pancreatitis, rapidly changes the physiologic response of the exocrine pancreas to a pathologic Ca^{2+}-signaling pattern. This pathologic Ca^{2+} signaling is associated with premature digestive enzyme activation and the onset of pancreatitis, both of which can be prevented by administration of an intracellular calcium chelator. We and others believe that alterations in calcium signaling and the premature activation of digestive proteases represent critical events in the onset of pancreatitis.

Mechanisms of pancreatic autodigestion

The exocrine pancreas synthesizes and secretes more protein per cell than any other exocrine organ. Much of its protein secretion consists of digestive proenzymes called zymogens that require proteolytic cleavage of an activation peptide to become active. After entering the small intestine, the pancreatic zymogen trypsinogen is first activated to trypsin by an intestinal protease, enterokinase (enteropeptidase). Trypsin then proteolytically processes other pancreatic enzymes to their active forms. Under physiologic conditions pancreatic proteases thus remain inactive during synthesis, intracellular transport, secretion from acinar cells, and transit through the pancreatic duct. They are activated only when reaching the lumen and brush border of the small intestine. About a century ago, the pathologist Hans Chiari [9] suggested that the pancreas of a patient who had died during an episode of acute necrotizing pancreatitis "had succumbed to its own digestive properties," and he created the term autodigestion to describe the underlying pathophysiologic disease mechanism. Since then, many attempts have been made to prove or disprove the role of premature intracellular zymogen activation as an initial or initiating event in the course of acute pancreatitis. Only recent advances in biochemical and molecular techniques have allowed investigators to address some of these questions conclusively.

Experimental models for intrapancreatic protease activation

Much of our current knowledge regarding the onset of pancreatitis was not gained from studies involving the human pancreas or patients with pancreatitis but came from animal and isolated cell models. There are several reasons these models are being used. (1) The pancreas is an inaccessible organ because of its anatomic location in the retroperitoneal space. Biopsies of the human pancreas are difficult to obtain for ethical and medical reasons. (2) Patients who are admitted to the hospital with acute pancreatitis already have passed through the initial stages of the disease when these events could have been studied. (3) The autodigestive process that characterizes this disease is a particularly significant impediment for investigations that address initiating pathophysiologic events using autopsy or surgical specimens. The issue of premature protease activation therefore has been studied mostly in animal models of the disease [10,11]. These models can be controlled experimentally, are highly reproducible, and recapitulate many of the cellular events that are associated with the clinical disease.

Cellular site of pancreatitis onset

The questions of where pancreatitis begins and through what mechanisms the disease is initiated were not easily resolved. Early hypotheses were based on autopsy studies of patients who had died in the course of pancreatitis. One of these early theories based on human autopsy material suggested that peripancreatic fat necrosis represents the initial event from which all later alterations arise [12]. This hypothesis was attractive because it implicated pancreatic lipase as the culprit for pancreatic necrosis. Lipase is secreted from acinar cells in its active form and does not require activation by limited proteolysis. Another hypothesis suggested that periductal cells represented the site of initial damage and that the extravasation of pancreatic juice from the ductal system is responsible for initiating the disease onset [13]. Subsequent controlled studies performed in animal models that simulate the human disease have demonstrated that the acinar cell is the initial site of morphologic damage [2]. The conclusion that pancreatitis begins in exocrine acinar cells, as opposed to the pancreatic ducts or some poorly defined extracellular space, is important because it represented a shift from earlier mechanistic and histopathologic interpretations of the disease onset and permitted researchers to enter into cell biologic investigations of the underlying causes of pancreatitis. The concept of acinar cells as the primary site of disease onset also is supported by recent clinical and genetic data [14,15] that are summarized in later discussion.

Pathophysiologic significance of digestive protease activation

Trypsinogen and other pancreatic proteases are synthesized by acinar cells as inactive proenzyme precursors and stored in membrane-confined zymogen granules. After activation in the small intestine, trypsin converts other pancreatic zymogens, such as chymotrypsinogen, proelastase, procarboxypeptidase, or prophospholipase A2, to their active forms [16]. Although small amounts of trypsinogen probably are activated within the pancreatic acinar cell under physiologic conditions, two protective mechanisms normally prevent cell damage from proteolytic activity. (1) Pancreatic secretory trypsin inhibitor (PSTI), the product of the SPINK1 gene, is co-secreted with pancreatic zymogens. PSTI can inhibit up to 20% of potential trypsin activity in humans [16], but this number may vary considerably among species. The fact that mutations in the SPINK1 gene are associated with certain forms of human pancreatitis [17–21] indicates that this protective mechanism may play a role in pancreatic pathophysiology. The implications of SPINK1 overexpression in a disease model of pancreatitis are discussed in more detail by Liddle elsewhere in this issue. (2) Cell biologic experiments using living rodent acini provided evidence that trypsin limits its own activity by autodegradation under conditions that mimic pancreatitis (see later discussion) [22]. Furthermore, certain mutations associated with human hereditary pancreatitis stabilize cationic trypsin against autolysis [23–26], suggesting that autodegradation might play a role in safeguarding the human pancreas against excess intrapancreatic trypsin activity. Although not demonstrated experimentally yet, logic would suggest that other pancreatic proteases might participate in a similar protective mechanism. In humans, mesotrypsin has been labeled a candidate for this function [27,28]. This minor trypsin isoform constitutes less than 5% of total secreted trypsinogens. Because of a Gly198→Arg substitution (Gly193→Arg in chymotrypsin numbering), this isoform is inhibited poorly by PSTI, which led to the suggestion that mesotrypsin might participate in degradation of other zymogens and proteases [29,30]. Mesotrypsin, however, is grossly defective not only in inhibitor binding but also in cleaving protein substrates [31]. A pathophysiologic role of mesotrypsin in intracellular protease degradation and a protective function in pancreatitis therefore is somewhat unlikely. The jury is still out on the pathophysiologic role of mesotrypsin, however, because its properties (eg, in signaling through protease-activated receptors) differ markedly from other trypsins, such as the cationic and anionic varieties [32].

The presence of another unknown enzyme activity effective in degrading protease zymogens also was observed in human pancreatic juice. This uncharacterized activity was named Enzyme Y and was proposed as one of the protective factors against pancreatitis [33]. Unfortunately, 15 years after its initial description this enzyme has remained just as elusive because no matching protein or gene ever was identified.

Theoretically, premature activation of large amounts of trypsinogen could overwhelm these protective mechanisms, leading to damage of the zymogen-confining membranes and the release of activated proteases into the cytosol. Moreover, the release of large amounts of calcium from zymogen granules into the cytosol might activate calcium-dependent proteases, such as calpains, which in turn could contribute to cell injury.

The suggestion that prematurely activated digestive enzymes play a central role in the pathogenesis of pancreatitis is based on the following observations: (1) the activity of pancreatic trypsin and elastase increases early in the course of experimental pancreatitis [34,35]; (2) the activation peptides of trypsinogen and carboxypeptidase A_1, which are cleaved from the respective proenzyme during the process of activation, are released into either the pancreatic tissue or the serum early in the course of acute pancreatitis [16,36–40]; (3) pretreatment with gabexate mesylate, a serine protease inhibitor, reduces the incidence of endoscopic retrograde cholangiopancreatography (ERCP)–induced pancreatitis [41]; (4) serine protease inhibitors reduce injury in experimental pancreatitis [42]; (5) hereditary pancreatitis often is associated with various mutations in the cationic trypsinogen gene that could render trypsinogen more prone to premature activation or may render active trypsin more resistant to degradation by other proteases [25]; (6) mutations in the SPINK1 gene that might render PSTI less effective are associated with certain forms of chronic pancreatitis [17–21].

In clinical and experimental studies that investigated the time course of pancreatitis it was found that zymogen activation occurs early in the disease course. One study that used the caerulein model of acute pancreatitis reported a biphasic pattern of trypsin activity that reached an early peak after 1 hour and a later second peak after several hours [40]. This suggests that more than one mechanism may be involved in the activation of pancreatic zymogens and the second peak may require the infiltration of inflammatory cells into the pancreas [40,43,44]. Taken together these observations represent compelling evidence that premature intracellular zymogen activation plays a critical role in initiating acute pancreatitis.

Subcellular site of initial protease activation

Identification of the subcellular site where pancreatitis begins is critical for understanding the pathophysiologic mechanisms involved in premature intrapancreatic protease activation. This question was addressed by three different approaches. Using a fluorogenic cell permeant substrate specific for trypsin fluorescence microscopy could localize trypsinogen activation clearly to the secretory compartment in acinar cells within minutes after supramaximal secretagogue stimulation [45]. When subcellular fractions containing different classes of secretory vesicles were subjected to density-gradient centrifugation it was found that trypsinogen activation does not arise initially in mature zymogen granules but in membrane-confined vesicles of lesser density that most likely correspond to immature condensing secretory vacuoles [45]. In experiments in which antibodies directed against the activation peptide of trypsin (TAP) were used for ultrastructural immunocytochemistry electron microscopy confirmed that the initial site of TAP generation and thus trypsinogen activation is the secretory pathway during experimental pancreatitis. Again, within minutes of pancreatitis induction TAP was found in membrane-confined secretory vesicles that were much less condensed than mature zymogen granules [45,46]. Taken together these data not only confirm that digestive protease activation begins within pancreatic acinar cells, as opposed to the pancreatic ducts or the interstitial space, but also indicate that mature zymogen granules in which digestive proteases are highly condensed are not necessarily the primary site of this activation. The first trypsin activity in acinar cells following a pathologic stimulus is detectable clearly in membrane-confined secretory vesicles in which trypsinogen and lysosomal enzymes (see later discussion) are present physiologically.

Clinical evidence for digestive protease activation

Several recent studies involving patients have contributed to understanding the role of zymogen activation in pancreatitis. In patients who underwent ERCP, an interventional medical procedure that requires cannulation of the pancreatic duct and is associated with a significant complication rate for pancreatitis, the prophylactic administration of a small molecular weight protease inhibitor reduced the incidence of pancreatitis [41]. Although protease inhibitors have not been found to be effective when used therapeutically in patients with clinically established pancreatitis [47], the result of the prophylactic study supports the conclusion that activation of pancreatic proteases is an inherent feature of the disease onset. Moreover, since reasonably specific antibodies have become available that detect TAP but do not cross-react with either active trypsin or inactive trypsinogen [48], the presence of TAP in serum and urine of patients with acute pancreatitis provides direct evidence for an activation of trypsinogen during pancreatitis. The amount of TAP released also seems to correlate with the disease severity [49].

Evidence from genetic studies

A different line of evidence comes from studies in which the genetic basis of pancreatitis was elucidated. Most patients in whom a genetic risk factor for pancreatitis has been identified carry point mutations in either the PRSS1 gene encoding cationic trypsinogen [14,50,51] or in the SPINK1 gene, which encodes PSTI [17–21]. The fact that the most common disease-associated mutations found in pancreatitis patients so far involve either trypsin(ogen) or its inhibitor suggests that trypsin plays a central role in the onset of human pancreatitis. Although trypsinogen clearly undergoes activation during pancreatitis and all reported protease mutations associated with hereditary pancreatitis exclusively affect trypsin(ogen), its ultimate role in the disease onset may be more complex than previously assumed.

Cathepsin B in premature digestive protease activation

Several lines of evidence have suggested a possible role for the lysosomal cysteine protease cathepsin B in the premature and intrapancreatic activation of digestive enzymes [52,53]. The largely circumstantial evidence for this cathepsin B hypothesis is based on the following observations: (1) CTSB has been shown to activate trypsinogen in vitro [54], (2) during the initial phase of acute pancreatitis in several animal models a redistribution of CTSB into a zymogen granule–containing subcellular compartment was detected by density gradient centrifugation [55], (3) in the same pancreatitis models lysosomal enzymes were detected by immunogold electron microscopy in secretory organelles that also contained digestive enzymes (eg, trypsinogen) [56]. Experimental approaches to show an essential role of CTSB in premature zymogen activation by inhibition of this lysosomal enzyme with synthetic inhibitors rendered contradictory results either increasing [57] or decreasing premature zymogen activation [58], or failing to improve the course of experimental pancreatitis [59]. To test the cathepsin B hypothesis more directly and to overcome the shortcomings of lysosomal enzyme inhibitors, which have only limited specificity for CTSB, a CTSB-deficient mouse strain that was generated by targeted disruption of the *ctsb* gene was studied in experimental pancreatitis [60]. The results of these studies were unequivocal: 90% of intrapancreatic trypsinogen activation during pancreatitis depends on the presence of cathepsin B [60]. Although the reduction in local and systemic complications of pancreatitis that were conveyed by the deletion of *ctsb* were not nearly as impressive, the experiments answered the question about the potential role of CTSB in premature digestive enzyme activation during experimental pancreatitis with a resounding yes and settled all arguments about this issue.

The relevance for human disease remained another matter, however. First attempts to establish the relevance of the cathepsin B pancreatitis hypothesis in humans focused on the capacity of the lysosomal enzyme to activate human trypsinogen, and specifically varieties of human trypsinogen into which disease-relevant mutations had been introduced that were identified in the context of hereditary pancreatitis studies. Hereditary pancreatitis, as mentioned above, is a disease that follows an autosomal dominant inheritance pattern, is associated with an early onset of chronic pancreatitis (usually in children and young adults), and is associated with various germline mutations in the cationic trypsinogen gene (*prss1*) [14,15]. When recombinant trypsinogen with hereditary pancreatitis mutations was subjected to activation by CTSB in vitro it was indeed found that some trypsins behaved differently from their wild-type counterpart [26,61], an observation that supported clearly the cathepsin B hypothesis of pancreatitis. On the other hand, the most common PRSS1 mutations, such as R122H and N29I, did not vary convincingly from wild-type trypsin in their activation kinetics by CTSB [62]. The same study further demonstrated that CTSB is secreted abundantly from the human exocrine pancreas, plentifully contained in pancreatic secretory zymogen granules (rather than in lysosomes), and active within the secretory pathway [62]. All cellular conditions for the cathepsin B pancreatitis hypothesis to be operative in humans thus were met. Moreover, the proposed requirement for a subcellular redistribution of CTSB into the secretory compartment [55] finally could be put to rest because most CTSB in the pancreas was found to reside in the secretory compartment already under physiologic conditions [62,63] rather than having to be redistributed there from lysosomes. Nevertheless, no direct evidence for an active involvement of CTSB in the onset of human pancreatitis—at least not in hereditary pancreatitis caused by the most common trypsin mutations—could be produced from these studies.

The production of evidence finally has been achieved in a recent study in which a group from India has sequenced the entire coding region of the *ctsb* gene from 51 South Indian patients with tropical pancreatitis and speculated that *ctsb* germline changes may explain the disease onset [64]. When they compared their *ctsb* sequencing data with that of 25 healthy controls they found 23 different polymorphisms. They went on to increase the number of patients to 140 (and that of controls to 155) to genotype all of them for 4 of these polymorphism. They found a significant difference between patients and controls only for a C76G polymorphism that results in a leucine to valine mutation at amino acid 26 (allele frequency in patients 0.46 versus 0.30 in controls). To rule out a chance finding they went farther south in India and recruited a second cohort of tropical pancreatitis patients (n = 166) and controls (n = 175) from Calicut and genotyped them for the same 4 polymorphism as the first group. Again, the Leu26Val mutation was about twice as common among patients as among controls.

So far the data would suggest that carrying a C76G polymorphism in the *ctsb* gene (ie, a leucine 26 to valine mutation in the CTSB protein) would double one's risk for developing tropical pancreatitis provided one is ethnically Drawidian and hails from Southern India. The study then went further. The fact that the most common *spink1* mutation associated with tropical pancreatitis (N34S) has no measurable effect on the trypsin-inhibiting capacity of the SPINK1/PSTI protein [65] lead to the speculation that rather than causing tropical pancreatitis in India [66] and idiopathic pancreatitis elsewhere [17–21], SPINK1 may act as a modifier gene for other genetic changes. That this was not the case for mutations in the cationic trypsinogen (*prss1*) gene had been shown already [21], but Mahurkar and colleagues also tested it for *ctsb*. As previously shown for trypsin, no differences in phenotype of pancreatitis or genotype in regard to N34S-positive and N34S-negative pancreatitis patients could be found for the L26V mutation. This phenomenon effectively demonstrates that whatever the effect of the CTSB mutation might be, it is unrelated to changes in SPINK1.

Other polymorphisms, those that do not lead to amino acid exchanges and were equally distributed between patients and controls, varied between N34S carriers and non-carriers in further subgroup analyses, but nothing in the study could exclude that this was a chance finding. Hard evidence therefore was only presented for a twofold pancreatitis risk in carriers of the L26V mutation in CTSB.

It remains unknown presently what the effect of this mutation on the cellular level could be. Because no functional data are available presently, structural consideration must serve as a surrogate and the interpretation necessarily remains speculative. The L26V mutation affects the propeptide region of CTSB, which makes it unlikely to have an effect on the catalytic center and thus on enzymatic activity of CTSB. The most that could be expected therefore from a mutation at this site would be an effect on CTSB trafficking, but that may be sufficient to be disease relevant because it matters greatly whether the mannose-6-phosphate–dependent sorting of CTSB ends up in a lysosome or in a zymogen granule where dangerous substrates, such as trypsinogens, reside. Furthermore, some lysosomal cysteine proteinases, including CTSB, are inhibited by their own propeptides [67] and that inhibitory mechanism could be speculated to be a target of the L26V mutation. An exchange of leucine by valine, however, should not produce a sizable change in the conformation of the propeptide. In any case, rat CTSB carries a valine in position 26 of the wild type [68], which is interesting because all initial animal studies that have established the mechanism of CTSB-induced trypsinogen activation and subcellular redistribution of lysosomal enzymes were performed in rats [55–58]. These studies therefore might be more representative for a 26 valine CTSB variety than for the human wild type.

Absent of recombinant enzyme studies little can be learned from the actual polymorphism either; a leucine to valine exchange is about as unexciting as a mutation can get, replacing one nonpolar amino acid with another that only differs in one CH_2 group. The most attractive explanation we could hope to emerge from functional studies would be that the mutation affects the capacity of CTSB to activate mesotrypsin, a trypsin variant that degrades SPINK1 [29], which in turn can inhibit cationic trypsin, which in turn has an established role in at least one variety of pancreatitis. As this complicated and hypothetic chain of events indicates, any assumption about the role of the newly detected *ctsb* polymorphism in the context of pancreatitis must remain wildly speculative. Even a role of CTSB in pancreatitis that is completely unrelated to the activation of trypsin must be considered, just as the function of SPINK1 in the pancreas was found in knockout animal studies to involve embryonic pancreas development and not at all, to the surprise of many, the premature activation of trypsinogen during pancreatitis [69]. Functional studies that look into the biochemistry, cell biology, and interaction with other proteins for different CTSB variants ultimately have to provide that answer. Whether other more common varieties of pancreatitis are associated equally with genetic *ctsb* changes also has to be determined.

All of the above data suggest that cathepsin B–induced protease activation is a critical component in the onset of pancreatitis and the time has finally arrived for evidence from human studies to emerge in support of this hypothesis. Several additional issues regarding the cathepsin hypothesis of pancreatitis remain to be addressed, however. (1) Different lysosomal cathepsins (eg, B, H, L, and so forth) may have vastly different roles in digestive protease activation or degradation. (2) The conditions under which two physiologically colocalized classes of enzymes begin to activate or degrade each other remain unknown and may have important therapeutic implications. (3) The cellular basis of the subcellular redistribution phenomenon of lysosomal enzymes remains poorly understood and could involve either protein sorting or vesicular fusion events. (4) If either the ratio of lysosomal cathepsins and digestive proteases or the processing of lysosomal cathepsins itself were to vary from one class of vesicular compartment to the next, or even within the same compartment, this may change the interpretation of the role of cathepsins in pancreatitis and therefore needs to be explored.

Role of trypsin in premature digestive protease activation

Our present understanding regarding the role of trypsin in the initial events of pancreatitis have come from two different approaches: (1) cell biology studies on isolated rat pancreatic acini, and (2) biochemical studies on recombinant human trypsinogens with hereditary pancreatitis-associated mutations. Unfortunately, these two approaches sometimes lead to seemingly incompatible conclusions, indicating that the role of trypsin in the disease onset is more complex than has been appreciated previously. The salient findings of these two approaches are summarized below.

In the absence of animal models in which wild-type rodent trypsinogens are replaced with mutant human trypsinogens—a daunting task because several genes need to be exchanged—isolated pancreatic acini and lobules offer an alternative to study the role of trypsin in pancreatitis. In a recent study that used a specific cell permeant and reversible trypsin inhibitor it was found that complete inhibition of trypsin activity does not prevent or even reduce the conversion of trypsinogen to trypsin [22]. A cell permeant cathepsin B inhibitor, on the other hand, prevented trypsinogen activation completely. In inhibitor washout experiments it was determined that following hormone-induced trypsinogen activation in pancreatic acinar cells 80% of the active trypsin immediately and directly is inactivated by trypsin itself. Taken together, these experiments suggest that trypsin activity is neither required nor involved in trypsinogen activation, that trypsinogen does not autoactivate in living pancreatic acinar cells, and that its most prominent role is in autodegradation [22]. This in turn suggests that intracellular trypsin activity might have a role in the defense against other potentially more harmful digestive proteases. Consequently, structural alterations that impair the function of trypsin in hereditary pancreatitis would eliminate a protective mechanism rather than generate a triggering event for pancreatitis [70]. Whether these experimental observations obtained from rodent pancreatic acini and lobules have any relevance to human hereditary pancreatitis is unknown presently because human cationic trypsinogen may have different activation and degradation characteristics in vivo. An important advantage of studies using isolated pancreatic acini and lobules to investigate the biologic role of trypsin is the fact that information is obtained on a cellular level rather than in vitro, and pancreatic enzymes can be studied in their physiologic environment. A disadvantage of this approach is the difficulty involved in obtaining human material and the limitations in distinguishing between different varieties and isoforms of trypsin.

The question of why structural changes in the cationic trypsinogen gene caused by germline mutations would lead to the onset of hereditary pancreatitis also has been a matter of debate. Because trypsin is one of the oldest known digestive enzymes, and because trypsin can activate several other digestive proteases in the gut and in vitro, and because pancreatitis is regarded as a disease caused by proteolytic autodigestion of the pancreas, it would seem reasonable to assume that pancreatitis is caused by a trypsin-dependent protease cascade within the pancreas itself. If this hypothesis is correct, the trypsinogen mutations that are found in association with hereditary pancreatitis should confer a gain of enzymatic function [14,15], and mutant trypsinogen would be more readily activated inside acinar cells, or alternatively, active trypsin would be less rapidly degraded inside acinar cells. Both events would lead to a prolonged or increased enzymatic action of trypsin within the cellular environment. On the other hand, several arguments can be raised against the gain-of-trypsin-function hypothesis of hereditary pancreatitis. Statistically, most hereditary disorders, including most autosomal-dominant diseases, are associated with loss-of-function mutations that either render a specific protein defective or impair its intracellular processing and targeting [71]. Moreover, a total of 16 amino acid mutations in the cationic trypsinogen protein, scattered over the various regions of the molecule, have been reported to be associated with pancreatitis or hereditary pancreatitis. It seems unlikely that such a great number of mutations located in entirely different regions of the PRSS1 gene all would have the same effect on trypsinogen and result in a gain of enzymatic function. A loss of enzymatic function in vivo accordingly would be a much simpler and more consistent explanation for the pathophysiologic role of hereditary pancreatitis mutations. To investigate the two alternative hypotheses, in vitro studies were performed that analyzed the biochemistry of recombinant human trypsinogens into which pancreatitis-associated mutations were introduced. Several studies found that either facilitated trypsinogen autoactivation or extended trypsin activity can result under defined experimental conditions [24,25,61,72]. Whether these in vitro conditions reflect the highly compartmentalized situation under which intracellular protease activation begins in vivo [73,74] is presently unknown, but the findings to date strongly favor a gain of trypsin function as a consequence of several trypsinogen mutations.

With respect to a loss-of-function mechanism, recently reported kindreds with hereditary pancreatitis that carry a novel R122C mutation [26,75,76] are interesting. The single nucleotide exchange in these families is located only one position upstream from the one found in the most common variety of hereditary pancreatitis and leads to an amino acid exchange at the same codon (R122C versus R122H). Biochemical studies revealed that enterokinase-induced activation, cathepsin B–induced activation, and autoactivation of Cys-122 trypsinogen are reduced significantly by 60% to 70% compared with the wild-type proenzyme. A possible interpretation of these results is that Cys-122 trypsinogen misfolds by forming mismatched disulfide bridges under intracellular in vivo conditions, resulting in a dramatic loss of trypsin function that cannot be compensated for by increased autoactivation. If this scenario reflects the in vivo conditions within the pancreas, it would represent the first direct evidence from a human study for a potential protective role of trypsin activity in pancreatitis [26]. A second trypsin mutation

(E79K) that was detected to be disease relevant by another group [77] also was found to result in approximately 90% loss of function as far as trypsin autoactivation is concerned.

The question of whether the gain-of-function hypothesis or the loss-of-function hypothesis correctly explains the pathophysiology of hereditary pancreatitis presently cannot be resolved completely, short of direct access to living human acini from carriers of PRSS1 mutations or a transgenic animal model into which the human PRSS1 mutations have been introduced; data for the latter are now forthcoming. Although most of in vitro biochemical studies indicate that increased trypsinogen activation is crucial in the onset of pancreatitis, the data from rodent studies suggest that the role of trypsin may be more complex than previously assumed and that other proteases are more directly involved in the proteolytic damage during pancreatitis against which trypsin could serve as a safeguard [78].

The ultimate proof that trypsin plays a similar role in human pancreatitis would be a hereditary pancreatitis family in which a significant deletion in the cationic trypsinogen gene, preferably affecting the enzyme's active site, would be found to segregate with the disease phenotype. This piece of evidence, however, is conspicuously missing so far.

Novel functions of trypsin

It generally is assumed that an increased intrapancreatic trypsin activity is involved in the onset of pancreatitis because trypsin cleaves specific protein substrates. On the other hand, recent evidence suggests that the role of trypsin in pancreatitis may involve functions that are completely unrelated to its digestive protease activity. In a recent study, the role of the Arg122–Val123 peptide bond was investigated in human cationic trypsinogen [79]. This bond previously was postulated to be a critical site of autocatalytic degradation (autolysis). Unexpectedly, it was found that trypsin-induced cleavage of its Arg122–Val123 bond did not proceed to completion and was not followed by gross degradation. Because of a trypsin-catalyzed resynthesis in vitro a dynamic equilibrium was established between intact trypsin(ogen) and its cleaved, double-chain form. When double-chain trypsinogen was isolated and incubated at 37°C, a rapid resynthesis of the Arg122–Val123 peptide bond was observed in vitro and a single-chain, intact trypsin(ogen) was generated. These observations demonstrate that trypsin has not only digestive but also synthetic activity for certain specialized substrates. A similar phenomenon was observed under extended incubation (weeks in some experiments!) of trypsin with canonical trypsin inhibitors and cleavage of the reactive site bond was found to occur until an equilibrium was reached between the intact and the cleaved protein forms [80]. Although cleavage and synthesis of the Arg122–Val123 bond in trypsinogen occurs at much faster rate and time-scale, the properties of this bond are analogous conceptually to the reactive site bond of trypsin inhibitors, suggesting that the surface loop containing Arg122 might serve as a low-affinity inhibitor of trypsin. This inhibitory activity indeed could be confirmed experimentally, yielding an estimated K_i of 80 µM. Although the physiologic role of either a synthetic activity of trypsin or the inhibitory activity of its Arg122–Val123 bond remains unclear at present, the hereditary pancreatitis-associated mutations R122H and R122C eliminate Arg122 and thus could abolish not only an important cleavage site of trypsin but also trypsinogen-mediated trypsin inhibition.

Role of pH in premature pancreatic protease activation

Changes in pH have a profound impact on autoactivation and autodigestion of trypsinogen. At acidic pH (3.0 or 3.5) pancreatic zymogens, as opposed to cathepsins, are stable and neither autoactivation nor autodegradation occur to any significant degree [81,82]. When pH is raised in either pancreatic juice or purified trypsinogen solutions, autoactivation becomes more rapid up to a maximum between pH 5 and pH 6. At neutral or slightly alkaline pH in the absence of Ca^{2+} the rate of autoactivation declines, whereas autodegradation becomes prevalent. In the presence of Ca^{2+} (see earlier discussion), autoactivation is maximal at slightly alkaline pH with minimal autodegradation. Inside the acinar cell the pH is regulated in a much more narrowly controlled range than used in in vitro experiments. We assume today that the pH within the lysosomal compartment is held within a range between 4.5 and 5.5 [83], whereas it is maintained between 6 and 7 in the secretory compartment [84]. The cytoplasmic vacuoles that arise during pancreatitis also appear to be acidic [42,85]. Maximal and supramaximal stimulation of pancreatic acinar cells leads to a slight increase (0.1–0.3) in intracellular pH but this process again depends on the presence of intracellular calcium [86]. In studies in which the acidic pH inside the vesicular compartments of acinar cells was neutralized by exposure to weak cell-permeable bases the premature protease activation induced by supramaximal hormone stimulation was found to be blocked [57,73]. This finding indicates that an acidic environment is required for premature protease activation to occur. On the other hand, when the same agents were used to neutralize the acinar cell compartments in vivo, experimental pancreatitis still was found to occur and neither its onset nor its course was affected [85]. This finding indicates that the role of the intracellular pH in premature zymogen activation is complex. A shift of the intracellular pH to conditions less favorable for a premature activation of procarboxypeptidase [57] and trypsinogen [73] by trypsin may optimize the conditions for a premature activation by cathepsin B. In this context activation of human cationic trypsinogen by cathepsin B exhibits sharp pH dependence in the acidic range. Between pH 4.0 and 5.2 a 100-fold decrease in activity was observed, suggesting that minor changes in intravesicular pH can have profound effects on cathepsin B–mediated trypsinogen activation in acinar cells [62]. Determining which of these mechanisms plays the critical role in the onset or subsequent course of acute clinical pancreatitis requires additional studies.

Summary

Recent advances in cell biologic and molecular techniques have permitted investigators to address the intracellular pathophysiology in a much more direct manner than previously was considered possible. Initial studies that have used these techniques have delivered several surprising results that appear to be incompatible with long-standing dogmas and paradigms of pancreatic research. Some of these insights will lead to new and testable hypotheses that will bring us closer to understanding the pathogenesis of pancreatitis. Only progress in elucidating the intracellular and molecular mechanisms involved in the disease onset will permit the development of effective strategies for the prevention and cure of this debilitating and still somewhat enigmatic disease.

References

[1] Lerch MM, Saluja AK, Runzi M, et al. Pancreatic duct obstruction triggers acute necrotizing pancreatitis in the opossum. Gastroenterology 1993;104:853–61.

[2] Lerch MM, Saluja AK, Dawra R, et al. Acute necrotizing pancreatitis in the opossum: earliest morphological changes involve acinar cells. Gastroenterology 1992;103:205–13.

[3] Hernandez CA, Lerch M. M. sphincter stenosis and gallstone migration through the biliary tract. Lancet 1993;341:1371–3.

[4] Lerch MM, Weidenbach H, Hernandez CA, et al. Pancreatic outflow obstruction as the critical event for human gall stone induced pancreatitis. Gut 1994;35:1501–3.

[5] Pohle T, Konturek JW, Domschke W, et al. Spontaneous flow of bile through the human pancreatic duct in the absence of pancreatitis: nature's human experiment. Endoscopy 2003;35:1072–5.

[6] Mooren FC, Hlouschek V, Finkes T, et al. Early changes in pancreatic acinar cell calcium signaling after pancreatic duct obstruction. J Biol Chem 2003;278:9361–9.

[7] Ward JB, Sutton R, Jenkins SA, et al. Progressive disruption of acinar cell calcium signaling is an early feature of cerulein-induced pancreatitis in mice. Gastroenterology 1996;111:481–91.

[8] Bragado MJ, San Roman JI, Gonzalez A, et al. Impairment of intracellular calcium homoeostasis in the exocrine pancreas after caerulein-induced acute pancreatitis in the rat. Clin Sci 1996;91:365–9.

[9] Chiari H. Über die Selbstverdauung des menschlichen Pankreas. Z Heilk 1896;17:69–96.

[10] Lerch MM, Adler G. Experimental pancreatitis. Curr Opin Gastroenterol 1993;9:752–9.

[11] Lerch MM, Adler G. Experimental animal models of acute pancreatitis. Int J Pancreatol 1994;15:159–70.

[12] Kloppel G, Dreyer T, Willemer S, et al. Human acute pancreatitis: its pathogenesis in the light of immunocytochemical and ultrastructural findings in acinar cells. Virchows Arch 1986;409:791–803.

[13] Foulis AK. Histological evidence of initiating factors in acute necrotizing pancreatitis in man. J Clin Path 1980;33:1125–31.

[14] Whitcomb DC, Gorry MC, Preston RA, et al. Hereditary pancreatitis is caused by a mutation on the cationic trypsinogen gene. Nat Genet 1996;14:141–5.

[15] Whitcomb DC. Genes means pancreatitis. Gut 1999;44:150.

[16] Rinderknecht H. Activation of pancreatic zymogens: normal activation, premature intra-pancreatic activation, protective mechanisms against inappropriate activation. Dig Dis Sci 1986;31:314–21.

[17] Witt H, Luck W, Hennies HC, et al. Mutations in the gene encoding the serine protease inhibitor, Kazal type 1 are associated with chronic pancreatitis. Nat Genet 2000;25: 213–6.

[18] Pfützer RH, Barmada MM, Brunskill AP, et al. SPINK1/PSTI polymorphisms act as disease modifiers in familial and idiopathic chronic pancreatitis. Gastroenterology 2000;119:615–23.

[19] Threadgold J, Greenhalf W, Ellis I, et al. The N34S mutation of SPINK1 (PSTI) is associated with a familial pattern of idiopathic chronic pancreatitis but does not cause the disease. Gut 2002;50:675–81.

[20] Weiss FU, Simon P, Bogdanova N, et al. Complete cystic fibrosis transmembrane conductance regulator gene sequencing in patients with idiopathic chronic pancreatitis and controls. Gut 2005;54:1456–60.

[21] Weiss FU, Simon P, Witt H, et al. SPINK1 mutations and phenotype expression in patients with trypsinogen mutation-associated pancreatitis. J Med Genet 2003;40:e1–5.

[22] Halangk W, Krüger B, Ruthenburger M, et al. Trypsin activity is not involved in premature, intrapancreatic trypsinogen activation. Am J Physiol Gastrointest Liver Physiol 2002;282: G367–74.

[23] Várallyay E, Pál G, Patthy A, et al. Two mutations in rat trypsin confer resistance against autolysis. Biochem Biophys Res Commun 1998;243:56–60.

[24] Sahin-Tóth M, Tóth M. Gain-of-function mutations associated with hereditary pancreatitis enhance autoactivation of human cationic trypsinogen. Biochem Biophys Res Commun 2000;278:286–9.

[25] Sahin-Tóth M. Human cationic trypsinogen: role of Asn-21 in zymogen activation and implications in hereditary pancreatitis. J Biol Chem 2000;275:22750–5.

[26] Simon P, Weiss FU, Sahin-Tóth M, et al. Hereditary pancreatitis caused by a novel PRSS1 mutation (Arg-122 → Cys) that alters autoactivation and autodegradation of cationic trypsinogen. J Biol Chem 2002;277:5404–10.

[27] Rinderknecht H, Renner IG, Abramson SB. Mesotrypsin: a new inhibitor-resistant protease from a zymogen in human pancreatic tissue and fluid. Gastroenterology 1984;86:681–92.

[28] Nyaruhucha CN, Kito M, Fukuoka SI. Identification and expression of the cDNA-encoding human mesotrypsin(ogen), an isoform of trypsin with inhibitor resistance. J Biol Chem 1997; 272:10573–8.

[29] Szmola R, Kukor Z, Sahin-Toth M. Human mesotrypsin is a unique digestive protease specialized for the degradation of trypsin inhibitors. J Biol Chem 2003;278:48580–9.

[30] Sahin-Toth M. Human mesotrypsin defies natural trypsin inhibitors: from passive resistance to active destruction. Protein Pept Lett 2005;12:457–64.

[31] Katona G, Berglund GI, Hajdu J, et al. Crystal structure reveals basis for the inhibitor resistance of human brain trypsin. J Mol Biol 2002;315:1209–18.

[32] Grishina Z, Ostrowska E, Halangk W, et al. Activity of recombinant trypsin isoforms on human proteinase-activated receptors (PAR): mesotrypsin cannot activate epithelial PAR-1, -2, but weakly activates brain PAR-1. Br J Pharmacol 2005;146:990–9.

[33] Rinderknecht H, Adham NF, Renner IG, et al. A possible zymogen self-destruct mechanism preventing pancreatic autodigestion. Int J Pancreatol 1988;3:33–44.

[34] Bialek R, Willemer S, Arnold R, et al. Evidence of intracellular activation of serine proteases in acute cerulein-induced pancreatitis in rats. Scand J Gastroenterol 1991;26:190–6.

[35] Luthen R, Niederau C, Grendell JH. Intrapancreatic zymogen activation and levels of ATP and glutathione during caerulein pancreatitis in rats. Am J Physiol 1995;268:G592–604.

[36] Schmidt J, Fernandez-del Castillo C, Rattner DW, et al. Trypsinogen-activation peptides in experimental rat pancreatitis: prognostic implications and histopathologic correlates. Gastroenterology 1992;103:1009–16.

[37] Appelros S, Thim L, Borgstorm A. Activation peptide of carboxypeptidase B in serum and urine in acute pancreatitis. Gut 1998;42:97–102.

[38] Gudgeon AM, Heath DI, Hurley P, et al. Trypsinogen activation peptides assay in the early prediction of severity of acute pancreatitis. Lancet 1990;335:4–8.

[39] Mithofer K, Fernandez-del Castillo C, Rattner D, et al. Subcellular kinetic of early typsinogen activation in acute rodent pancreatitis. Am J Physiol 1998;274:G71–9.

[40] Gukovskaya AS, Vaquero E, Zaninovic V, et al. Neutrophils and NADPH oxidase mediate intrapancreatic trypsin activation in murine experimental acute pancreatitis. Gastroenterology 2002;122:974–84.

[41] Cavallini G, Tittobello A, Frulloni L, et al. Gabexate for the prevention of pancreatic damage related to endoscopic retrograde cholaniopancreatography. N Engl J Med 1996;335: 919–23.

[42] Niederau C, Grendell JH. Intracellular vacuoles in experimental acute pancreatitis in rats and mice are an acidified compartment. J Clin Invest 1988;81:229–36.

[43] Schnekenburger J, Mayerle J, Buchwalow I, et al. PTP-kappa and PTP SHP-1 are involved in the regulation of cell-cell contacts at adherens junctions in the exocrine pancreas. Gut 2005;54:1445–55.

[44] Mayerle J, Schnekenburger J, Krüger B. Extracellular shedding of E-cadherin by leukocyte elastase during experimental pancreatitis. Gastroenterology 2005;129:1251–67.

[45] Krüger B, Lerch MM, Tessenow W. Direct detection of premature proteases activation in living pancreatic acinar cells. Lab Invest 1998;78:763–4.

[46] Hofbauer B, Saluja AK, Lerch MM, et al. Intra-acinar cell activation of trypsinogen during caerulein-induced pancreatitis in rats. Am J Physiol 1998;275:G352–62.

[47] Büchler M, Malfertheiner P, Uhl W, et al. Gabexate mesilate in human acute pancreatitis. German Pancreatitis Study Group. Gastroenterology 1993;104:1165–70.

[48] Hurley PR, Cook A, Jehanli A, et al. Development of radioimmunoassays for free tetra-L-aspartyl-L-lysine trypsinogen activation peptides (TAP). J Immunol Methods 1988;111: 195–203.

[49] Neoptolemos JP, Kemppainen EA, Mayer JM, et al. A multicentre study of early prediction of severity in acute pancreatitis by urinary trypsinogen activation peptide. Lancet 2000;355: 1955–60.

[50] Teich N, Mössner J, Keim V. Mutations of the cationic trypsinogen in hereditary pancreatitis. Hum Mutat 1998;12:39–43.

[51] Simon P, Weiss FU, Zimmer KP, et al. Spontaneous and sporadic trypsinogen mutations in idiopathic pancreatitis. JAMA 2002;288:2122.

[52] Steer ML, Meldolesi J. The cell biology of experimental pancreatitis. N Engl J Med 1987;316: 144–50.

[53] Gorelick F, Matovcik L. Lysosomal enzymes and pancreatitis. Gastroenterology 1995;109: 620–5.

[54] Figarella C, Miszczuk-Jamska B, Barrett A. Possible lysosomal activation of pancreatic zymogens: activation of both human trypsinogens by cathepsin B and spontaneous acid activation of human trypsinogen-1. Biol Chem Hoppe Seyler 1988;369:293–8.

[55] Saluja A, Hashimoto S, Saluja M, et al. Subcellular redistribution of lysosomal enzymes during caeruleun-induced pancreatitis. Am J Physiol 1987;253:G508–16.

[56] Watanabe O, Baccino FM, Steer ML, et al. Supramaximal caeruleun stimulation and ultrastructure of rat pancreatic acinar cell: early morphological changes during development of experimental pancreatitis. Am J Physiol 1984;246:G457–67.

[57] Leach SD, Modlin IM, Scheele GA, et al. Intracellular activation of digestive zymogens in rat pancreatic acini: stimulation by high does of cholecystokinin. J Clin Invest 1991;87: 362–6.

[58] Saluja AK, Donovan EA, Yamanaka K, et al. Cerulein-induced in vitro activation of trypsinogen in rat pancreatic acini is mediated by cathepsin B. Gastroenterology 1997;113: 304–10.

[59] Steer ML, Saluja AK. Experimental acute pancreatitis: studies of the early events that lead to cell injury. In: Go VLW, DiMagno EP, Gardner JD, et al, editors. The pancreas: biology, pathobiology, and disease. New York: Raven Press; 1993. p. 489–500.

[60] Halangk W, Lerch MM, Brandt-Nedelev B, et al. Role of cathepsin B in intracellular trypsinogen activation and the onset of acute pancreatitis. J Clin Invest 2000;106:773–81.

[61] Szilágyi L, Kenesi E, Katona G. Comparative in vitro studies on native and recombinant human cationic trypsins. Cathepsin B is a possible pathological activator of trypsinogen in pancreatitis. J Biol Chem 2001;276:24574–80.

[62] Kukor Z, Mayerle J, Kruger B, et al. Presence of cathepsin B in the human pancreatic secretory pathway and its role in trypsinogen activation during hereditary pancreatitis. J Biol Chem 2002;277:21389–96.

[63] Tooze J, Hollinshead M, Hensel G, et al. Regulated secretion of mature cathepsin B from rat exocrine pancreatic cells. Eur J Cell Biol 1991;56:187–200.

[64] Mahurkar S, Idris MM, Reddy DN, et al. Association of cathepsin B gene polymorphisms with tropical calcific pancreatitis. Gut In press.

[65] Kuwata K, Hirota M, Shimizu H, et al. Functional analysis of recombinant pancreatic secretory trypsin inhibitor protein with amino-acid substitution. J Gastroenterol 2002;37: 928–34.

[66] Chandak GR, Idris MM, Reddy DN, et al. Mutations in the pancreatic secretory trypsin inhibitor gene (PSTI/SPINK1) rather than the cationic trypsinogen gene (PRSS1) are significantly associated with tropical calcific pancreatitis. J Med Genet 2002;39:347–51.

[67] Quraishi O, Nagler DK, Fox T, et al. The occluding loop in cathepsin B defines the pH dependence of inhibition by its propeptide. Biochemistry 1999;38:5017–23.

[68] Takio K, Towatari T, Katunuma N, et al. Homolgy of amino acid sequences of rat liver cathepsins B and H with that of papain. Proc Natl Acad Sci U S A 1983;80:3666–70.

[69] Ohmuraya M, Hirota M, Araki M, et al. Autophagic cell death of pancreatic acinar cells in serine protease inhibitor Kazal type 3-deficient mice. Gastroenterology 2005;129:696–705.

[70] Lerch MM, Gorelick FS. Trypsinogen activation in acute pancreatitis. Med Clin North Amer 2000;84:549–63.

[71] Scriver CR. Mutation analysis in metabolic (and other genetic) disease: how soon, how useful. Eur J Pediatr 2000;159:243–5.

[72] Teich N, Ockenga J, Hoffmeister A, et al. Chronic pancreatitis associated with an activation peptide mutation that facilitates trypsin activation. Gastroenterology 2000;119:461–5.

[73] Krüger B, Albrecht E, Lerch MM. The role of intracellular calcium signaling in premature protease activation and the onset of pancreatitis. Am J Pathol 2000;157:43–50.

[74] Krüger B, Weber IA, Albrecht E, et al. Effect of hyperthermia on premature intracellular trypsinogen activation in the exocrine pancreas. Biochem Biophys Res Commun 2001; 282:159–65.

[75] Le Marechal C, Chen JM, Quere I, et al. Discrimination of three mutational events that result in a disruption of the R122 primary autolysis site of the human cationic trypsinogen (PRSS1) by denaturing high performance liquid chromatography. BMC Genet 2001; 2:19.

[76] Pfützer R, Myers E, Applebaum-Shapiro S, et al. Novel cationic trypsinogen (PRSS1) N29T and R122C mutations cause autosomal dominant hereditary pancreatitis. Gut 2002;50: 271–2.

[77] Teich N, Le Marechal C, Kukor Z, et al. Interaction between trypsinogen isoforms in genetically determined pancreatitis: mutation E79K in cationic trypsin (PRSS1) causes increased transactivation of anionic trypsinogen (PRSS2). Hum Mutat 2004;23:22–31.

[78] Ruthenbürger M, Krüger B, Halangk W, et al. Intracellular trypsinogen activation is not involved in acinar cell necrosis but may have a protective role. Pancreatology 2001;1:176–7.

[79] Kukor Z, Tóth M, Pál G, et al. Human cationic trypsinogen. Arg(117) is the reactive site of an inhibitory surface loop that controls spontaneous zymogen activation. J Biol Chem 2002; 277:6111–7.

[80] Laskowski M Jr, Qasim MA. What can the structures of enzyme-inhibitor complexes tell us about the structures of enzyme substrate complexes? Biochim Biophys Acta 2000;1477: 324–37.

[81] Colomb E, Figarella C, Guy O. The two human trypsinogens: evidence of complex formation with basic pancreatic trypsin inhibitor—proteolytic activity. Biochim Biophys Acta 1979;570:397–405.

[82] Colomb E, Figarella C. Comparative studies on the mechanism of activation of the two human trypsinogens. Biochim Biophys Acta 1979;571:343–51.

[83] Maxfield FR. Measurement of vacuolar pH and cytoplasmic calcium in living cells using fluorescence microscopy. Methods Enzymol 1989;173:745–71.

[84] Orci L, Ravazzola M, Anderson R. The condensing vacuole of exocrine cells is more acidic than the mature secretory vesicle. Nature 1987;326:77–9.

[85] Lerch MM, Saluja AK, Dawra R. The effect of chloroquine administration on two experimental models of acute pancreatitis. Gastroenterology 1993;104:1768–79.

[86] Carter KJ, Rutledge PL, Steer ML, et al. Secretagogue-induced changes in intracellular pH and amylase release in mouse pancreatic acini. Am J Physiol 1987;253:G690–6.

ELSEVIER
SAUNDERS

Endocrinol Metab Clin N Am
35 (2006) 333–343

ENDOCRINOLOGY
AND METABOLISM
CLINICS
OF NORTH AMERICA

Biochemistry and Biology of SPINK-PSTI and Monitor Peptide

Rolf Graf, PhD*, Daniel Bimmler, MD

*Pancreatitis Research Laboratory, Department of Visceral and Transplantation Surgery,
University Hospital Zürich, DL 34, Rämistrasse 100, Zürich 8091, Switzerland*

The pancreas synthesizes and secretes digestive enzymes that are delivered to the intestine. To protect the pancreas from autodigestion, several protective mechanisms have evolved: (1) the pancreas, site of synthesis and secretion, is separated from the site of digestive activity; (2) most pancreatic enzymes are produced as inactive precursors (ie, zymogens), which are activated only on entry into the duodenum; and (3) the pancreas synthesizes an inhibitor of trypsin, the so-called "pancreatic secretory trypsin inhibitor" (PSTI). Trypsin is required for the activation of other zymogens (eg, chymotrypsinogen or proelastase). PSTI plays an important role in the equilibrium of protection in the pancreas and digestion in the duodenum: although it is important to inhibit premature activation of trypsin in the former, it is just as essential to allow trypsin activation and hence activation of all zymogens in the latter.

This article summarizes functional aspects of PSTI-SPINK. In addition, the role of monitor peptide (ie, PSTI-I in the rat) is discussed. Further articles deal with the pathophysiology in pancreatitis [1] and genetic alterations in the SPINK gene [2].

Pancreatic secretory trypsin inhibitor

With the development of trypsin biochemistry, the search for specific inhibitors led to the discovery of a number of animal and plant inhibitors. First, a basic pancreatic trypsin inhibitor from bovine pancreas was purified and characterized. This so-called "Kunitz-type inhibitor" inhibits both trypsin and chymotrypsin [3] and is not secreted. In contrast, a secretory form

---

* Corresponding author.
E-mail address: rolf.graf@usz.ch (R. Graf).

0889-8529/06/$ - see front matter © 2006 Elsevier Inc. All rights reserved.
doi:10.1016/j.ecl.2006.02.005

produced by the pancreatic acinar cell was separately identified by Kazal and coworkers [4] and characterized later by Greene and coworkers [5]: this inhibitor is specific to trypsin and is called Kazal-type. Its genetic nomenclature, SPINK, reflects this: serine protease inhibitor Kazal-type 1. SPINK-PSTI is found in a number of species including humans, rodents, bovines, cats, dogs, and birds. Presumably, all animals with a pancreas have evolved a system of checks and balances that contributes to the equilibrium of activation and protection.

Structure

The amino acid composition and sequence of bovine and human PSTI have been solved by conventional chemistry in the 1960s and 1970s [5,6]. The conserved part consists of 56 amino acids with a high homology across species. The location of six cysteines is spaced and according to the human numeration Cys9-Cys38, Cys16-Cys35, and Cys24-Cys56 each form a disulfide bridge resulting in a highly folded globular peptide. For a sequence comparison see Table 1.

Identification of the reactive site [7] of the bovine trypsin inhibitor was performed at acidic pH by exposure to trypsin. A limited cleavage at residue 18/19 of the bovine PSTI was observed and it was suggested that this is the primary site of interaction with trypsin [8]. This basic residue at position 18 (Arg, Lys) provides a substrate that reaches into the active site of trypsin. Amino acids surrounding this site seem negatively to influence the activity of trypsin, hence reducing the catalytic velocity. This results in an inhibitory effect. On extended incubation of PSTI and trypsin, however, activity reappears. This was recognized a long time ago and was termed "temporary inhibition" [9]. After cleavage of the primary site, additional basic residues are cleaved at positions 42/43 and 52/53. The cleavage of these residues render the inhibitor inactive. To demonstrate further that the specificity is in the N-terminal area at amino acids 18 to 21 recombinant PSTI was modified with Lys18Leu, Ile19Glu, and Asn21Arg to simulate a potential chymotrypsin inhibitory site. Indeed, there was an interaction with chymotrypsin as demonstrated by crystallization of the complex PSTI-chymotrypsinogen [10].

To understand the structure-function relationship and later the exploration of genetic variances putatively involved in the etiology of chronic pancreatitis, the efficient production of synthetic PSTI by recombinant technology was required. Several groups reported on recombinant PSTI [11,12] over the years.

Kikuchi and coworkers [13] performed a study with recombinant human PSTI and introduced several mutations to determine the mode of inhibition and inactivation of PSTI. The basic residues at position 42 to 44 were changed to serines or threonines. They came to the conclusion that the inhibitory activity of PSTI was predominantly caused by residue Arg44-Gln45

Table 1
Sequence comparison of the pancreatic secretory trypsin inhibitor from species indicated on the left

Species	Sequence comparison					
		*	A			
Human	DSLGRW	AK**C**YNELNG**C**	TKIYDPV**C**GT	DGNTYPNE**C**V	L**C**FENRKRQT	SILIQKSGP**C**
Dog	NNMLQRQ	AN**C**NLKVNG**C**	NKIYNPI**C**GS	DGITYANE**C**L	L**C**LENKKRQT	SILVEKSGP**C**
Pig	TSPQRE	AT**C**TSEVSG**C**	PKIYNPV**C**GT	DGITYSNE**C**V	L**C**SENKKRQT	PVLIQKSGP**C**
Cow	NIIGRE	AK**C**TNEVNG**C**	PRIYNPV**C**GT	DGVTYSNE**C**L	L**C**MENKERQT	PVLIQKSGP**C**
Mouse	KVTGKE	AS**C**HDAVAG**C**	PRIYDPV**C**GT	DGITYANE**C**V	L**C**FENRKRIE	PVLIRKGGP**C**
Rat I	GNPPAEVNGKT	PN**C**PKQIMG**C**	PRIYDPV**C**GT	NGITYPSE**C**S	L**C**FENRKFGT	SIHIQRRGT**C**
Rat II	KVIGKK	AN**C**PNTLVG**C**	PRDYDPV**C**GT	DGKTYANE**C**I	L**C**FENRKFGT	SIRIQRRGL**C**
Basic	RPDF**C**LEPP	YTGP**C**KARMI	RYFYNAKAGL	**C**QPFVYGG**C**R	AKRNNFKSAE	D**C**MRT**C**GGA

Cysteines are printed in bold face.
A, The basic residue as part of the trypsin binding site.
At the bottom, the sequence of the basic pancreatic trypsin inhibitor (bovine, aprotinin) is shown for comparison.
* Human asparagine mutated to serine.

and that inactivation of PSTI was a result of the removal of the dipeptide Arg42-Lys43. This study is somewhat contradictory to a similar investigation into the structure-function relationship of rat monitor peptide. Homologous amino acids were mutated and it was shown that inhibition of trypsin activity was strongly impaired if the Arg23-Ile24 (homologue to human Arg18-Ile19) was changed to Met-Asn. Furthermore, mutation of the dipeptide Arg57-Arg58 (homologue to human Lys52-Ser53) abolished inhibitory activity [14].

Identification of a mutant PSTI (N34S) involved in the cause of chronic pancreatitis [2] demonstrated that this inhibitor may be directly responsible for pathophysiologic changes leading to disease. Further investigation to prove that the mutation was functionally different used recombinant technology to change the codon at N34S. There were, however, no obvious functional differences when interacting with trypsin, leading to the conclusion that the genetic effect might be on the level of splicing [15].

Szmola and coworkers [16] could demonstrate that mesotrypsinogen, the least abundant of the trypsin isoforms, preferentially deactivates PSTI. They hypothesize that the PSTI pool might be reduced through premature activation of mesotrypsinogen. It was furthermore shown that mesotrypsinogen is a preferred substrate of cathepsin B, which was implied in mediating early damage in acinar cells [17].

Tissue distribution

PSTI is expressed in the acinar cell of the pancreas, whereas duct cells do not show any immunoreactivity. Moreover, PSTI is found in epithelial cells throughout the gastrointestinal tract. In the stomach and in small intestine and rectum, PSTI is found both during fetal development and in adult individuals. Other organs, such as the kidney and lung, also produce PSTI. The functional role in these organs is unclear [18]. PSTI has been associated with wound repair, predominantly in intestinal lesions [19]. Independent investigations have shown that PSTI is localized to Paneth cells [20] in the intestine and that the same cell type synthesizes trypsin [21]. Purification and characterization of PSTI from porcine intestine led to the conclusion that the intestinal inhibitor is identical to the pancreatic product [22]. It was concluded that Paneth cells resemble pancreatic acinar cells [20,22].

In a number of predominantly neoplastic diseases a trypsin inhibitor was identified in the tumors and called "tumor-associated trypsin inhibitor" (TATI) [23]. Its role in tumor development remains unclear but after its characterization it was clear that it is identical to PSTI. Based on sequence analysis, which indicated a homology to epidermal growth factor, it was speculated that TATI and PSTI might play a growth-promoting role in tumor development. One study showed enhancement of cell proliferation. For a review on TATI and its potential role in tumor growth see the review by Stenman [24].

Functional aspects

Protection from premature activation

It is widely accepted that PSTI is a protective molecule in the pancreas. Compelling experimental evidence suggests that during acute pancreatitis, trypsinogen is prematurely activated. The process of activation has been debated among a number of groups. One hypothesis is based on the observation that during supramaximal stimulation of the pancreas with cerulein, lysosomal enzymes are in contact with trypsinogen. This idea was derived from morphologic observations that included a rearrangement of cellular compartments. It was hypothesized that lysosomes and zymogens may fuse. Cathepsin B was then suggested to be an activator of trypsinogen [17,25]. Indeed, cathepsin inhibitors could suppress trypsinogen activation in isolated acini [17] and could reduce the severity of cerulein-induced pancreatitis [26]. Furthermore, experiments with knockout mice for cathepsin B supported this concept because in these animals cerulein-induced pancreatitis was milder and less intra-acinar trypsin was detected [27]. In further studies, cathepsin B was also found in apposition with trypsinogen in zymogen granules indicating that a fusion of lysosomes and zymogens is not even necessary [28]. On the basis of these experimental observations, the role of PSTI as an inhibitor of trypsinogen activation is a key issue. It is unclear whether cathepsin B–activated trypsinogen can be inhibited by PSTI. Furthermore, in the densely packed zymogen granule, molecular movement may be restricted.

PSTI from several species have been investigated to determine the inhibitory activity toward trypsin. The determination of ki as an indicator of affinity was 10 to 11 M for human PSTI, 10 to 14 M for basic pancreatic trypsin inhibitor, and in the range of 6×10 to 9 M for rat PSTI-I. Because of the coevolution of PSTI and trypsin, however, determinations of affinity with the commonly used bovine trypsin might not reflect the actual inhibitory capacity in individual species. Porcine PSTI does not seem to inhibit human trypsin. Furthermore, within one species, trypsinogen isoforms may respond differently. A sound experiment would include a test of all trypsin isoforms from the same species of the inhibitor. This is often not feasible because purification of isoforms is tricky and for experimental purposes not practical. The most prominent research animals, mice and rats, secrete up to 10 different isoforms of trypsinogen. Not all isoforms are inhibited by PSTI: mesotrypsinogen [29], a minor form which comprises about 5% to 10% of all trypsinogen, is not affected by this inhibitor. It has been suggested that mesotrypsinogen is part of the protective system in the pancreas. The role of PSTI-I in the rat is of particular interest: in addition to having trypsin inhibitory capacity, PSTI-I is involved in the feedback regulation in the duodenum (see monitor peptide next). The question arose whether this "inhibitor" had a bona fide function in the pancreas or whether it was functionally adapted for its role in the duodenum. In experiments with bovine and rat trypsin, the authors found that this inhibitor had a lower affinity with a ki of 6×10 to 9 M. This apparently lower ki indicated a potential loss of the enzyme inhibitor role. Experiments were designed to test whether activation of pancreatic juice could be prevented. A small amount of enteropeptidase added to juice was able to activate trypsin and subsequently chymotrypsin quickly. After addition of PSTI, this activation could be almost completely suppressed. Residual activity could be caused by mesotrypsinogen. Rat PSTI-I was capable of preventing premature activation [30].

This raises the question why trypsin activation can be observed in the pancreas and whether it is indeed a pathophysiologic factor in the development of pancreatitis. The pathophysiologic role of trypsin remains a matter of debate, but several studies showed that experimental pancreatitis could be ameliorated by application of trypsin inhibitors before induction [31,32]. It was hoped that commercially available inhibitors (eg, Foy or Trasylol) might prevent or reduce the course of pancreatitis. Unfortunately, acute pancreatitis is a very fast process, and application of these inhibitors after the onset of pancreatitis was conceivably too late.

Monitor peptide

Several laboratories [33–35] independently investigated the feedback regulation of pancreatic enzyme secretion [36,37]. It was recognized that components of the intestinal secretion [35] and of pancreatic juice [33] are involved, and that trypsin is an important regulatory factor. Cholecystokinin (CCK), which is released into the bloodstream from intestinal cells, seemed to mediate the feedback control of pancreatic secretion. Several other factors are involved in this feedback regulation, including monitor peptide, luminal CCK-releasing factor [38], and diazepam binding inhibitor [39]. The following focuses on PSTI-I, which was termed "monitor peptide." The roles of the other factors are discussed elsewhere [40].

The role of PSTI-I as a feedback regulator was recognized more than 20 years ago. In essence, a bioassay was used to determine whether the presence of PSTI-I in the lumen of the duodenum and small intestine had any effect on the secretory activity of the pancreas [33,41]. It was shown that free PSTI-I induced a strong secretion of pancreatic protein. The identification of PSTI-I from whole bile-pancreatic juice demonstrated that this molecule is actively involved and partially responsible for a feedback regulation [33,41]. PSTI-I furthermore elicited a specific response (ie, the induction of CCK secretion in intestinal cells) [42]. The following working hypothesis was formulated: in the presence of nutritional protein in the duodenum, activated pancreatic trypsin is involved in digestion of these proteins, particularly if the proteins are in excess. PSTI-I is then free to bind to intestinal epithelial cells and induce CCK-release, which enhances pancreatic secretion. As soon as all nutritional protein is digested, PSTI-I is bound by trypsin and subsequently degraded. The reduction in free PSTI-I results in a decreasing CCK-release and in a subsequent reduction of pancreatic secretion. Hence, in the presence of nutrional protein PSTI-I is free and promotes secretion, in the absence of proteins PSTI-I is degraded and cannot stimulate CCK-secretion. Although human PSTI can bind to isolated rat intestinal cells [14], there was no stimulatory effect on pancreatic secretion in conscious rats [43]. Furthermore, no effect has been found in segments of the human intestine, suggesting the lack of a PSTI binding protein–receptor in man.

The binding protein–receptor has been demonstrated in two independent investigations. Initially, the protein was identified as a 45-kd protein in mucosal cells scraped from the intestinal wall [14]. The receptor binds PSTI-I and with a similar affinity human PSTI. Other protease inhibitors (eg, Foy or Soy bean inhibitor) do not bind to the receptor. To further investigate the mechanism of signal transduction of monitor peptide, isolated mucosal cells from the duodenum were used. It was shown that calcium ionophore in the presence of extracellular calcium could induce a CCK release. When monitor peptide was used to stimulate CCK-release, calcium was required in the extracelluar medium. This demonstrated that monitor peptide signaling was calcium dependent [14,42,44]. The authors have demonstrated with a chemically synthesized PSTI-I that one and the same molecule inhibits trypsin, binds to membrane fractions from the intestine, and evokes an increase in trypsinogen secretion by a duodenal feedback loop. The authors own preparation exhibited interaction with a protein of about 35 kd. Trypsin and the binding protein–receptor seem to compete for PSTI [30]. Monitor peptide binding sites are not restricted to the intestine. Binding was also observed in the liver. In both organs, binding could not be blocked by excess epidermal growth factor and GTPγS, suggesting that the binding protein–receptor was neither an epidermal growth factor–like receptor nor a G-protein coupled receptor [45].

Growth factor

The establishment of the amino acid sequence of PSTI led to the search for sequence homologies. It was observed that PSTI shared a low but significant sequence homology with growth factors, particularly epidermal growth factor [46]. Because the distribution of PSTI was not restricted to the pancreas, research into functional analysis took other roles into consideration: beside the protection against premature trypsin activity and activation, mitogenic activity is conceivable. The association of PSTI (TATI) with tumor growth and its low but significant homology were the basis for subsequent experiments to prove an active role of PSTI in growth promotion. A mitogenic activity was demonstrated for several cell lines [47–51]. It is unclear whether this mitogenic activity is mediated through an epidermal growth factor–like receptor [52] or by a PSTI-specific receptor of 140,000 kd [53]. It has been suggested that PSTI is involved in mucosal repair, because it is expressed in Paneth cells. For a discussion of this topic see the review by Marchbank and coworkers [19].

Tumor-associated trypsin inhibitor and clinical approaches

In 1982, Stenman and coworkers [54] identified a urinary peptide from a patient with ovarian cancer. This peptide was called "tumor-associated trypsin inhibitor" and it turned out to be secreted from a number of cancers and cancer cell lines. In the same year, it was shown that this peptide was identical to PSTI [23]. Besides biologic implications, TATI-PSTI was investigated as a potential marker for the presence of tumors. To facilitate studies on TATI-PSTI, sensitive diagnostic reagents (ie, antibodies and radioimmunoassay) were developed to quantitate this peptide in tissue, serum, and other body fluids [55]. In a number of studies various cancers were investigated including ovarian, bladder, kidney, pancreatic, colorectal tumors, and adenocarcinoma of the lung [56–60]. TATI seems to be a prognostic marker of ovarian, bladder, and kidney cancer as summarized in a current review [24]. Clinical investigations demonstrated that serum levels of PSTI increase in acute pancreatitis [55] and that they do so in endoscopic retrograde cholangiopancreatography–induced pancreatitis within 2 hours of the intervention [61], whereas it was reduced in pancreatic juice [62] of patients with pancreatic cancer. In patients with pancreas transplantations, perioperatively high levels returned to normal after a few days in patients with a favorable course, whereas in acute rejection episodes a strong increase was found [63].

Based on the diverse biologic roles of this trypsin inhibitor, SPINK-PSTI will receive future attention. In recent observations concerning the pathophysiology of acute and chronic pancreatitis, PSTI seems to be a new factor that may play a crucial role in the development of these inflammatory diseases.

References

[1] Nathan JD, Romac J, Peng RY, et al. Transgenic expression of pancreatic secretory trypsin inhibitor-I ameliorates secretagogue-induced pancreatitis in mice. Gastroenterology 2005; 128:717–27.

[2] Witt H, Luck W, Hennies HC, et al. Mutations in the gene encoding the serine protease inhibitor, Kazal type 1 are associated with chronic pancreatitis. Nat Genet 2000;25:213–6.

[3] Kassell B, Radicevic M, Berlow S, et al. The Basic Trypsin Inhibitor of Bovine Pancreas. I. An Improved Method of Preparation and Amino Acid Composition. J Biol Chem 1963;238: 3274–9.

[4] Kazal LA, Spicer DS, Brahisnky RA. Isolation of a crystalline trypsin inhibitor-anticoagulant from the pancreas. J Am Chem Soc 1948;70:304–40.

[5] Greene LJ, Rigbi M, Fackre DS. Trypsin inhibitor from bovine pancreatic juice. J Biol Chem 1966;241:5610–8.

[6] Bartelt DC, Greene LJ. The primary structure of the porcine pancreatic secretory trypsin inhibitor. I. Amino acid sequence of the reduced S-aminoethylated protein. J Biol Chem 1971; 246:2218–29.

[7] Ozawa K, Laskowski M Jr. The reactive site of trypsin inhibitors. J Biol Chem 1966;241: 3955–61.

[8] Rigbi M, Greene LJ. Limited proteolysis of the bovine pancreatic secretory trypsin inhibitor at acid pH. J Biol Chem 1968;243:5457–64.

[9] Laskowski M, Wu FC. Temporary inhibition of trypsin. J Biol Chem 1953;204:797–805.

[10] Hecht HJ, Szardenings M, Collins J, et al. Three-dimensional structure of the complexes between bovine chymotrypsinogen A and two recombinant variants of human pancreatic secretory trypsin inhibitor (Kazal-type). J Mol Biol 1991;220:711–22.

[11] Maywald F, Boldicke T, Gross G, et al. Human pancreatic secretory trypsin inhibitor (PSTI) produced in active form and secreted from Escherichia coli. Gene 1988;68:357–69.

[12] Kikuchi N, Nagata K, Horii T, et al. Production of recombinant human pancreatic secretory trypsin inhibitor by Escherichia coli. J Biochem (Tokyo) 1987;102:607–12.

[13] Kikuchi N, Nagata K, Shin M, et al. Site-directed mutagenesis of human pancreatic secretory trypsin inhibitor. J Biochem (Tokyo) 1989;106:1059–63.

[14] Yamanishi R, Kotera J, Fushiki T, et al. A specific binding of the cholecystokinin-releasing peptide (monitor peptide) to isolated rat small-intestinal cells. Biochem J 1993;14:57–63.

[15] Kuwata K, Hirota M, Shimizu H, et al. Functional analysis of recombinant pancreatic secretory trypsin inhibitor protein with amino-acid substitution. J Gastroenterol 2002;37:928–34.

[16] Szmola R, Kukor Z, Sahin-Toth M. Human mesotrypsin is a unique digestive protease specialized for the degradation of trypsin inhibitors. J Biol Chem 2003;278:48580–9.

[17] Saluja AK, Donovan EA, Yamanaka K, et al. Cerulein-induced in vitro activation of trypsinogen in rat pancreatic acini is mediated by cathepsin B. Gastroenterology 1997;113:304–10.

[18] Fukayama M, Hayashi Y, Koike M, et al. Immunohistochemical localization of pancreatic secretory trypsin inhibitor in fetal and adult pancreatic and extrapancreatic tissues. J Histochem Cytochem 1986;34:227–35.

[19] Marchbank T, Freeman TC, Playford RJ. Human pancreatic secretory trypsin inhibitor. Digestion 1998;59:167–74.

[20] Bohe M, Lindstrom C, Ohlsson K. Immunohistochemical demonstration of pancreatic secretory proteins in human paneth cells. Scand J Gastroenterol Suppl 1986;126:65–8.

[21] Bohe M, Borgstrom A, Lindstrom C, et al. Trypsin-like immunoreactivity in human Paneth cells. Digestion 1984;30:271–5.

[22] Agerberth B, Ostenson CG, Efendic S, et al. Pancreatic secretory trypsin inhibitor (PSTI) isolated from pig intestine. Influence on insulin and somatostatin release. FEBS Lett 1991; 281:227–30.

[23] Huhtala ML, Pesonen K, Kalkkinen N, et al. Purification and characterization of a tumor-associated trypsin inhibitor from the urine of a patient with ovarian cancer. J Biol Chem 1982;257:13713–6.

[24] Stenman UH. Tumor-associated trypsin inhibitor. Clin Chem 2002;48:1206–9.

[25] Yamaguchi H, Kimura T, Mimura K, et al. Activation of proteases in cerulein-induced pancreatitis. Pancreas 1989;4:565–71.

[26] Van Acker GJ, Saluja AK, Bhagat L, et al. Cathepsin B inhibition prevents trypsinogen activation and reduces pancreatitis severity. Am J Physiol Gastrointest Liver Physiol 2002;283: G794–800.

[27] Halangk W, Lerch MM, Brandt-Nedelev B, et al. Role of cathepsin B in intracellular trypsinogen activation and the onset of acute pancreatitis. J Clin Invest 2000;106:773–81.

[28] Kukor Z, Mayerle J, Kruger B, et al. Presence of cathepsin B in the human pancreatic secretory pathway and its role in trypsinogen activation during hereditary pancreatitis. J Biol Chem 2002;277:21389–96.

[29] Rinderknecht H, Renner IG, Abramson SB, et al. Mesotrypsin: a new inhibitor-resistant protease from a zymogen in human pancreatic tissue and fluid. Gastroenterology 1984;86:681–92.

[30] Graf R, Klauser S, Fukuoka S-I, et al. The bifunctional rat pancreatic secretory trypsin inhibitor/monitor peptide provides protection against premature activation of pancreatic juice. Pancreatology 2003;3:195–206.

[31] Ito T, Kimura T, Furukawa M, et al. Protective effects of gabexate mesilate on acute pancre-
      atitis induced by tacrolimus (FK-506) in rats in which the pancreas was stimulated by caer-
      ulein. J Gastroenterol 1994;29:305–13.
[32] Satoh H, Harada M, Tashiro S, et al. The effect of continuous arterial infusion of gabexate
      mesilate (FOY-007) on experimental acute pancreatitis. J Med Invest 2004;51:186–93.
[33] Fukuoka S, Tsujikawa M, Fushiki T, et al. Stimulation of pancreatic enzyme secretion by
      a peptide purified from rat bile-pancreatic juice. J Nutr 1986;116:1540–6.
[34] Lu L, Louie D, Owyang C. A cholecystokinin releasing peptide mediates feedback regulation
      of pancreatic secretion. Am J Physiol 1989;256:G430–5.
[35] Miyasaka K, Guan DF, Liddle RA, et al. Feedback regulation by trypsin: evidence for intra-
      luminal CCK-releasing peptide. Am J Physiol 1989;257:G175–81.
[36] Green GM, Olds BA, Matthews G, et al. Protein, as a regulator of pancreatic enzyme secre-
      tion in the rat. Proc Soc Exp Biol Med 1973;142:1162–7.
[37] Green GM, Lyman RL. Feedback regulation of pancreatic enzyme secretion as a mechanism
      for trypsin inhibitor-induced hypersecretion in rats. Proc Soc Exp Biol Med 1972;140:6–12.
[38] Spannagel AW, Green GM, Guan D, et al. Purification and characterization of a luminal
      cholecystokinin-releasing factor from rat intestinal secretion. Proc Natl Acad Sci U S A
      1996;93:4415–20.
[39] Owyang C, Louie DS, Tatum D. Feedback regulation of pancreatic enzyme secretion. Sup-
      pression of cholecystokinin release by trypsin. J Clin Invest 1986;77:2042–7.
[40] Owyang C. Discovery of a cholecystokinin-releasing peptide: biochemical characterization
      and physiological implications. Chin J Physiol 1999;42:113–20.
[41] Fushiki T, Fukuoka S, Iwai K. Stimulatory effect of an endogenous peptide in rat pancreatic
      juice on pancreatic enzyme secretion in the presence of atropine: evidence for different mode
      of action of stimulation from exogenous trypsin inhibitors. Biochem Biophys Res Commun
      1984;118:532–7.
[42] Guan D, Ohta H, Tawil T, et al. CCK-releasing activity of rat intestinal secretion: effect of
      atropine and comparison with monitor peptide [published erratum appears in Pancreas 1991
      May;6(3):373]. Pancreas 1990;5:677–84.
[43] Miyasaka K, Funakoshi A. Stimulatory effect of synthetic luminal cholecystokinin releasing
      factor (LCRF) fragment (1-35) on pancreatic exocrine secretion in conscious rats. Pancreas
      1997;15:310–3.
[44] Bouras EP, Misukonis MA, Liddle RA. Role of calcium in monitor peptide-stimulated cho-
      lecystokinin release from perifused intestinal cells. Am J Physiol 1992;262:G791–6.
[45] McVey DC, Romac JM, Clay WC, et al. Monitor peptide binding sites are expressed in the
      rat liver and small intestine. Peptides 1999;20:457–64.
[46] Scheving LA. Primary amino acid sequence similarity between human epidermal growth
      factor-urogastrone, human pancreatic secretory trypsin inhibitor, and members of porcine
      secretin family. Arch Biochem Biophys 1983;226:411–3.
[47] Fukuoka S, Fushiki T, Kitagawa Y, et al. Growth stimulating activity on 3T3 fibroblasts of
      the molecular weight 6,500-peptide purified from rat pancreatic juice. Biochem Biophys Res
      Commun 1986;139:545–50.
[48] Ogawa M, Tsushima T, Ohba Y, et al. Stimulation of DNA synthesis in human fibroblasts by
      human pancreatic secretory trypsin inhibitor. Res Commun Chem Pathol Pharmacol 1985;
      50:155–8.
[49] McKeehan WL, Sakagami Y, Hoshi H, et al. Two apparent human endothelial cell growth
      factors from human hepatoma cells are tumor-associated proteinase inhibitors. J Biol Chem
      1986;261:5378–83.
[50] Freeman TC, Curry BJ, Calam J, et al. Pancreatic secretory trypsin inhibitor stimulates the
      growth of rat pancreatic carcinoma cells. Gastroenterology 1990;99:1414–20.
[51] Fukuda M, Fujiyama Y, Sasaki M, et al. Monitor peptide (rat pancreatic secretory trypsin
      inhibitor) directly stimulates the proliferation of the nontransformed intestinal epithelial cell
      line, IEC-6. Digestion 1998;59:326–30.

[52] Fukuoka S, Fushiki T, Kitagawa Y, et al. Competition of a growth stimulating-/cholecysto-kinin (CCK) releasing-peptide (monitor peptide) with epidermal growth factor for binding to 3T3 fibroblasts. Biochem Biophys Res Commun 1987;145:646–50.

[53] Niinobu T, Ogawa M, Murata A, et al. Identification and characterization of receptors specific for human pancreatic secretory trypsin inhibitor. J Exp Med 1990;172:1133–42.

[54] Stenman UH, Huhtala ML, Koistinen R, et al. Immunochemical demonstration of an ovarian cancer-associated urinary peptide. Int J Cancer 1982;30:53–7.

[55] Kitahara T, Takatsuka Y, Fujimoto KI, et al. Radioimmunoassay for human pancreatic secretory trypsin inhibitor: measurement of serum pancreatic secretory trypsin inhibitor in normal subjects and subjects with pancreatic diseases. Clin Chim Acta 1980;103:135–43.

[56] Satake K, Inui A, Sogabe T, et al. The measurement of serum immunoreactive pancreatic secretory trypsin inhibitor in gastrointestinal cancer and pancreatic disease. Int J Pancreatol 1988;3:323–31.

[57] Higashiyama M, Monden T, Ogawa M, et al. Immunohistochemical study on pancreatic secretory trypsin inhibitor (PSTI) in gastric carcinomas. Am J Clin Pathol 1990;93:8–13.

[58] Higashiyama M, Monden T, Tomita N, et al. Expression of pancreatic secretory trypsin inhibitor (PSTI) in colorectal cancer. Br J Cancer 1990;62:954–8.

[59] Ohmachi Y, Murata A, Matsuura N, et al. Specific expression of the pancreatic-secretory-trypsin-inhibitor (PSTI) gene in hepatocellular carcinoma [published erratum appears in Int J Cancer 1994 Apr 1;57(1):139]. Int J Cancer 1993;55:728–34.

[60] Pasanen PA, Eskelinen M, Partanen K, et al. Tumour-associated trypsin inhibitor in the diagnosis of pancreatic carcinoma. J Cancer Res Clin Oncol 1994;120:494–7.

[61] Lempinen M, Stenman UH, Halttunen J, et al. Early sequential changes in serum markers of acute pancreatitis induced by endoscopic retrograde cholangiopancreatography. Pancreatol 2005;5:157–64.

[62] Marks WH, Ohlsson K, Wehlin L, et al. Pancreatic secretory trypsin inhibitor, cathodal trypsin, and pancreatic elastase in pancreatic juice collected at endoscopic retrograde cholangiopancreatography. Curr Surg 1985;42:26–8.

[63] Suzuki Y, Kuroda Y, Sollinger HW, et al. Plasma pancreatic secretory trypsin inhibitor as a marker of pancreas graft rejection after combined pancreas-kidney transplantation. Transplantation 1991;52:504–7.

ELSEVIER
SAUNDERS

Endocrinol Metab Clin N Am
35 (2006) 345–356

ENDOCRINOLOGY
AND METABOLISM
CLINICS
OF NORTH AMERICA

Pathophysiology of SPINK Mutations in Pancreatic Development and Disease

Rodger A. Liddle, MD

*Department of Medicine, Duke University and Durham VA Medical Centers,
Box 3913, Durham, NC 27710, USA*

A central feature of pancreatitis is inappropriate activation of proteolytic enzymes within the pancreas that leads to autodigestion, inflammation, and necrosis of the gland. The most important of these enzymes is trypsin, because it has the ability to activate other pancreatic proenzymes. Two mechanisms seem to protect the pancreas against premature enzyme activation. The first defense is inhibition of trypsin by an endogenous pancreatic trypsin inhibitor that is produced and stored with zymogens in acinar cells. The second defense is the ability of trypsin to autoinactivate because trypsin can cleave specific basic amino acid residues, rendering other trypsin molecules inactive. Under normal conditions, protease activity within the pancreas is limited by safeguards that either inhibit or destroy trypsin. This article summarizes a body of work related to the role of the endogenous pancreatic trypsin inhibitor in pancreatic physiology and disease, including genetic associations with pancreatitis.

Role of enzyme activation in pancreatitis

The exocrine portion of the pancreas, which comprises 90% of the gland, synthesizes, stores, and secretes digestive enzymes. Pancreatic enzymes are packaged in zymogen granules and are released into the pancreatic duct on stimulation of the gland. Most pancreatic enzymes are synthesized as proenzymes and it is only on reaching the duodenum that they become converted to their active forms. This activation occurs by exposure to enterokinase, which cleaves trypsinogen to trypsin, which in turn activates other proenzymes. In the duodenum, enzymes facilitate the digestion of food.

This work was supported by grant numbers DK 064213 and DK 38626 from the National Institutes of Health.

E-mail address: liddl001@mc.duke.edu

Inadvertent activation of trypsin within the pancreas, however, has the potential to cause premature activation of other proenzymes. Liberation of proteolytic enzymes within the pancreas can lead to extensive damage through a process of autodigestion caused by uninhibited enzymatic destruction of normal cellular proteins. If not blocked, a cascade of enzymatic activation occurs that amplifies this self-destructive process leading to the pathophysiologic sequelae known as "pancreatitis." Consequently, it is extremely difficult to inhibit pancreatitis once it has been initiated.

It has long been believed that trypsin activation plays a central role in the pathogenesis of pancreatitis. This concept has been supported by substantial experimental evidence. Visual evidence was provided by electron microscopic studies showing fusion of zymogen granules (containing trypsinogen and other proenzymes) with lysosomal vesicles to form large membrane-bound organelles [1]. Biochemical evidence has shown that colocalization of zymogens with lysosomal enzymes, such as cathepsin B, converts trypsinogen to trypsin within the acinar cell [2–4]. Zymogen-lysosome colocalization can occur by two processes: missorting of vesicles during their formation or fusion of existing vesicles. Either process can produce premature enzyme activation. Although it is not believed to be extensive, colocalization of zymogens with lysosomal enzymes has been observed in normal acinar cells [5,6]. Because these occur in a nonpathologic setting, there must be mechanisms within the pancreas to limit enzyme activation and prevent uncontrolled enzyme activation that otherwise leads to pancreatitis.

Pancreatic trypsin inhibitor

An endogenous trypsin inhibitor was first purified from pancreas in 1948 [7] and has been commonly known as "pancreatic secretory trypsin inhibitor." It is in the serine protease family of inhibitors and was subsequently named *s*erine *p*rotease *in*hibitor of the *K*azal type (SPINK). Although there are various forms in different species, the human form is known as SPINK1. SPINK1 is synthesized in acinar cells where it is packaged and stored in zymogen granules and secreted into pancreatic juice along with enzymes. By virtue of its trypsin inhibitor activity, it has long been thought that the function of SPINK is to inhibit trypsin should it become inadvertently activated within the pancreas. This mechanism prevents pancreatic autodigestion by uncontrolled trypsin activity.

The human SPINK1 gene is located on chromosome 5 and is comprised of approximately 7.5 kilobases, which contain four exons [8]. This gene encodes for a single polypeptide of 79 amino acids including a 23–amino acid signal peptide [9]. The mature SPINK1 protein is 56 amino acids long and contains six cysteine residues, which form three disulfide bridges. This conformation produces a heat- and acid-stable, three-loop, clover-leaf configuration that is similar to other proteins found in the lumen of the gut, such as trefoils. The tertiary structure is believed to stabilize the molecule in the harsh enzymatic environment of the intestine.

Pancreatic trypsin inhibitors of different species are highly homologous. They all share a common (Lys-Ile) region that is a specific binding site for trypsin [9]. When incubated together, SPINK and trypsin form a stable interaction caused by a covalent bond between the carboxyl group of the reactive lysine of SPINK and the catalytic serine residue of trypsin. This interaction is reversible, however, and enzymatic trypsin activity can be recovered from the SPINK-trypsin complex following prolonged incubation [10]. It has been proposed that this association and dissociation has physiologic relevance. Should trypsin become activated within the pancreas, it can bind SPINK. Together, the SPINK-trypsin complex is secreted into pancreatic juice, where on reaching the small intestine the inhibitor can dissociate or be degraded. In this manner, trypsin activity is only temporarily inhibited and may be reactivated in the intestine where it can facilitate digestion.

Importantly, human SPINK does not inhibit mesotrypsin or chymotrypsin and SPINKs from other species do not inhibit human trypsin effectively.

Trypsinogen mutations and hereditary pancreatitis

Hereditary pancreatitis is a familial disease characterized by recurrent attacks of acute pancreatitis that ultimately results in chronic pancreatitis with both exocrine and endocrine pancreatic insufficiency. The disease was initially described in 1952 in a family with an apparent autosomal-dominant inheritance pattern with disease penetrance of approximately 80% [11,12]. It was not until 1996 when the gene defect responsible for hereditary pancreatitis was discovered, however, that clinicians gained substantial and novel insights into the pathogenesis of the disorder [13]. Mutations in the PRSS1 (*protease serine* 1) gene, which encodes cationic trypsinogen, have been found in multiple different families with hereditary pancreatitis. The most common mutation is R122H, which alters a trypsin-sensitive site that stabilizes the molecule against autoinactivation. It is believed that should trypsinogen become activated within the pancreas, trypsin can limit zymogen activation by self-hydrolysis at the arginine residue at position 122, which destroys its enzymatic activity. The mutated trypsin molecule is resistant to such autoinactivation. Two other mutations, N29I and A16V, may increase the frequency of autoactivation or affect trypsinogen translocation, respectively, as mechanisms predisposing to pancreatitis. Other PRSS1 mutations have also been associated with hereditary pancreatitis [14–16]; however, the mechanisms by which these alter trypsinogen function are still under investigation. It is worth noting that a pathogenic role for a mutated trypsinogen gene in development of chronic pancreatitis was not suspected before discovery of the hereditary pancreatitis gene defect.

Two factors led to the search for other gene mutations that may cause hereditary pancreatitis. First, there are many families in whom pancreatitis seems to be inherited, but mutations in the PRSS1 gene are lacking. In addition, approximately one third of patients with chronic pancreatitis have no discernible cause for their disease. Second, once trypsin was implicated as playing a major role in the development of hereditary pancreatitis, it seemed logical to envision that alterations in pancreatic trypsin inhibitor could also reduce the protective barrier against pancreatic autodigestion. For these reasons, investigators began to look for mutations in the SPINK1 gene in patients with chronic pancreatitis.

Idiopathic chronic pancreatitis and mutations in the SPINK1 gene

In 2000, a mutational analysis of the SPINK1 gene in patients with chronic pancreatitis and hereditary pancreatitis lacking the PRSS1 mutation identified an A → G transition producing an N34S mutation [17]. Because the variant did not segregate with the disease and the mutation was found in 3 of 400 control chromosomes, however, it was excluded as a disease-causing mutation. In addition, a C → T transition producing a P55S mutation was also noted in this study population, but it too was discounted because it was found in 2 of 400 control chromosomes. It was not until Witt and coworkers [18] screened 96 unrelated children and adolescents with idiopathic chronic pancreatitis who did not have PRSS1 mutations and found the N34S mutation in 23% of patients, that it was clear that mutations in the SPINK1 gene were associated with pancreatitis. Four other sequence variants in the SPINK1 gene (M1T, L14P, -53C → T, IVS3 + 2T) also were found in single patients. The N34S mutation was found in one heterozygous carrier. A transmission disequilibrium test indicated that SPINK1 mutations were potentially causative of pancreatitis. The authors proposed that the N34S mutation, which is located near the Lys-Ile site of SPINK1, might lead to decreased trypsin inhibitory capacity within the pancreas. Reduced inhibitor activity disrupts the balance between trypsin (should trypsinogen become inadvertently activated) and its inhibitor, predisposing to zymogen activation and subsequent autoactivation and pancreatitis. This hypothesis is supported by extrapolation from other species in which asparagine at position 34 is not fully conserved between species [19]. It has been demonstrated experimentally that porcine trypsin inhibitor, which has a serine at this position, is not an effective inhibitor of human trypsin [9]. With this study alone, however, it was unclear whether pancreatitis associated with SPINK1 mutations represented an autosomal-recessive disease caused by SPINK1 mutations per se, or was caused by SPINK1 mutations in combination with unidentified genes or other factors.

Subsequently, Pfutzer and coworkers [20] sequenced the entire SPINK1 gene in 112 patients with sporadic or familial chronic pancreatitis who lacked PRSS1 mutations. The N34S mutation was detected in 26% of patients, confirming the observations of Witt and coworkers [18], and several additional genetic variants were identified in the SPINK1 gene (D50E, IVS3 + 125 C → A, and IVS3 + 184 T → A). Of 380 control alleles, three N34S and two P55S mutations were found. The ages of onset of pancreatitis and disease severity were similar between heterozygous and homozygous patients. It was clear that SPINK1 mutations were associated with pancreatitis, but were relatively common in the normal population. These data suggest that SPINK1 mutations are disease modifying, but in and of themselves, do not cause pancreatitis. The authors speculated that SPINK1 mutations may lower the threshold for pancreatitis from other genetic or environmental factors.

The association between SPINK1 mutations and chronic pancreatitis has been confirmed in a number of subsequent studies [21–34]. Taken together several conclusions can be drawn. First, SPINK1 mutations segregate in families with pancreatitis, perhaps in a complex pattern with another pancreatitis-related gene. Second, the N34S mutation is common, occurring in approximately 2% of control individuals. Third, the common SPINK1 mutations seem to decrease the age of onset of pancreatitis in affected individuals.

SPINK1 mutations have been investigated in three other pancreatitis-related conditions: (1) tropical pancreatitis, (2) alcoholic pancreatitis, and (3) idiopathic chronic pancreatitis associated with mutations in the cystic fibrosis transmembrane regulator (CFTR) gene. Each of these conditions is discussed next.

SPINK1 mutations in tropical pancreatitis

Tropical pancreatitis is a form of chronic pancreatitis that occurs in tropical countries but the etiology is unknown. It has been divided into subcategories known as either "tropical calcific pancreatitis" or "fibrocalculous pancreatic diabetes" based on the absence or presence of diabetes mellitus early in the development of chronic pancreatitis. SPINK1 mutations have been found in both types of tropical pancreatitis. In a population from Bangladesh, 15 of 37 patients with tropical pancreatitis were found to have the N34S mutation [35]. In addition, another SPINK1 mutation (Y54H) was found in a patient lacking the N34S mutation. Other studies also have indicated a high rate of SPINK1 mutations in tropical pancreatitis [36–38] suggesting that they play a role in the development of the disease.

SPINK1 mutations and alcoholic chronic pancreatitis

It has long been recognized that chronic excessive alcohol ingestion is associated with pancreatitis. Although a familial pattern has been suggested by some, a genetic basis for alcoholic chronic pancreatitis has not been identified. With the discovery that SPINK1 mutations may predispose to pancreatitis, it was logical to search for similar mutations in patients with alcoholic pancreatitis. Several studies have reported a weak association [21,28,31,39,40]. In the largest study, the N34S mutation was found in 16 (5.8%) of 274 alcoholic patients compared with 4 (0.8%) of 540 of control individuals [21]. Although the incidence was low, this was a statistically significant difference, and it is conceivable that SPINK1 mutations contribute to the pathogenesis of chronic pancreatitis in alcoholic patients even though the precise mechanism is currently unknown.

SPINK1 and cystic fibrosis transmembrane conductance regulator mutations in idiopathic chronic pancreatitis

Idiopathic chronic pancreatitis is the most common cause of chronic pancreatitis in nonalcoholic patients. Most cases of idiopathic chronic pancreatitis are sporadic and it was not suspected that idiopathic chronic pancreatitis may have a genetic basis until two groups reported an association between idiopathic chronic pancreatitis and mutations in the cystic fibrosis gene, which encodes the cystic fibrosis transmembrane conductance regulator (CFTR) [41,42]. These two studies showed that approximately 20% of patients with idiopathic chronic pancreatitis had cystic fibrosis–causing mutations. The risk of developing idiopathic chronic pancreatitis was increased approximately fivefold in cystic fibrosis carriers and was even higher in compound heterozygotes.

Despite carrying CFTR mutations, however, most compound heterozygotes do not develop idiopathic chronic pancreatitis, indicating that other factors are involved in the genesis of pancreatitis. Following identification of SPINK1 mutations, investigators tested their cystic fibrosis carriers with idiopathic chronic pancreatitis for SPINK1 mutations [27,30]. It was found that the N34S mutation was associated with idiopathic chronic pancreatitis in both children and adults. Moreover, higher than expected numbers of SPINK1 mutations were found in idiopathic chronic pancreatitis patients with CFTR mutations indicating that the risk of idiopathic chronic pancreatitis was increased in individuals carrying mutations of these two separate genes. By combining the two studies, SPINK1 mutations were found in 6 of 36 patients with pancreatitis with at least one CFTR mutation and in 3 of 15 CFTR compound heterozygotes. These data indicate that the risk of idiopathic chronic pancreatitis is increased by approximately 10-fold by having a SPINK1 mutation, approximately 40-fold in CFTR compound heterozygotes, and by approximately 500-fold by having both genotypes [43].

It has been reported that *SPINK1* and *CFTR* mutations are frequent among patients infected with HIV suffering from acute pancreatitis [44]. The authors suggested that these mutations increase the susceptibility to pancreatitis when patients are exposed other environmental risk factors including drugs or infectious causes.

Other associations

The combination of a SPINK1 N34S mutation together with a mutation in the calcium-sensing receptor was reported in a family with familial chronic pancreatitis [45]. The importance of this dual mutation in the inheritance pattern and severity of pancreatitis requires further investigation.

SPINK1 and trypsin inhibitor activity

Despite the association between SPINK1 mutations and increased risk of chronic pancreatitis, the mechanisms by which SPINK1 mutations predispose to pancreatitis are not well understood. SPINK1 is a potent protease inhibitor that is stored in zymogen granules of the acinar cell. Both of these attributes suggest that SPINK1 is capable of inhibiting trypsin should it become activated within the pancreas. Because trypsin activation is believed to be an important and perhaps necessary step in the pathogenesis of pancreatitis, it seems likely that reduced SPINK1 activity could predispose to pancreatitis. Conversely, it is conceivable that increased SPINK1 activity may reduce the likelihood or severity of pancreatitis.

The N34S mutation, which is the most common SPINK1 mutation linked to pancreatitis, was initially thought to reduce trypsin inhibitor activity of the SPINK1 protein [18]. It was proposed that the asparagine residue at position 34 is important for inhibiting human trypsin because porcine trypsin has a serine in this position and is less effective than human SPINK1 in inhibiting human trypsin [19,46,47]. To test this hypothesis, a possible functional defect in the N34S mutant SPINK1 molecule was examined using structural modeling [20]. The lysine residue located at position 41 in the SPINK1 molecule is recognized by the specificity pocket of trypsin. The structural orientation of this region was analyzed by computer modeling for both normal and mutated SPINK1 molecules. The authors demonstrated that the N34S region is in close proximity to the active pocket of trypsin and that amino acid substitutions of the N34S type changed the orientation of the inhibitor with the enzyme pocket of trypsin. The investigators proposed that the N34S conversion was substantial enough to alter the interaction of SPINK1 with trypsin perhaps leading to weaker binding and weaker enzyme inhibition.

These provocative studies led the way to functional testing of the N34S SPINK1 mutant protein for alterations in trypsin inhibitor activity. Surprisingly, in in vitro assays under various experimental conditions, the trypsin inhibitory activities of recombinant wild-type SPINK1 and the N34S mutant were identical [48]. Moreover, the susceptibility of the N34S mutant to trypsin digestion was not increased and the binding kinetics of the N34S mutant and wild-type SPINK1 proteins were also indistinguishable from one another. These studies did not identify any abnormalities in the biochemical function of the N34S SPINK1 mutant protein. These data do not prove, however, that the mutant protein is not defective in some other way, such as enhanced susceptibility to digestion by enzymes other than trypsin or abnormal cellular trafficking that could affect local trypsin inhibitor activity [49].

Animal models

SPINK deficiency

Although very strong genetic evidence indicates that a SPINK1 defect leads to chronic pancreatitis, the mechanism by which this occurs is unknown. The lack of biochemical impairment in the predominant N34S mutant of SPINK1 was a surprise to investigators in the field. If trypsin activity is central to the pathogenesis of pancreatitis, as is widely believed, then pancreatitis may occur under conditions in which trypsin activation exceeds trypsin inhibitor capacity. To evaluate this relationship, the role of SPINK1 in pancreatic development was assessed in mice with genetic deletion of the SPINK gene [50]. The mouse SPINK homolog is SPINK3. *SPINK3*-deficient (*SPINK3−/−*) mice were generated by gene targeting in embryonic stem cells. In (*SPINK3−/−*) mice, the pancreas developed normally until embryonic day 15.5; however, by day 16.5 pancreatic acinar cells (but not islets or duct cells) underwent autophagic degeneration. There was limited inflammatory cell infiltration in the pancreas and no sign of apoptosis. Within a few days of birth, rapid pancreatic cell death occurred; mice failed to gain weight and died by 2 weeks of age. In contrast to homozygous (*SPINK3−/−*) knockout mice, the pancreas in heterozygous (*SPINK3+/−*) mice developed normally, mice gained weight, and exhibited no discernible abnormal phenotypic features.

The absence of inflammation, necrosis, and apoptosis in *SPINK3−/−* mice indicated this is not a model of pancreatitis, although it clearly represents a destructive process within the pancreas. Although it was thought that absence of SPINK3 may result in greater activation of trypsin and subsequent activation of other pancreatic enzymes, trypsin activity was similar in homozygous (*SPINK3−/−*), heterozygous (*SPINK3+/−*), and wild-type mice suggesting that trypsin was not significantly activated in *SPINK3−/−* mice. Interestingly, trypsin mRNA expression (detected at day 15.5) coincided with the onset of autophagy within acinar cells. Even though it was not possible to demonstrate increased trypsin activity in *SPINK3−/−* mice, this does not mean the contribution of SPINK3 to cellular autophagy is independent of a trypsin inhibitor effect. The authors suggest that autophagy plays a more important role in pancreatitis than previously recognized and raise the intriguing possibility that pancreatitis is caused by an autophagic process and not by trypsin activation [50].

Increased pancreatic trypsin inhibitor activity and pancreatitis

The amount of endogenous trypsin inhibitor present in the pancreas is sufficient to inhibit approximately 20% of the trypsin in the gland should all of the trypsinogen become prematurely activated [46]. It is quite logical to expect that endogenous pancreatic trypsin inhibitor may limit enzyme activation and subsequent damage from inappropriately activated trypsin. To test the hypothesis that endogenous trypsin inhibitor confers protection against pancreatitis, a recent study used a transgenic mouse model to increase trypsin inhibitor levels in the pancreas [51]. Rat pancreatic secretory trypsin inhibitor I (a homolog of SPINK1) was targeted to pancreatic acinar cells by creating a minigene driven by the mouse elastase enhancer-promoter. This targeted expression increased trypsin inhibitor capacity by 190% in transgenic mice compared with nontransgenic mice. In a model of cerulein-induced pancreatitis, mice expressing the trypsin inhibitor transgene developed much less severe pancreatitis. Interestingly, there was no difference in trypsinogen activation peptide levels between cerulein-treated transgenic and nontransgenic mice, indicating that trypsin inhibitor expression did not prevent trypsin activation. Trypsin activity was substantially lower in transgenic mice versus nontransgenic mice receiving cerulein, however, suggesting that trypsin inhibitor overexpression prevented pancreatitis by inhibiting the activity of trypsin. This study demonstrated that the severity of pancreatitis could be ameliorated by increasing pancreatic levels of trypsin inhibitor. This finding is consistent with the concept that endogenous trypsin inhibitor protects against pancreatitis by limiting protease activity and thereby reducing pancreatic injury.

Summary

The genetic predisposition of SPINK1 mutations causing pancreatitis has been known only for approximately 5 years. Over this brief time, however, a number of important observations have been made by investigators in the field. It has been confirmed that SPINK plays an important role in protecting the pancreas against pancreatitis. There is clear evidence that SPINK1 mutations are associated with development of both acute and chronic pancreatitis. The N34S mutation is the most frequent SPINK1 variant associated with chronic pancreatitis, even though it is commonly observed in the general population. These findings, however, indicate that in most patients with SPINK1 mutations, the genetic variants do not cause the disease independently, but may act in concert with genetic or environmental factors. The associations of *SPINK1* with *PRSS1* (cationic trypsinogen) or *CFTR* mutations suggest that pancreatitis-associated susceptibility genes may be additive, greatly increasing the risk of developing pancreatitis.

Despite these advances there is much that is not known about SPINK1 in pancreatic physiology and pancreatitis. First, multiple different genetic variants of SPINK1 have been associated with pancreatitis, but it has yet to be determined how any of these actually cause pancreatitis. Second, it has been speculated that SPINK1 must act in combination with other genetic or environmental factors but these factors remain undefined. Third, little is known about the regulation of SPINK1 gene and protein expression and whether it is subject to manipulation. These are major issues that require thoughtful and thorough investigation and, hopefully, will lead to novel diagnostic, prognostic, and even therapeutic approaches for patients with pancreatitis.

References

[1] Scheele G, Adler G, Kern H. Exocytosis occurs at the lateral plasma membrane of the pancreatic acinar cell during supramaximal secretagogue stimulation. Gastroenterology 1987;92:345–53.

[2] Bialek R, Willemer S, Arnold R, et al. Evidence of intracellular activation of serine proteases in acute cerulein-induced pancreatitis in rats. Scand J Gastroenterol 1991;26:190–6.

[3] Hofbauer B, Saluja AK, Lerch MM, et al. Intra-acinar cell activation of trypsinogen during caerulein-induced pancreatitis in rats. Am J Physiol 1998;275:G352–62.

[4] Steer ML. Frank Brooks memorial Lecture: the early intraacinar cell events which occur during acute pancreatitis. Pancreas 1998;17:31–7.

[5] Saluja A, Saluja M, Villa A, et al. Pancreatic duct obstruction in rabbits causes digestive zymogen and lysosomal enzyme colocalization. J Clin Invest 1989;84:1260–6.

[6] Luthen R, Niederau C, Niederau M, et al. Influence of ductal pressure and infusates on activity and subcellular distribution of lysosomal enzymes in the rat pancreas. Gastroenterology 1995;109:573–81.

[7] Kazal LA, Spicer DS, Brahinsky RA. Isolation of crystalline trypsin inhibitor-anticoagulant protein from the pancreas. J Am Chem Soc 1948;70:304–40.

[8] Horii A, Kobayashi T, Tomita N, et al. Primary structure of human pancreatic secretory trypsin inhibitor (PSTI) gene. Biochem Biophys Res Commun 1987;149:635–41.

[9] Bartelt DC, Shapanka R, Greene LJ. The primary structure of the human pancreatic secretory trypsin inhibitor: amino acid sequence of the reduced S-aminoethylated protein. Arch Biochem Biophys 1977;179:189–99.

[10] Laskowski M, Wu FC. Temporary inhibition of trypsin. J Biol Chem 1953;204:797–805.

[11] Comfort MW, Steinberg AG. Pedigree of a family with hereditary chronic relapsing pancreatitis. Gastroenterology 1952;21:54–63.

[12] McElroy R, Christiansen PA. Hereditary pancreatitis in a kinship associated with portal vein thrombosis. Am J Med 1972;52:228–41.

[13] Whitcomb DC, Gorry MC, Preston RA, et al. Hereditary pancreatitis is caused by a mutation in the cationic trypsinogen gene. Nat Genet 1996;14:141–5.

[14] Ferec C, Raguenes O, Salomon R, et al. Mutations in the cationic trypsinogen gene and evidence for genetic heterogeneity in hereditary pancreatitis. J Med Genet 1999;36:228–32.

[15] Teich N, Ockenga J, Hoffmeister A, et al. Chronic pancreatitis associated with an activation peptide mutation that facilitates trypsin activation. Gastroenterology 2000;119:461–5.

[16] Pfutzer R, Myers E, Applebaum-Shapiro S, et al. Novel cationic trypsinogen (PRSS1) N29T and R122C mutations cause autosomal dominant hereditary pancreatitis. Gut 2002;50:271–2.

[17] Chen JM, Mercier B, Audrezet MP, et al. Mutational analysis of the human pancreatic secretory trypsin inhibitor (PSTI) gene in hereditary and sporadic chronic pancreatitis. J Med Genet 2000;37:67–9.

[18] Witt H, Luck W, Hennies HC, et al. Mutations in the gene encoding the serine protease inhibitor, Kazal type 1 are associated with chronic pancreatitis. Nat Genet 2000;25:213–6.

[19] Marchbank T, Freeman TC, Playford RJ. Human pancreatic secretory trypsin inhibitor: distribution, actions and possible role in mucosal integrity and repair. Digestion 1998;59:167–74.

[20] Pfutzer RH, Barmada MM, Brunskill AP, et al. SPINK1/PSTI polymorphisms act as disease modifiers in familial and idiopathic chronic pancreatitis. Gastroenterology 2000;119:615–23.

[21] Witt H, Luck W, Becker M, et al. Mutation in the SPINK1 trypsin inhibitor gene, alcohol use, and chronic pancreatitis. JAMA 2001;285:2716–7.

[22] Chen JM, Mercier B, Audrezet MP, et al. Mutations of the pancreatic secretory trypsin inhibitor (PSTI) gene in idiopathic chronic pancreatitis. Gastroenterology 2001;120:1061–4.

[23] Ockenga J, Dork T, Stuhrmann M. Low prevalence of SPINK1 gene mutations in adult patients with chronic idiopathic pancreatitis. J Med Genet 2001;38:243–4.

[24] Kaneko K, Nagasaki Y, Furukawa T, et al. Analysis of the human pancreatic secretory trypsin inhibitor (PSTI) gene mutations in Japanese patients with chronic pancreatitis. J Hum Genet 2001;46:293–7.

[25] Kuwata K, Hirota M, Sugita H, et al. Genetic mutations in exons 3 and 4 of the pancreatic secretory trypsin inhibitor in patients with pancreatitis. J Gastroenterol 2001;36:612–8.

[26] Plendl H, Siebert R, Steinemann D, et al. High frequency of the N34S mutation in the SPINK1 gene in chronic pancreatitis detected by a new PCR-RFLP assay. Am J Med Genet 2001;100:252–3.

[27] Noone PG, Zhou Z, Silverman LM, et al. Cystic fibrosis gene mutations and pancreatitis risk: relation to epithelial ion transport and trypsin inhibitor gene mutations. Gastroenterology 2001;121:1310–9.

[28] Threadgold J, Greenhalf W, Ellis I, et al. The N34S mutation of SPINK1 (PSTI) is associated with a familial pattern of idiopathic chronic pancreatitis but does not cause the disease. Gut 2002;50:675–81.

[29] Truninger K, Witt H, Kock J, et al. Mutations of the serine protease inhibitor, Kazal type 1 gene, in patients with idiopathic chronic pancreatitis. Am J Gastroenterol 2002;97:1133–7.

[30] Audrezet MP, Chen JM, Le Marechal C, et al. Determination of the relative contribution of three genes-the cystic fibrosis transmembrane conductance regulator gene, the cationic trypsinogen gene, and the pancreatic secretory trypsin inhibitor gene-to the etiology of idiopathic chronic pancreatitis. Eur J Hum Genet 2002;10:100–6.

[31] Drenth JP, te Morsche R, Jansen JB. Mutations in serine protease inhibitor Kazal type 1 are strongly associated with chronic pancreatitis. Gut 2002;50:687–92.

[32] Gomez-Lira M, Bonamini D, Castellani C, et al. Mutations in the SPINK1 gene in idiopathic pancreatitis Italian patients. Eur J Hum Genet 2003;11:543–6.

[33] Schneider A, Barmada MM, Slivka A, et al. Clinical characterization of patients with idiopathic chronic pancreatitis and SPINK1 Mutations. Scand J Gastroenterol 2004;39:903–4.

[34] Le Marechal C, Chen JM, Le Gall C, et al. Two novel severe mutations in the pancreatic secretory trypsin inhibitor gene (SPINK1) cause familial and/or hereditary pancreatitis. Hum Mutat 2004;23:205.

[35] Schneider A, Suman A, Rossi L, et al. SPINK1/PSTI mutations are associated with tropical pancreatitis and type II diabetes mellitus in Bangladesh. Gastroenterology 2002;123:1026–30.

[36] Bhatia E, Choudhuri G, Sikora SS, et al. Tropical calcific pancreatitis: strong association with SPINK1 trypsin inhibitor mutations. Gastroenterology 2002;123:1020–5.

[37] Hassan Z, Mohan V, Ali L, et al. SPINK1 is a susceptibility gene for fibrocalculous pancreatic diabetes in subjects from the Indian subcontinent. Am J Hum Genet 2002;71:964–8.

[38] Chandak GR, Idris MM, Reddy DN, et al. Mutations in the pancreatic secretory trypsin inhibitor gene (PSTI/SPINK1) rather than the cationic trypsinogen gene (PRSS1) are significantly associated with tropical calcific pancreatitis. J Med Genet 2002;39:347–51.

[39] Schneider A, Pfutzer RH, Barmada MM, et al. Limited contribution of the SPINK1 N34S mutation to the risk and severity of alcoholic chronic pancreatitis: a report from the United States. Dig Dis Sci 2003;48:1110–5.

[40] Perri F, Piepoli A, Stanziale P, et al. Mutation analysis of the cystic fibrosis transmembrane conductance regulator (CFTR) gene, the cationic trypsinogen (PRSS1) gene, and the serine protease inhibitor, Kazal type 1 (SPINK1) gene in patients with alcoholic chronic pancreatitis. Eur J Hum Genet 2003;11:687–92.

[41] Cohn JA, Friedman KJ, Noone PG, et al. Relation between mutations of the cystic fibrosis gene and idiopathic pancreatitis. N Engl J Med 1998;339:653–8.

[42] Sharer N, Schwarz M, Malone G, et al. Mutations of the cystic fibrosis gene in patients with chronic pancreatitis. N Engl J Med 1998;339:645–52.

[43] Cohn JA, Mitchell RM, Jowell PS. The impact of cystic fibrosis and PSTI/SPINK1 gene mutations on susceptibility to chronic pancreatitis. Clin Lab Med 2005;25:79–100.

[44] Felley C, Morris MA, Wonkam A, et al. The role of CFTR and SPINK-1 mutations in pancreatic disorders in HIV-positive patients: a case-control study. AIDS 2004;18:1521–7.

[45] Felderbauer P, Hoffmann P, Einwachter H, et al. A novel mutation of the calcium sensing receptor gene is associated with chronic pancreatitis in a family with heterozygous SPINK1 mutations. BMC Gastroenterol 2003;3:34.

[46] Rinderknecht H. Pancreatic secretory enzymes. In: Go VLW, DiMagno JD, Gardner JD, et al, editors. The pancreas: biology, pathophysiology, and disease. New York: Raven Press; 1993. p. 219–51.

[47] Figarella C, Negri GA, Guy O. The two human trypsinogens. Inhibition spectra of the two human trypsins derived from their purified zymogens. Eur J Biochem 1975;53:457–63.

[48] Hirota M, Kuwata K, Ohmuraya M, et al. From acute to chronic pancreatitis: the role of mutations in the pancreatic secretory trypsin inhibitor gene. JOP 2003;4:83–8.

[49] Szmola R, Kukor Z, Sahin-Toth M. Human mesotrypsin is a unique digestive protease specialized for the degradation of trypsin inhibitors. J Biol Chem 2003;278:48580–9.

[50] Ohmuraya M, Hirota M, Araki M, et al. Autophagic cell death of pancreatic acinar cells in serine protease inhibitor Kazal type 3-deficient mice. Gastroenterology 2005;129:696–705.

[51] Nathan JD, Romac J, Peng RY, et al. Transgenic expression of pancreatic secretory trypsin inhibitor-I ameliorates secretagogue-induced pancreatitis in mice. Gastroenterology 2005; 128:717–27.

ELSEVIER
SAUNDERS

Endocrinol Metab Clin N Am
35 (2006) 357–369

ENDOCRINOLOGY
AND METABOLISM
CLINICS
OF NORTH AMERICA

Genes of Type 2 Diabetes in β Cells

Mirko Trajkovski[a], Hassan Mziaut[a], Peter E. Schwarz[b],
Michele Solimena[a,b,*]

[a]Experimental Diabetology, Carl Gustav Carus Medical School,
Dresden University of Technology, Fetscherstrasse 74, 01307 Dresden, Germany
[b]III° Medical Clinic, Carl Gustav Carus Medical School, Dresden University of Technology,
Fetscherstrasse 74, 01307 Dresden, Germany

Diabetes mellitus is a complex metabolic disorder of epidemic proportions. It currently affects 170 million people worldwide, and its prevalence is rising dramatically. Diabetes develops when the insulin production and secretion are not sufficient to satisfy the metabolic demands of the organism. The insulin hormone lowers the blood glucose levels, and any insufficiency in the insulin secretion or action leads to hyperglycemia and diabetes. According to the American Diabetes Association, diabetes can be classified as type 1 diabetes, type 2 diabetes, gestational diabetes, and other specific types of diabetes that cannot be included in any of the previous forms, such as maturity-onset diabetes of the young (MODY) [1]. In addition, an intermediate group of prediabetic subjects is recognized whose glucose levels, although not meeting the criteria for diabetes, are still too high to be considered normal. This group is classified as impaired glucose tolerance and impaired fasting glucose (Table 1).

Type 2 diabetes is the most common form of diabetes, accounting for approximately 90% of all patients. Its frequent association with other metabolic disorders has given rise to the so-called "metabolic syndrome" [2] the concept of which has developed in the last 80 years [3,4] but recently has been questioned [5,6]. Although the definitions of metabolic syndrome by the World Health Organization WHO [7] and the National Cholesterol Education Program's Adult Treatment Panel III [8] are different, there is wide agreement that its essential components include glucose intolerance, obesity, hypertension, and dyslipidemia. Many factors contribute to the development of type 2 diabetes. Often environmental and behavioral factors and obesity contribute to its pathogenesis [9]. Genetic factors, however, also have been shown to play a key role in the development of diabetes.

* Corresponding author.
E-mail address: michele.solimena@mailbox.tu-dresden.de (M. Solimena).

Table 1
Criteria for diagnosis of diabetes

Normoglycemia	Pre-diabetic	Diabetes mellitus
FPG < 100 mg/dL	[a]FPG ≥ 100 mg/dL and <126 mg/dL	FPG ≥ 126 mg/dL
2 h PG < 140 mg/dL	[b]2 h PG ≥ 140 mg/dL and <200 mg/dL	2 h PG ≥ 200 mg/dL

Abbreviations: FPG, fasting plasma glucose; PG, post 75 g glucose load.
[a] Impaired fasting glucose.
[b] Impaired glucose tolerance.

Sixty percent of the offspring of diabetic patients is estimated to have abnormal glucose tolerance by the age of 60 years [10]. In MODYs the mutation of a single gene that is inherited as an autosomal-dominant trait causes diabetes. In recent years most MODY genes have been identified. The genetic background of type 2 diabetes, which is the most common form of the disease, is only partially known. From a genetic point of view, type 2 diabetes is a complex polygenic disorder associated with polymorphisms of multiple genes, the frequency of which varies among different ethnic groups [11]. Many of these genes are involved in glucose sensing or insulin secretion and action, whereas others are associated with increased susceptibility to metabolic conditions, such as obesity and lipid disorders, which in turn promote diabetes development. This review provides first a brief overview of the genes that confer susceptibility to type 2 diabetes primarily by affecting β cells, with emphasis on their function. For those genes that do not appear to impair β-cell function directly, such as peroxisome proliferating receptor-gamma, beta-3-adrenergic receptor, or adiponectin , the reader is referred to specific reviews on the topic [12,13]. The second part of this review summarizes recent advances in our understanding of insulin gene expression, which could be related to the association between polymorphisms in the calpain 10 gene (CAPN10) and the increased susceptibility to type 2 diabetes [14].

Type 2 diabetes susceptibility genes of β cells

Glucose transporter 2

This transporter is mostly responsible for the entry of glucose in β cells. It is constitutively expressed at their surface and in liver and intestinal cells. Because its capacity to transport glucose is high, its opening enables the equilibrium between extracellular and intracellular glucose to be reached rapidly. Glucose transporter 2 (GLUT2) is encoded by the SLC2A2 gene that is located on human chromosome 3 and contains 11 exons. Its product is a peptide with 12 membrane-spanning domains containing several sites for glucose binding. A single nucleotide polymorphism (SNP) that replaces threonine 110 with isoleucine within the second membrane-spanning domain is increased modestly in type 2 diabetic patients. Mutation of valine 197 to isoleucine in the fifth membrane-spanning domain impairs glucose transport and has been found in a diabetic patient [15–17].

Glucokinase

Once it is inside the cytosol of β cells, glucose is phosphorylated to glucose-6-phosphate by an atypical member of the hexokinase family called glucokinase (GCK, or hexokinase IV). The gene GCK is located on human chromosome 7, contains 12 exons, and acts as the glucose sensor of β cells. Activation of GCK only occurs when glucose concentrations are greater than 5 mmol/L [18]. Contrary to the other members of the hexokinase family, GCK is not inhibited by its product, thus enabling GCK to remain active while glucose is abundant. This enzyme regulates the metabolic flux of glucose into β cells, therefore, and is the rate-limiting step for glycolysis. This key metabolic pathway produces ATP from the anaerobic and aerobic oxidation of glucose metabolites, and eventually induces the secretion of insulin. The importance of GCK in glucose homeostasis and diabetes is highlighted by the identification of many GCK mutations that alter the threshold for glucose-stimulated insulin release. On one hand, activating mutations can lower the threshold for insulin release to 1.5 mmol/L, thereby causing persistent hyperinsulinemic hypoglycemia of infancy (PHHI) [19]. Inactivating mutations on both GCK alleles, on the other hand, increase the levels of glucose required to stimulate insulin secretion, hence leading to permanent neonatal diabetes (diabetes at birth) [20]. Inheriting inactivating mutations on a single GCK allele is responsible instead for mild hyperglycemia and MODY2 [21].

Insulin

Insulin was the first hormone to be identified [22]. Most animals have a single copy of the insulin gene, which in humans is located on the short arm of chromosome 11. Rodents have two nonallelic insulin genes (I and II) that encode identical polypeptide chains, but differ in the number of introns and chromosomal location [23]. The initial translation product of the insulin mRNA is preproinsulin, which is converted into proinsulin following the cotranslational removal of its signal peptide. After its exit from the Golgi complex and sorting into secretory granules (SGs), proinsulin is cleaved by two Ca^{2+}-dependent converting proteases termed protein convertase 1/3 PC1/3 [24–27] and 2 PC2 [28]. These cleavages separate proinsulin into three polypeptides named chain A (21 amino acids), chain B (30 amino acids), and the intervening C-peptide, respectively. Chains A and B remain associated by two disulfide bridges and together form insulin. Several SNPs and mutations have been identified within the insulin gene that are associated with an increased risk for type 2 diabetes. The phenylalanine at position 24 is highly conserved and its aromatic ring is believed to be important for anchoring insulin to the insulin receptor (IR, see later discussion). Mutations affecting this residue are associated with diabetes [29]. Another point mutation that converts arginine 65 into histidine prevents proinsulin cleavage, thereby causing increased proinsulin secretion and diabetes [30,31].

ATP-sensitive K$^+$ channels

ATP production from glycolysis increases the ATP/ADP ratio within β cells, hence favoring the binding of ATP to ATP-sensitive K$^+$ channels (K$_{ATP}$ channels) [32] and their closure. This phenomenon causes the depolarization of β-cell membranes [33], the opening of voltage-gated Ca^{2+} channels, and the entry of Ca^{2+}. Ca^{2+} in turn acts as a second messenger that triggers the exocytosis of insulin SGs. Insulin is secreted in two temporally distinct phases in response to glucose stimulation. The first phase of insulin secretion has its peak approximately 2 to 4 minutes after glycemia has reached the threshold value of approximately 5.5 mmol/L and generally lasts up to 10 minutes. The second phase begins approximately 20 minutes after glucose stimulation, reaches its plateau within 15 minutes, and usually does not last longer than 60 minutes. Among several pathways inducing glucose-stimulated insulin secretion, the K$_{ATP}$ channel-dependent or triggering pathway is the one responsible for the first phase of insulin secretion, which results from the exocytosis of insulin SGs that are already docked to the plasma membrane.

Most K$_{ATP}$ channels consist of two subunits, Kir6.2 and SUR1. Kir6.2 and SUR1 genes are adjacent to each other in the short arm of human chromosome 11. K$_{ATP}$ channels are believed to be a complex including four SUR1 and four Kir6.2 proteins. SUR1 is a member of the ATP-binding cassette transporter family of proteins that use the energy of ATP to transport molecules across membranes, and typically contain two ATP-binding domains, also know as nucleotide binding folds (NBF 1 and 2), and two transmembrane domains. Mutations in Kir6.2 or SUR1 can alter the nucleotide sensitivity and closure probability of K$_{ATP}$ channels. There are mutations reported for NBF1 and NBF2 in SUR1 that favor the closure of the K$_{ATP}$ channel and are associated with increased insulin release and PHHI [34–36]. Especially frequent in Kir6.2 is the replacement of glutamic acid 23 to lysine (E23K), which decreases insulin release [37–39]. A SUR1 variant, which is often linked to Kir6.2 E23K, has an alanine instead of a serine at position 1369 (S1369A) and also is associated with defects in insulin release and diabetes.

Insulin receptor

The gene encoding the IR is located on human chromosome 19. It contains 23 exons and it is expressed primarily in insulin target cells, including hepatocytes, muscle cells, adipocytes, and β cells. The receptor is a heterotetrameric tyrosine kinase consisting of two insulin-binding extracellular α subunits and two predominantly intracellular β subunits [40], linked by disulfide bridges. Insulin binding elicits the kinase activity of the IR, which autophosphorylates first its β subunits and then insulin receptor substrates 1 (IRS1) and 2 (IRS2), which bind the phosphorylated receptor. Phosphorylated IRS1 and IRS2, in turn, act as adaptor proteins for the recruitment of factors associated with two distinct signaling pathways. One pathway is Ras-dependent and leads to the activation of MAP kinases, which are primarily responsible for the mitogenic effect of insulin. The other pathway is Ras-independent and prompts the activation of the serine/threonine kinase AKT/PKB following the generation of phosphatidylinositol 3-phosphates by phosphatidylinositol 3-kinase (PI3K). Among other functions, AKT/PKB triggers the translocation of the glucose transporter GLUT4 to the plasma membrane, thereby allowing glucose uptake by hepatocytes, muscle cells, and adipocytes. In β cells the IR signaling is relevant mostly to sustain β-cell mass and insulin secretion [41,42].

Mutations of the insulin receptor are responsible for leprechaunism, severe insulin resistance [43] with diabetes, acanthosis nigricans [44], and polycystic ovary syndrome [45]. Knockout of mouse IR in β cells was sufficient to reduce the first phase of insulin secretion and led to glucose intolerance [41]. Polymorphisms in the IR gene do not appear to be a common trait among most patients who have type 2 diabetes.

Insulin receptor substrate 1

The gene encoding IRS1 is located on human chromosome 2. There are several missense variants of the IRS1 gene characterized by amino acid replacement, namely G81R, P512A, S892G, and G972R, which have been suggested to be more common among type 2 diabetes patients than in control subjects [46,47]. Glycine 972 in particular is located in close proximity to the two tyrosine phosphorylation sites that are involved in the binding of PI3K. Its replacement into arginine therefore could impair insulin by affecting the PI3K/AKT pathway [47].

Phosphoinositide 3-kinase

PI3K has a catalytic and regulatory subunit. The gene encoding the regulatory PI3K subunit is located on human chromosome 5. This subunit contains two SH2 domains that bind tyrosine phosphorylated residues in motifs that are present in IR (two) and in IRS1 (four). The full activation of the PI3K requires both SH2 domains to bind the tyrosine-phosphorylated motifs present in the IRS1. The PI3K missense variant M326I and the intronic variant SNP42 are associated with increased diabetes risk and have been proposed to affect glucose homeostasis [48–50].

Hepatocyte nuclear factor 1-α

Hepatocyte nuclear factor 1-α (HNF1α) is a transcription factor that plays a key role in the development and function of the pancreatic β cells by regulating the expression of many genes, including insulin and HNF4α [51]. In addition to β cells, it is highly expressed in liver and kidney. The HNF1α gene is located on human chromosome 12. The HNF1α protein is active as a homodimer, which is stabilized by the dimerization cofactor of HNF-1 alpha (DCOH) [52]. A subset of mutations that destabilize the formation of HNF1α dimers accounts for the deficient insulin production and secretion in MODY3 [53,54]. Because of its role in β-cell development, there is growing evidence that HNF1α missense variations also may play a role in the development of type 2 diabetes. Common HNF1α missense variants A98V, S319G, and P447L are associated with lower insulin secretion [55], whereas the I27L variant is linked to reduced insulin sensitivity. Recent meta-analysis studies, however, have suggested that common HNF1α variants, with the exception of the rare V98 allele, only play a minor role in type 2 diabetes unless associated with other genetic or environmental predisposing factors [56,57].

Hepatocyte nuclear factor 4-α

The gene encoding hepatocyte nuclear factor 4-α (HNF4α) is located on human chromosome 20. It regulates gene expression in liver, pancreatic β cells, kidney, and intestine during embryonic development and in adult life. Specifically, it controls the expression of insulin, GLUT2, mitochondrial uncoupling protein-2, and other genes linked to insulin secretion [58]. Mutations of this gene cause insulinopenia, thereby indicating that reduced levels of HNF4α lead to β-cell dysfunction [59–61].

In particular, coding genetic variants of HNF4α have been identified in MODY1 patients. Other genetic variants associated with MODY1 and type 2 diabetes are found in the HNF4α alternative promoter region called P2, where HNF1α binds [51,62–64].

NEUROD1

NEUROD1 is a basic helix-loop-helix (bHLH) transcription factor that is important for cell fate determination during neurogenesis [65]. The NEUROD1 gene is mapped on human chromosome 2 and is highly expressed in brain and in the precursor of several islet cells, including β cells. Specifically, it regulates insulin gene expression by binding to a critical E-box motif in the insulin promoter [66]. Accordingly, NEUROD1 knockout mice display an abnormal pancreatic islet morphogenesis and diabetes [66]. Insertion of a cytosine at position 206 in NEUROD1 generates a truncated polypeptide lacking the C-terminal transactivation domain and is responsible for impaired insulin secretion and MODY6. Replacement of arginine 111 with leucine (R111L) within the bHLH domain, which is responsible for DNA binding, instead is associated with type 2 diabetes.

Calpain 10

Unlike the above-mentioned type 2 diabetes susceptibility genes, CAPN10 was not identified using a candidate gene approach, but through a unique positional cloning strategy following a genome-wide scanning in diabetic sibling pairs [14,67]. In particular, linkage studies in the Mexican American population localized a major susceptibility locus for type

2 diabetes on a region of chromosome 2q, which contains the CAPN10 gene. Subsequent analyses revealed that an intronic G/A polymorphism in CAPN10 termed SNP-43 was linked to type 2 diabetes. The association of SNP-43 with the disease was weak [14], however, except in Pima Indians [68] and African Americans [69]. Inclusion of two additional intronic SNPs, defined as SNP-19 and SNP-63, allowed the further identification of two major CAPN10 haplotypes, termed 112 and 121, the combination of which is associated with type 2 diabetes among multiple ethnic groups [14,70–77]. The 112/121 haplotype has a variable population frequency and correlates with reduced levels of CAPN10 mRNA in muscle cells and insulin resistance [14,68,71].

Calpains are cytosolic cysteine proteases that catalyze the endoproteolytic cleavage of a wide array of substrates, including cytoskeletal proteins, kinases, phosphatases, and transcription factors [78,79]. The human genome includes 14 calpain genes. Most information about calpains has been gathered through studies on calpain-1 and calpain-2, which are expressed ubiquitously and are activated in vitro by low and high levels of Ca^{2+}, respectively. Calpains preferentially recognize bonds between protein domains, thereby leading to the generation of large peptide fragments that retain functionally intact domains. Calpains are regarded as biomodulators, therefore, because the properties of substrate proteins often are modified after calpain hydrolysis [79–82]. In addition to type 2 diabetes, deficits in calpain activity have been associated with the development of autosomal recessive limb-girdle muscular dystrophy type 2A (LGMD2A), cataracts, and age-related hypertension [83].

How is CAPN10 contributing to the development of type 2 diabetes? Until today there is no clear answer to this question, especially because the specific function of CAPN10 remains to be elucidated. Inhibition of CAPN10 activity originally was associated with an approximately 60% decrease in insulin-stimulated glucose uptake into cultured mouse adipocytes because of impaired translocation of glucose transporter 4 (GLUT4)–containing vesicles to the plasma membrane [84]. Recent studies, however, have shown that deficits of GLUT4 vesicle translocation resulted from the inhibition of proteasome cysteine proteases, rather than calpains [85]. In β cells CAPN10 activation is required for promoting apoptosis in response to ryanodine, fatty acids, and low glucose [86]. Increasing evidence indicates that calpains also can regulate β-cell secretion. Exposure of mouse islets to calpain inhibitors leads to increased glucose-dependent insulin release [87], possibly by acting on proteins involved in the exocytosis of the insulin-containing secretory granules. Conversely, calpain inhibition decreased insulin secretion from rat insulinoma cells [88]. This diminution may result from the reduced proteolysis of SNAP-25 [89], a protein implicated in the fusion of secretory granules with the plasma membrane. These inhibitors, however, can affect other calpains in addition to CAPN10. Recent studies in particular have pointed to the role of calpain-1 (Fig. 1) in the upregulation of insulin

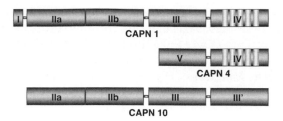

Fig. 1. CAPN1, CAPN4, and CAPN10 domain structure.

production through the cleavage of the receptor tyrosine phosphatase-like protein ICA512/IA-2 [90]. ICA512 is enriched in the membrane of insulin secretory granules [91] and is involved in the regulation of insulin secretion [92]. On secretory granule exocytosis, ICA512 is transiently inserted into the plasma membrane where its cytoplasmic domain is proteolyzed by calpain-1. The ICA512 cytosolic fragment resulting from this cleavage is then targeted to the nucleus, where it upregulates the expression of insulin [90] and other secretory granule components (our unpublished observations) (Fig. 2). Through this novel pathway β-cells could adjust directly the production of secretory granules to their consumption. It would be interesting to determine whether ICA512 also is cleaved by CAPN10, and if so, whether this process is linked to the increased susceptibility to type 2 diabetes in carriers of the 112/121 haplotype.

Summary

Diabetes and its complications represent one of the major threats to public health worldwide. Increasing evidence in human and animal models

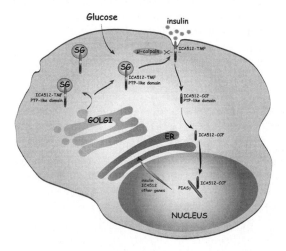

Fig. 2. The ICA512 signaling pathway.

indicates that deficient β-cell function is an essential factor for the development of the disease. Genetic studies have led to the identification of numerous susceptibility genes for type 2 diabetes, most of which regulate β-cell glucose metabolism, gene expression, or insulin secretion. The need to elucidate further the physiology of β cells in normal and pathologic conditions and alleviate the burden of diabetes could not be more compelling.

References

[1] American Diabetes Association. Diagnosis and classification of diabetes mellitus. Diabetes Care 2004;27(Suppl 1):S5–10.
[2] Eckel RH, Grundy SM, Zimmet PZ. The metabolic syndrome. Lancet 2005;365:1415–28.
[3] Grundy SM, Cleeman JI, Daniels SR, et al. Diagnosis and management of the metabolic syndrome: an American Heart Association/National Heart, Lung, and Blood Institute scientific statement. Circulation 2005;112:2735–52.
[4] Grundy SM, Cleeman JI, Daniels SR, et al. Diagnosis and management of the metabolic syndrome: an American Heart Association/National Heart, Lung, and Blood Institute scientific statement: executive summary. Circulation 2005;112:e285–90.
[5] Kahn R, Buse J, Ferrannini E, et al. The metabolic syndrome: time for a critical appraisal: joint statement from the American Diabetes Association and the European Association for the Study of Diabetes. Diabetes Care 2005;28:2289–304.
[6] Kahn R, Buse J, Ferrannini E, et al. The metabolic syndrome: time for a critical appraisal. Joint statement from the American Diabetes Association and the European Association for the Study of Diabetes. Diabetologia 2005;48:1684–99.
[7] Alberti KG, Zimmet PZ. Definition diagnosis and classification of diabetes mellitus and its complications. Part 1: diagnosis and classification of diabetes mellitus provisional report of a WHO consultation. Diabet Med 1998;15:539–53.
[8] Executive summary of the third report of the National Cholesterol Education Program (NCEP) expert panel on detection, evaluation, and treatment of high blood cholesterol in adults (Adult Treatment Panel III). JAMA 2001;285:2486–97.
[9] Zimmet P, Alberti KG, Shaw J. Global and societal implications of the diabetes epidemic. Nature 2001;414:782–7.
[10] Tattersal RB, Fajans SS. Prevalence of diabetes and glucose intolerance in 199 offspring of thirty-seven conjugal diabetic parents. Diabetes 1975;24:452–62.
[11] Permutt MA, Wasson J, Cox N. Genetic epidemiology of diabetes. J Clin Invest 2005;115:1431–9.
[12] Parikh H, Groop L. Candidate genes for type 2 diabetes. Rev Endocr Metab Disord 2004;5:151–76.
[13] Barroso I. Genetics of type 2 diabetes. Diabet Med 2005;22:517–35.
[14] Horikawa Y, Oda N, Cox NJ, et al. Genetic variation in the gene encoding calpain-10 is associated with type 2 diabetes mellitus. Nat Genet 2000;26:163–75.
[15] Katagiri H, Asano T, Shibasaki Y, et al. Substitution of leucine for tryptophan 412 does not abolish cytochalasin B labeling but markedly decreases the intrinsic activity of GLUT1 glucose transporter. J Biol Chem 1991;266:7769–73.
[16] Ishihara H, Asano T, Katagiri H, et al. The glucose transport activity of GLUT1 is markedly decreased by substitution of a single amino acid with a different charge at residue 415. Biochem Biophys Res Commun 1991;176:922–30.
[17] Garcia JC, Strube M, Leingang K, et al. Amino acid substitutions at tryptophan 388 and tryptophan 412 of the HepG2 (Glut1) glucose transporter inhibit transport activity and targeting to the plasma membrane in Xenopus oocytes. J Biol Chem 1992;267:7770–6.
[18] Matschinsky FM. Regulation of pancreatic beta-cell glucokinase: from basics to therapeutics. Diabetes 2002;51(Suppl 3):S394–404.

[19] Gloyn AL. Glucokinase (GCK) mutations in hyper- and hypoglycemia: maturity-onset diabetes of the young, permanent neonatal diabetes, and hyperinsulinemia of infancy. Hum Mutat 2003;22:353–62.

[20] Njolstad PR, Sagen JV, Bjorkhaug L, et al. Permanent neonatal diabetes caused by glucokinase deficiency: inborn error of the glucose-insulin signaling pathway. Diabetes 2003;52: 2854–60.

[21] Katagiri H, Asano T, Ishihara H, et al. Nonsense mutation of glucokinase gene in late-onset non-insulin-dependent diabetes mellitus. Lancet 1992;340:1316–7.

[22] Banting FG, Best CH. Pancreatic extracts. 1922. J Lab Clin Med 1990;115:254–72.

[23] Soares MB, Schon E, Henderson A, et al. RNA-mediated gene duplication: the rat preproinsulin I gene is a functional retroposon. Mol Cell Biol 1985;5:2090–103.

[24] Seidah NG, Gaspar L, Mion P, et al. cDNA sequence of two distinct pituitary proteins homologous to Kex2 and furin gene products: tissue-specific mRNAs encoding candidates for pro-hormone processing proteinases. DNA Cell Biol 1990;9:415–24.

[25] Smeekens SP, Avruch AS, LaMendola J, et al. Identification of a cDNA encoding a second putative prohormone convertase related to PC2 in AtT20 cells and islets of Langerhans. Proc Natl Acad Sci U S A 1991;88:340–4.

[26] Smeekens SP, Chan SJ, Steiner DF. The biosynthesis and processing of neuroendocrine peptides: identification of proprotein convertases involved in intravesicular processing. Prog Brain Res 1992;92:235–46.

[27] Smeekens SP, Montag AG, Thomas G, et al. Proinsulin processing by the subtilisin-related proprotein convertases furin, PC2, and PC3. Proc Natl Acad Sci U S A 1992;89:8822–6.

[28] Rhodes CJ, Lincoln B, Shoelson SE. Preferential cleavage of des-31,32-proinsulin over intact proinsulin by the insulin secretory granule type II endopeptidase: implication of a favored route for prohormone processing. J Biol Chem 1992;267:22719–27.

[29] Hua QX, Shoelson SE, Inouye K, et al. Paradoxical structure and function in a mutant human insulin associated with diabetes mellitus. Proc Natl Acad Sci U S A 1993;90:582–6.

[30] Shibasaki Y, Kawakami T, Kanazawa Y, et al. Posttranslational cleavage of proinsulin is blocked by a point mutation in familial hyperproinsulinemia. J Clin Invest 1985;76:378–80.

[31] Barbetti F, Raben N, Kadowaki T, et al. Two unrelated patients with familial hyperproinsulinemia due to a mutation substituting histidine for arginine at position 65 in the proinsulin molecule: identification of the mutation by direct sequencing of genomic deoxyribonucleic acid amplified by polymerase chain reaction. J Clin Endocrinol Metab 1990;71:164–9.

[32] Cook DL, Hales CN. Intracellular ATP directly blocks K + channels in pancreatic B-cells. Nature 1984;311:271–3.

[33] Ashcroft FM, Harrison DE, Ashcroft SJ. Glucose induces closure of single potassium channels in isolated rat pancreatic beta-cells. Nature 1984;312:446–8.

[34] Goksel DL, Fischbach K, Duggirala R, et al. Variant in sulfonylurea receptor-1 gene is associated with high insulin concentrations in non-diabetic Mexican Americans: SUR-1 gene variant and hyperinsulinemia. Hum Genet 1998;103:280–5.

[35] Thomas PM, Cote GJ, Wohllk N, et al. Mutations in the sulfonylurea receptor gene in familial persistent hyperinsulinemic hypoglycemia of infancy. Science 1995;268:426–9.

[36] Huopio H, Otonkoski T, Vauhkonen I, et al. A new subtype of autosomal dominant diabetes attributable to a mutation in the gene for sulfonylurea receptor 1. Lancet 2003;361: 301–7.

[37] Schwanstecher C, Meyer U, Schwanstecher M. K(IR)6.2 polymorphism predisposes to type 2 diabetes by inducing overactivity of pancreatic beta-cell ATP-sensitive K(+) channels. Diabetes 2002;51:875–9.

[38] Schwanstecher C, Neugebauer B, Schulz M, et al. The common single nucleotide polymorphism E23K in K(IR)6.2 sensitizes pancreatic beta-cell ATP-sensitive potassium channels toward activation through nucleoside diphosphates. Diabetes 2002;51(Suppl 3):S363–7.

[39] Schwanstecher C, Schwanstecher M. Nucleotide sensitivity of pancreatic ATP-sensitive potassium channels and type 2 diabetes. Diabetes 2002;51(Suppl 3):S358–62.

[40] White MF, Kahn CR. The insulin signaling system. J Biol Chem 1994;269:1–4.

[41] Kulkarni RN, Bruning JC, Winnay JN, et al. Tissue-specific knockout of the insulin receptor in pancreatic beta cells creates an insulin secretory defect similar to that in type 2 diabetes. Cell 1999;96:329–39.

[42] Otani K, Kulkarni RN, Baldwin AC, et al. Reduced beta-cell mass and altered glucose sensing impair insulin-secretory function in betaIRKO mice. Am J Physiol Endocrinol Metab 2004;286:E41–9.

[43] Taylor SI, Marcus-Samuels B, Ryan-Young J, et al. Genetics of the insulin receptor defect in a patient with extreme insulin resistance. J Clin Endocrinol Metab 1986;62:1130–5.

[44] Rudiger HW, Dreyer M, Kuhnau J, et al. Familial insulin-resistant diabetes secondary to an affinity defect of the insulin receptor. Hum Genet 1983;64:407–11.

[45] Leme CE, Wajchenberg BL, Lerario AC, et al. Acanthosis nigricans, hirsutism, insulin resistance and insulin receptor defect. Clin Endocrinol (Oxf) 1982;17:43–9.

[46] Almind K, Bjorbaek C, Vestergaard H, et al. Aminoacid polymorphisms of insulin receptor substrate-1 in non-insulin-dependent diabetes mellitus. Lancet 1993;342:828–32.

[47] Almind K, Inoue G, Pedersen O, et al. A common amino acid polymorphism in insulin receptor substrate-1 causes impaired insulin signaling: evidence from transfection studies. J Clin Invest 1996;97:2569–75.

[48] Hansen L, Zethelius B, Berglund L, et al. In vitro and in vivo studies of a naturally occurring variant of the human p85alpha regulatory subunit of the phosphoinositide 3-kinase: inhibition of protein kinase B and relationships with type 2 diabetes, insulin secretion, glucose disappearance constant, and insulin sensitivity. Diabetes 2001;50:690–3.

[49] Hansen T, Andersen CB, Echwald SM, et al. Identification of a common amino acid polymorphism in the p85alpha regulatory subunit of phosphatidylinositol 3-kinase: effects on glucose disappearance constant, glucose effectiveness, and the insulin sensitivity index. Diabetes 1997;46:494–501.

[50] Kawanishi M, Tamori Y, Masugi J, et al. Prevalence of a polymorphism of the phosphatidylinositol 3-kinase p85 alpha regulatory subunit (codon 326 Met → Ile) in Japanese NIDDM patients. Diabetes Care 1997;20:1043.

[51] Odom DT, Zizlsperger N, Gordon DB, et al. Control of pancreas and liver gene expression by HNF transcription factors. Science 2004;303:1378–81.

[52] Mendel DB, Hansen LP, Graves MK, et al. HNF-1 alpha and HNF-1 beta (vHNF-1) share dimerization and homeo domains, but not activation domains, and form heterodimers in vitro. Genes Dev 1991;5:1042–56.

[53] Hua QX, Zhao M, Narayana N, et al. Diabetes-associated mutations in a beta-cell transcription factor destabilize an antiparallel "mini-zipper" in a dimerization interface. Proc Natl Acad Sci U S A 2000;97:1999–2004.

[54] Byrne MM, Sturis J, Menzel S, et al. Altered insulin secretory responses to glucose in diabetic and nondiabetic subjects with mutations in the diabetes susceptibility gene MODY3 on chromosome 12. Diabetes 1996;45:1503–10.

[55] Chiu KC, Chuang LM, Ryu JM, et al. The I27L amino acid polymorphism of hepatic nuclear factor-1alpha is associated with insulin resistance. J Clin Endocrinol Metab 2000;85:2178–83.

[56] Winckler W, Burtt NP, Holmkvist J, et al. Association of common variation in the HNF1alpha gene region with risk of type 2 diabetes. Diabetes 2005;54:2336–42.

[57] Weedon MN, Owen KR, Shields B, et al. A large-scale association analysis of common variation of the HNF1alpha gene with type 2 diabetes in the UK Caucasian population. Diabetes 2005;54:2487–91.

[58] Wang H, Maechler P, Antinozzi PA, et al. Hepatocyte nuclear factor 4alpha regulates the expression of pancreatic beta -cell genes implicated in glucose metabolism and nutrient-induced insulin secretion. J Biol Chem 2000;275:35953–9.

[59] Stoffel M, Duncan SA. The maturity-onset diabetes of the young (MODY1) transcription factor HNF4alpha regulates expression of genes required for glucose transport and metabolism. Proc Natl Acad Sci U S A 1997;94:13209–14.

[60] Shih DQ, Dansky HM, Fleisher M, et al. Genotype/phenotype relationships in HNF-4alpha/MODY1: haploinsufficiency is associated with reduced apolipoprotein (AII), apolipoprotein (CIII), lipoprotein(a), and triglyceride levels. Diabetes 2000;49:832–7.

[61] Barroso I, Luan J, Middelberg RP, et al. Candidate gene association study in type 2 diabetes indicates a role for genes involved in beta-cell function as well as insulin action. PLoS Biol 2003;1:E20.

[62] Thomas H, Jaschkowitz K, Bulman M, et al. A distant upstream promoter of the HNF-4alpha gene connects the transcription factors involved in maturity-onset diabetes of the young. Hum Mol Genet 2001;10:2089–97.

[63] Love-Gregory LD, Wasson J, Ma J, et al. A common polymorphism in the upstream promoter region of the hepatocyte nuclear factor-4 alpha gene on chromosome 20q is associated with type 2 diabetes and appears to contribute to the evidence for linkage in an ashkenazi jewish population. Diabetes 2004;53:1134–40.

[64] Silander K, Mohlke KL, Scott LJ, et al. Genetic variation near the hepatocyte nuclear factor-4 alpha gene predicts susceptibility to type 2 diabetes. Diabetes 2004;53:1141–9.

[65] Lee JE, Hollenberg SM, Snider L, et al. Conversion of Xenopus ectoderm into neurons by NeuroD, a basic helix-loop-helix protein. Science 1995;268:836–44.

[66] Naya FJ, Huang HP, Qiu Y, et al. Diabetes, defective pancreatic morphogenesis, and abnormal enteroendocrine differentiation in BETA2/neuroD-deficient mice. Genes Dev 1997;11:2323–34.

[67] Hanis CL, Boerwinkle E, Chakraborty R, et al. A genome-wide search for human non-insulin-dependent (type 2) diabetes genes reveals a major susceptibility locus on chromosome 2. Nat Genet 1996;13:161–6.

[68] Baier LJ, Permana PA, Yang X, et al. A calpain-10 gene polymorphism is associated with reduced muscle mRNA levels and insulin resistance. J Clin Invest 2000;106:R69–73.

[69] Garant MJ, Kao WH, Brancati F, et al. SNP43 of CAPN10 and the risk of type 2 diabetes in African-Americans: the Atherosclerosis Risk in Communities Study. Diabetes 2002;51:231–7.

[70] Orho-Melander M, Klannemark M, Svensson MK, et al. Variants in the calpain-10 gene predispose to insulin resistance and elevated free fatty acid levels. Diabetes 2002;51:2658–64.

[71] Evans JC, Frayling TM, Cassell PG, et al. Studies of association between the gene for calpain-10 and type 2 diabetes mellitus in the United Kingdom. Am J Hum Genet 2001;69:544–52.

[72] Rasmussen SK, Urhammer SA, Berglund L, et al. Variants within the calpain-10 gene on chromosome 2q37 (NIDDM1) and relationships to type 2 diabetes, insulin resistance, and impaired acute insulin secretion among Scandinavian Caucasians. Diabetes 2002;51:3561–7.

[73] Cassell PG, Jackson AE, North BV, et al. Haplotype combinations of calpain 10 gene polymorphisms associate with increased risk of impaired glucose tolerance and type 2 diabetes in South Indians. Diabetes 2002;51:1622–8.

[74] Fingerlin TE, Erdos MR, Watanabe RM, et al. Variation in three single nucleotide polymorphisms in the calpain-10 gene not associated with type 2 diabetes in a large Finnish cohort. Diabetes 2002;51:1644–8.

[75] Sun HX, Zhang KX, Du WN, et al. Single nucleotide polymorphisms in CAPN10 gene of Chinese people and its correlation with type 2 diabetes mellitus in Han people of northern China. Biomed Environ Sci 2002;15:75–82.

[76] Tsai HJ, Sun G, Weeks DE, et al. Type 2 diabetes and three calpain-10 gene polymorphisms in Samoans: no evidence of association. Am J Hum Genet 2001;69:1236–44.

[77] Hegele RA, Harris SB, Zinman B, et al. Absence of association of type 2 diabetes with CAPN10 and PC-1 polymorphisms in Oji-Cree. Diabetes Care 2001;24:1498–9.

[78] Sorimachi H, Ishiura S, Suzuki K. Structure and physiological function of calpains. Biochem J 1997;328(Pt 3):721–32.

[79] Saido TC, Sorimachi H, Suzuki K. Calpain: new perspectives in molecular diversity and physiological-pathological involvement. FASEB J 1994;8:814–22.

[80] Carafoli E, Molinari M. Calpain: a protease in search of a function? Biochem Biophys Res Commun 1998;247:193–203.

[81] Sorimachi H, Suzuki K. The structure of calpain. J Biochem (Tokyo) 2001;129:653–64.

[82] Huang Y, Wang KK. The calpain family and human disease. Trends Mol Med 2001;7: 355–62.

[83] Zatz M, Starling A. Calpains and disease. N Engl J Med 2005;352:2413–23.

[84] Paul DS, Harmon AW, Winston CP, et al. Calpain facilitates GLUT4 vesicle translocation during insulin-stimulated glucose uptake in adipocytes. Biochem J 2003;376:625–32.

[85] Cooke DW, Patel YM. GLUT4 expression in 3T3–L1 adipocytes is repressed by proteasome inhibition, but not by inhibition of calpains. Mol Cell Endocrinol 2005;232:37–45.

[86] Johnson JD, Han Z, Otani K, et al. RyR2 and calpain-10 delineate a novel apoptosis pathway in pancreatic islets. J Biol Chem 2004;279:24794–802.

[87] Sreenan SK, Zhou YP, Otani K, et al. Calpains play a role in insulin secretion and action. Diabetes 2001;50:2013–20.

[88] Ort T, Voronov S, Guo J, et al. Dephosphorylation of beta2-syntrophin and Ca2 + /mu-calpain-mediated cleavage of ICA512 upon stimulation of insulin secretion. EMBO J 2001;20:4013–23.

[89] Marshall C, Hitman GA, Partridge CJ, et al. Evidence that an isoform of calpain-10 is a regulator of exocytosis in pancreatic beta-cells. Mol Endocrinol 2005;19:213–24.

[90] Trajkovski M, Mziaut H, Altkruger A, et al. Nuclear translocation of an ICA512 cytosolic fragment couples granule exocytosis and insulin expression in {beta}-cells. J Cell Biol 2004; 167:1063–74.

[91] Solimena M, Dirkx R Jr, Hermel JM, et al. ICA 512, an autoantigen of type I diabetes, is an intrinsic membrane protein of neurosecretory granules. EMBO J 1996;15:2102–14.

[92] Saeki K, Zhu M, Kubosaki A, et al. Targeted disruption of the protein tyrosine phosphatase-like molecule IA-2 results in alterations in glucose tolerance tests and insulin secretion. Diabetes 2002;51:1842–50.

ELSEVIER
SAUNDERS

Endocrinol Metab Clin N Am
35 (2006) 371–384

ENDOCRINOLOGY
AND METABOLISM
CLINICS
OF NORTH AMERICA

Genetic Basis of Maturity-Onset Diabetes of the Young

Martine Vaxillaire, PharmD, PhD[a,*],
Philippe Froguel, MD, PhD[a,b]

[a]CNRS UMR8090 Unit, Institute of Biology and Pasteur Institute of Lille,
1 rue du Professeur Calmette BP 245 59019, Lille, France
[b]Imperial College Genome Centre and Genomic Medicine, Hammersmith Hospital,
Du Cane Road, London, W12 0NN, United Kingdom

Type 2 diabetes mellitus (T2D) is a heterogeneous metabolic disease occurring with concomitant or interdependent defects of insulin secretion and action [1,2]. It generally is accepted that T2D results from a complex interplay of genetic and environmental factors influencing several intermediate traits of relevance to the diabetic phenotype (β-cell mass, insulin secretion, insulin action, fat distribution, obesity). T2D seems to result from several combined gene defects, the simultaneous action of several susceptibility alleles, or combinations of frequent variants at several loci that may have deleterious effects when predisposing environmental factors are present. T2D also is considered as a multigenic condition, meaning that many different combinations of gene defects may exist among diabetic patients. In fact, T2D seems to be composed of subtypes wherein genetic susceptibility is strongly associated with environmental factors at one end of the spectrum (common polygenic T2D forms) and highly genetic forms at the other end. Several monogenic forms of diabetes have been identified, such as maturity-onset diabetes of the young (MODY) and maternally inherited diabetes and deafness [3,4]. Moreover, retrospective studies showed that low birth weight was associated with insulin resistance and T2D in adulthood [5,6]. It has been proposed that this association results from a metabolic adaptation to poor fetal nutrition [7]. The identification of gene variants that contribute to variation in fetal growth and to the susceptibility to T2D, however, suggests that this metabolic programming also could be genetically determined in part [8].

* Corresponding author.
  E-mail address: martine.vaxillaire@good.ibl.fr (M. Vaxillaire).

0889-8529/06/$ - see front matter © 2006 Elsevier Inc. All rights reserved.
doi:10.1016/j.ecl.2006.02.009

The complex interactions between genes and environment complicate the task of identifying any single genetic susceptibility factor to T2D. Common T2D in adults is a complex polygenic disease that arises as predisposing environmental factors interact with many genetic variants (susceptibility alleles) interspersed through the genome. Each susceptibility allele, considered in isolation, confers only a small increased risk for disease (typically in the 1–1.5 fold range), implying the need to use large population-based samples and cases enriched for familiality and early onset to reliably detect such modest effects. Most of the diabetes-associated genes were discovered by studying the highly familial and monogenic forms of diabetes with young age of onset, such as MODY. In this article we review the clinical heterogeneity and genetic basis of the different MODY subtypes and also focus on the lessons that have emerged from these monogenic forms of diabetes.

Definition and diagnostic criteria for maturity-onset diabetes of the young

The term *maturity-onset diabetes of the young* was based on the old classification of diabetes into juvenile-onset and maturity-onset diabetes. The American Diabetes Association and the World Health Organization have introduced a revised, cause-based classification for diabetes. MODY is now defined as a genetic defect in β-cell function with subclassification according to the gene involved.

MODY is a familial form of non–insulin dependent diabetes with autosomal dominant inheritance that usually develops at childhood, adolescence, or young adulthood, and presents primary insulin-secretion defects [3]. The main diagnostic criteria for MODY are

- Early onset of diabetes, frequently diagnosed before age 25 years in at least one and ideally two family members. Anticipation or progressive reduction in the age of diagnosis in succeeding generations was reported in almost all reported MODY pedigrees, probably because of enhanced awareness of diabetes leading to earlier testing.
- Non–insulin dependence shown by absence of insulin treatment 5 years after diagnosis or significant C-peptide even in a patient on insulin treatment.
- Autosomal dominant inheritance (ie, vertical transmission of diabetes through at least two or ideally three generations, with a similar phenotype in diabetic family members).
- Rare association with obesity with the MODY phenotype (obesity not required for the development of this form of diabetes).
- Diabetes resulting from β-cell dysfunction. Insulin levels are often in the normal range, though inappropriately low for the degree of hyperglycemia.

The prevalence of MODY is estimated at less than 5% of patients who have T2D in most white populations [9].

Molecular genetics of maturity-onset diabetes of the young

The well-defined mode of inheritance with high penetrance and the early age of onset of diabetes allows the collection of multigenerational pedigrees, making MODY an attractive model for genetic studies. MODY is not a single entity but is a heterogeneous disease with regard to genetic, metabolic, and clinical features. Not all MODY genes have been identified, but heterozygous mutations in six genes cause most of the MODY cases (Table 1). These genes encode the enzyme glucokinase (GCK/*MODY2*) [10,11] and the transcription factors hepatocyte nuclear factor 4 alpha (HNF4α/*MODY1*) [12], hepatocyte nuclear factor 1 alpha (HNF1α/*MODY3*) [13,14], insulin promoter factor 1 (IPF1/*MODY4*) [15], hepatocyte nuclear factor 1 beta (HNF1β/*MODY5*) [16], and NeuroD1/Beta2 (*MODY6*) [17]. Moreover, additional *MODY* genes remain to be discovered, because there are families in which MODY cosegregates with markers outside the known *MODY* loci [18,19].

The relative prevalence of the different subtypes of MODY has been shown to vary greatly in studying British, French, German, and Spanish family cohorts [20–23]. MODY2 represents from 8% to 63% of cases (the most prevalent form in French families) and MODY3 from 21% to 64% of cases (the most prevalent form in British families). The other MODY subtypes are rare disorders in all these populations, having been described in only a few families, whereas additional unknown MODY loci (MODYX) represent 16% to 45% of the cases (the most prevalent form in German and Spanish families). These contrasting results may be because of differences in the genetic background of these populations, or may reflect, at least partly, ascertainment bias in the recruitment of families.

Glucokinase mutations and maturity-onset diabetes of the young, type 2

Glucokinase phosphorylates glucose to glucose-6-phosphate in pancreatic β cells and hepatocytes, and plays a major role in the regulation and integration of glucose metabolism [40]. More than 120 different GCK mutations have been observed to date [24]. The kinetic properties of recombinant GCK proteins have shown that the relative enzymatic activity of the mutant proteins was impaired, resulting in decreased glycolytic flux in pancreatic β cells [25]. This defect translates in vivo as a glucose-sensing defect leading to an increase in the blood glucose threshold that triggers insulin secretion [26], and a right shift in the dose–response curve of glucose-induced insulin secretion [27]. Decreased net accumulation of hepatic glycogen and increased hepatic gluconeogenesis following standard meals were observed in glucokinase-deficient subjects and contribute to the postprandial hyperglycemia of MODY2 patients [28]. Despite these multiple defects in the pancreas and the liver, the hyperglycemia associated with GCK mutations often is mild, with fewer than 50% of subjects presenting with overt diabetes. There is a lower prevalence of diabetes microvascular complications (retinopathy and proteinuria) in MODY2 than in other subtypes of MODY

Table 1
Subtypes of maturity-onset diabetes of the young and genes involved

MODY type	Gene locus	Gene name	Year of discovery [reference]	Distribution	Onset of diabetes	Primary defect	Severity of diabetes	Complications
MODY1	20q	*HNF4α*	1996 [12]	Rare	Adolescence Early adulthood	Pancreas/other	Severe	Frequent
MODY2	7p	*GCK*	1992 [11]	10%–65%[a]	Early childhood	Pancreas/liver	Mild	Rare
MODY3	12q	*TCF1*/*HNF1α*	1996 [13]	20%–75%[a]	Adolescence Early adulthood	Pancreas/kidney /other	Severe	Frequent
MODY4	13q	*IPF1*	1997 [15]	Rare	Early adulthood	Pancreas	Severe	Unknown
MODY5	17q	*TCF2*/*HNF1β*	1997 [16]	Rare	—	Kidney/pancreas	Severe	Kidney disease
MODY6	2q32	*NEUROD1*	1999 [17]	Rare	Early adulthood	Pancreas	Severe	Unknown

[a] Different distributions in different populations.

and late-onset T2D [29]. It was observed that GCK mutations in the fetus result in reduced birth weight, probably by affecting insulin-mediated fetal growth, whereas maternal GCK mutations indirectly increase the birth weight by increasing fetal insulin secretion, as a consequence of maternal hyperglycemia during fetal life. Neither of these effects persist into adult life, however [30,31]. There is growing evidence that common variants upstream of *GCK* (like −30 G/A in the β-cell promoter) influence fasting glucose levels, birth weight, and cardiovascular diseases [32].

Mutations in the transcription factor genes

Positional cloning of *MODY* loci and studies in candidate genes have led to the identification of mutations in five transcription factors: HNF1α, HNF4α, HNF1β, IPF1, and NeuroD1. Gene targeting experiments in animals have demonstrated that many of these islet-expressed genes have a key role in fetal pancreas development and neogenesis, and in β-cell differentiation and function [33].

Mutations in *HNF1α/TCF1* account for most of the MODY linked with a defect in nuclear factors. More than 150 different mutations located in the coding or promoter regions were found in various populations [24]. An insulin secretory defect in the absence of insulin resistance was observed in diabetic and nondiabetic carriers of *MODY3* mutations [34]. In contrast to the usually mild hyperglycemia attributable to glucokinase deficiency, MODY3 is a more severe form of diabetes, often evolving toward insulin dependency. Microvascular complications of diabetes are observed as frequently in MODY3 as in late age of onset diabetic subjects [35]. HNF1α is also expressed in the kidney, and a defect in the renal reabsorption of glucose often is associated with the pancreatic β-cell defect in MODY3 subjects [36]. Heterozygous knockout mice lacking one copy of HNF1α have a normal phenotype, whereas MODY3 subjects all are heterozygous for their mutations and fully express the diabetes phenotype [37]. Experimental data showed that only the mutations located in the transactivation domain of the protein exhibit a dominant negative effect on HNF1α transactivation potential [38]. The target genes associated with the β-cell defect of *MODY3*/HNF1α were partly characterized from knockout mice studies [39,40].

MODY1 is much less prevalent, and only a few kindred were described with HNF4α mutations associated with diabetes [24]. HNF4α is a member of the steroid/thyroid hormone receptor superfamily and initially known as an upstream regulator of HNF1α expression. It was demonstrated that long-chain fatty acids directly modulate the transcriptional activity of HNF4α by binding as acyl-CoA thioesters to the ligand binding domain of HNF4α [41]. This observation could contribute important data to the understanding of the role of dietary fats in the control of insulin secretion. Here again, a few target genes of HNF4α associated with β-cell defect have been defined in insulin secretion pathway and in glucose transport and metabolism [42,43]. The recent discovery of a genetic interaction between the two transcriptional regulators, HNF1α and HNF4α, that occurs specifically in differentiated pancreatic β cells can help model some molecular pathogenic events in the development of the MODY phenotype [44,45]. HNF4α controls the expression of HNF1α in embryonic endoderm, liver, and pancreatic cells, whereas the HNF1α control of HNF4α is restricted to pancreatic cells and in part to intestinal cells. This cellular specificity is explained by the existence of an alternate promoter of HNF4α known as P2. HNF1β and IPF1 may also regulate HNF4α through the P2 promoter in the pancreas. Furthermore, in a large MODY family, a nucleotide substitution in the IPF1 binding site that cosegregated with diabetes was shown to cause a threefold reduction in transcriptional activity [44]. Current evidence indicates that there is interdependence between HNF1α and HNF4α in a positive cross-regulatory loop specifically occurring in pancreatic cells and essential for the differentiated β-cell function. Such a model would propose that loss of one functional allele results in insufficient activator concentration required to elicit normal target gene responses in islets.

Mutations in *HNF1β/TCF2* were also described in a few families with early-onset diabetes consistent with MODY. In these pedigrees, *HNF1β* mutations are associated with diabetes and severe kidney disease, which may appear before the impairment of glucose tolerance. Polycystic renal disease or particular histologic abnormalities showing mega-nephrons are present in some subjects. This finding has led to the recognition of a discrete clinical syndrome associated with *HNF1β* mutations, the RCAD syndrome [46,47]. Indeed, this nuclear factor plays a major role in kidney development and nephron differentiation. In addition, internal genital abnormalities have been described in some female carriers [46]. Altogether, point mutations, small deletions or insertions, and large genomic rearrangements of TCF2 account for 70% of the cases of patients presenting with a clinical phenotype consistent with MODY5 [48].

All of these genetic defects in transcription factors lead to abnormalities of glucose homeostasis and thereby promote the development of chronic hyperglycemia through alterations in insulin secretion and possibly in the development of the pancreatic islets. In this regard, a deletion in the homeodomain transcription factor insulin promoter factor-1 (IPF1 or IDX1, STF1, PDX1), was found to cosegregate with MODY in a large kindred presenting a consanguineous link [15]. The phenotype of the subjects who are heterozygous for the mutation ranges from normal to impaired glucose tolerance to overt non–insulin-dependent diabetes. One child who is homozygous for the mutation was born with pancreatic agenesis, and suffers from diabetes and exocrine insufficiency. IPF1 is critical for the embryonic development of the pancreatic islets and for transcriptional regulation of endocrine pancreatic tissue-specific genes in adults, such as the insulin, glucose transporter-2 (GLUT2), and glucokinase genes in β cells, and the somatostatin gene in β cells. IPF1 is expressed normally in all cells of the pancreatic bud, and its absence in mice arrests development at the bud stage leading to pancreatic agenesis.

The transcription factor NeuroD1 is involved in the regulation of endocrine pancreas development. In *NeuroD1* null mice, pancreatic islet morphogenesis is abnormal and hyperglycemia develops, in part because of inadequate expression of the insulin gene. Mutations in *NeuroD1* were shown to cosegregate with early onset T2D and autosomal dominant–like transmission [17]. This observation suggests that NeuroD1 also might play an important role in endocrine pancreas development or insulin gene expression in humans.

Altogether, mutations in *GCK* and *HNF1α (TCF1)* account for around two thirds of all MODY cases, the other MODY subtypes being rare disorders described in only a few families [24]. These distinct molecular causes are associated with substantial differences in clinical course, explaining the clinical heterogeneity. Heterozygous *GCK* mutations cause fasting hyperglycemia, present from birth, which is only slowly progressive, usually responsive to diet, and leads to few complications. In contrast, *HNF1α* mutations are associated with diabetes onset in early adulthood and a more severe deterioration in glucose homeostasis. Patients who have *HNF1α* mutations also show a particular sensitivity to the hypoglycemic effects of sulfonylureas [49]. This pharmacogenetic effect is consistent with models of HNF1α deficiency, which show that the β-cell defect is upstream of the sulfonylurea receptor, and also highlights that definition of the genetic basis of hyperglycemia has strong implications for patient management.

It is important to identify these subtypes in patients presenting with early-onset diabetes, given that a precise molecular diagnosis may offer valuable prognostic and therapeutic benefits.

Other candidate genes for familial diabetes

In addition to the established MODY genes, mutations have implicated some additional genes in familial diabetes. A mutation in islet brain-1 (IB1) was found to be associated with diabetes in one family [50]. IB1 is a homologue of the c-jun amino-terminal kinase interacting protein 1 (JIP1), which plays a role in the modulation of apoptosis. IB1 also is a transactivator of the islet glucose transporter GLUT2. Because the mutant IB1 was found to be unable to prevent apoptosis in vitro, abnormal function of IB1 may render the β cells more susceptible to apoptotic stimuli, thus decreasing β-cell mass. A nonsense mutation (Q310X) in the gene *MAPK8IP1*, coding for another β-cell transcription factor, islet-1 (Is1), was described in a Japanese family with strong family history of diabetes [51].

Other genes encoding key components of insulin secretion pathways were tested as potential candidates for a role in the genetic susceptibility of T2D. The pancreatic β cell ATP-sensitive potassium channel (K_{ATP}) plays a central role in glucose-induced insulin secretion by linking signals derived from glucose metabolism to cell membrane depolarization and insulin exocytosis [52]. K_{ATP} is composed of two distinct subunits, an inwardly rectifying ion channel forming the pore (Kir6.2), and a regulatory subunit that is a sulfonylurea receptor (SUR1) belonging to the ATP-binding cassette (ABC) superfamily. The genes encoding these two subunits are located 4.5 kb apart on the human chromosome 11p15.1. Recessive mutations in each of these genes result in familial persistent hyperinsulinemic hypoglycemia in infancy, demonstrating their role in the regulation of insulin secretion [52]. Activating mutations in the Kir6.2/*KCNJ11* gene are also responsible for the extreme phenotype of neonatal diabetes [53,54]. A mild dominant form of hypoglycemia attributable to a mutation in the SUR1/*ABCC8* gene E1507K, which reduces channel activity, is reported to produce hyperinsulinism at an early age followed by a decreasing insulin-secretory capacity in early adulthood and diabetes in middle age [55]. This mutation represents a new subtype of autosomal dominant diabetes, which underlines close relationships between a progressive deterioration of insulin secretion and decrease in insulin sensibility involved in the pathogenesis and appearance of overt diabetes, thus leading to frank diabetes over time.

A missense mutation (N333S) in the active site of the enzyme transglutaminase 2 (TGase 2) was identified in a patient who has MODY and in his father who is diabetic and moderately overweight. Assessment of in vivo fast insulin release and glucose-stimulated insulin secretion from isolated islets of TGase 2 $^{-/-}$ mice revealed mild impairment of β cell insulin secretory ability [56]. Though the substitution is highly indicative of a role for TGase 2 in the disease and in keeping with the TGase 2 knockout mouse phenotype, the definitive involvement of the enzyme in the pathophysiology of MODY still requires further substantiation.

Contribution of maturity-onset diabetes of the young genes to multifactorial forms of type 2 diabetes

There now is increasing evidence that variants in the genes implicated in monogenic and syndromic forms of diabetes also are involved directly in susceptibility to more common multifactorial forms of the disease. Indeed, if major mutations (ie, causing a substantial functional defect and normally rare or absent in the general population) lead to a highly penetrant form of diabetes, it seems plausible that more subtle genetic changes affecting the structure or expression of proteins might play a role in determining (minor) susceptibility to T2D. Our current understanding of genetic variants influencing T2D strongly supports this hypothesis (Table 2) [24].

Mutations in *HNF1α* were identified in African Americans and Japanese subjects with atypical nonautoimmune diabetes with acute onset [65,66], and a common polymorphism in *HNF1α* was found to be associated with mild

Table 2
Human genes identified as responsible for monogenic type 2 diabetes and for which large or replicated case-control studies have shown association between common variants in or close to the gene and increased diabetes

Gene	Monogenic disease	OMIM	Polygenic type 2 diabetes	Reference
HNF4α	MODY1	125850	5′SNPs (P2 promoter) increased risk in Finnish (OR = 1.33) and Ashkenazim (OR = 1.4)	[58,68]
GCK	MODY2	125851	variant −30G/A (β-cell promoter) allele frequency: 20%	[32]
HNF1α/TCF1	MODY3	600496	G319S, OR = 1.97 in Oji-Cree	[67]
IPF1	MODY4	606392	5′SNPs (OR = 1.8) and coding variants increased risk in Caucasian population	[69]
TIEG2/KLF11	Early-onset T2D (T220M, A347S)	603301	G62R, OR = 1.29 in North European population	[61]
KCNJ11	Permanent neonatal diabetes mellitus (PNDM)	606176	E23K, OR = 1.2	[62,63]
ABCC8	CHI and dominant T2D	256450	L270V, OR = 1.15	[62,64]

Abbreviations: OMIM, Online Mendelian Inheritance in Man database; OR, odds ratio; SNP, single nucleotide polymorphism.

insulin-secretion defects [59]. In the Oji-Cree Native Canadian population the private G319S variant in *HNF1α/MODY3* gene accelerates the onset of T2D by seven years, and is found in 40% of diabetic patients [67]. Recently, several studies found that frequent variants in the *HNF1α* gene region are associated with T2D in different ethnic groups [57].

Moreover, mutations in *HNF4α* and *IPF1* genes also were identified in a few families with late-onset T2D. Previous mutation analyses of the coding exons of *HNF4α* have failed to identify frequent variants associated with T2D. Two more recent independent studies in Ashkenazim and Finnish populations, however, have reported convincing associations with common variants adjacent to the *HNF4α* P2 promoter [58,68]. Some of the diabetes-associated variants account for most of the evidence for linkage to chromosome 20q13 reported in these populations. Consistent with these results, genetic variation near the P2 region of *HNF4α* is associated with T2D in other Danish and United Kingdom populations, but not in French and other white populations [60], which argues for genetic heterogeneity with regard to the role of this gene. The causal variants affecting the expression or function of HNF4α are still unknown and could result in a combination of relative insulin deficiency and defective regulation of the hepatic gluconeogenesis.

There also are some indications that regulatory and coding variants in *IPF1/Pdx1* increase T2D risk (Martine Vaxillaire, unpublished results, 2005) [69]. *IPF1/Pdx1* has a dosage-dependent regulatory effect on the expression of β-cell–specific genes and therefore assists in the maintenance of euglycemia. As a consequence, frequent variants in the regulatory binding sequences controlling *IPF1/Pdx1* expression in the β cell or in the genes coding for transcription factors known to regulate *IPF1/Pdx1* could contribute to common T2D susceptibility.

We recently showed that three nonsynonymous mutations in the TGF-β–inducible transcription factor *KLF11/TIEG2* associate with monogenic early-onset (MODY-like diabetes) and polygenic middle age–onset T2D [61]. These mutations are responsible for altered KLF11 transcriptional regulation activity (eg, on insulin and Pdx1 expression). These results strongly suggest a role for the TGFβ signaling pathway in pancreatic diseases affecting endocrine islets (diabetes) or exocrine cells (cancer).

A major lesson learned from monogenic diabetes is the need to identify functional mutations cosegregating with early-onset diabetes as proof of the concept of a given gene's pivotal role in the establishment and maintenance of adequate β-cell functional capacity, as was revealed by the discovery of the IPF1–HNF regulatory network in β cells. Whether or not such genes also contribute to the genetic risk for multifactorial T2D is another issue, dealing with epidemiology and with the search for biomarkers for diabetes. It is likely that additional β-cell–expressed genes, when mutated, can increase the risk for the different genetic forms of T2D, and their identification should help lead to a better understanding of diabetes.

Summary

Currently, less than 15% of the genetic determinants of T2D have been unveiled. It is likely, however, that other genes contributing to the genetic risk for T2D soon will be discovered. The identification of T2D genes will improve our understanding of the molecular mechanisms that maintain glucose homeostasis and of the precise molecular defects leading to chronic hyperglycemia. A nosological classification of T2D based on primary pathophysiological mechanisms then will be possible. This classification could lead to the development of more specifically targeted antidiabetic drugs or even gene-based therapies. Moreover, pharmacogenetic testing might then be used to predict for each patient the therapeutic response to different classes of drugs. The identification of T2D genes also will provide the tools for the timely identification of high-risk individuals who might benefit from early behavioral or medical intervention for preventing the development of diabetes. An important reduction in diabetes-related morbidity and mortality then could be expected, along with a reduction in the costs of the treatment of diabetes and its complications.

References

[1] DeFronzo RA, Prato SD. Insulin resistance and diabetes mellitus. J Diabetes Complications 1996;10(5):243–5.

[2] Ferrannini E. Insulin resistance versus insulin deficiency in non-insulin-dependent diabetes mellitus: problems and prospects. Endocr Rev 1998;19(4):477–90.

[3] Froguel P, Velho G. Molecular genetics of maturity-onset diabetes of the young. Trends Endocrinol Metab 1999;10(4):142–6.

[4] van den Ouweland JM, Lemkes HH, Trembath RC, et al. Maternally inherited diabetes and deafness is a distinct subtype of diabetes and associates with a single point mutation in the mitochondrial tRNA(Leu(UUR)) gene. Diabetes 1994;43(6):746–51.

[5] Hales CN, Barker DJ, Clark PM, et al. Fetal and infant growth and impaired glucose tolerance at age 64. BMJ 1991;303(6809):1019–22.

[6] Lithell HO, McKeigue PM, Berglund L, et al. Relation of size at birth to non-insulin dependent diabetes and insulin concentrations in men aged 50-60 years. BMJ 1996;312(7028):406–10.

[7] Barker DJ. The fetal and infant origins of disease. Eur J Clin Invest 1995;25(7):457–63.

[8] Hattersley AT, Tooke JE. The fetal insulin hypothesis: an alternative explanation of the association of low birthweight with diabetes and vascular disease. Lancet 1999;353(9166):1789–92.

[9] Ledermann HM. Is maturity onset diabetes at young age (MODY) more common in Europe than previously assumed? Lancet 1995;345(8950):648.

[10] Froguel P, Vaxillaire M, Sun F, et al. Close linkage of glucokinase locus on chromosome 7p to early-onset non-insulin-dependent diabetes mellitus. Nature 1992;356(6365):162–4.

[11] Froguel P, Zouali H, Vionnet N, et al. Familial hyperglycemia due to mutations in glucokinase. Definition of a subtype of diabetes mellitus. N Engl J Med 1993;328(10):697–702.

[12] Yamagata K, Furuta H, Oda N, et al. Mutations in the hepatocyte nuclear factor-4alpha gene in maturity-onset diabetes of the young (MODY1). Nature 1996;384(6608):458–60.

[13] Vaxillaire M, Boccio V, Philippi A, Vigouroux C, Terwilliger J, Passa P, et al. A gene for maturity onset diabetes of the young (MODY) maps to chromosome 12q. Nat Genet 1995;9(4):418–23.

[14] Yamagata K, Oda N, Kaisaki PJ, et al. Mutations in the hepatocyte nuclear factor-1alpha gene in maturity-onset diabetes of the young (MODY3). Nature 1996;384(6608):455–8.

[15] Stoffers DA, Ferrer J, Clarke WL, et al. Early-onset type-II diabetes mellitus (MODY4) linked to IPF1. Nat Genet 1997;17(2):138–9.

[16] Horikawa Y, Iwasaki N, Hara M, et al. Mutation in hepatocyte nuclear factor-1 beta gene (TCF2) associated with MODY. Nat Genet 1997;17(4):384–5.

[17] Malecki MT, Jhala US, Antonellis A, et al. Mutations in NEUROD1 are associated with the development of type 2 diabetes mellitus. Nat Genet 1999;23(3):323–8.

[18] Frayling TM, Lindgren CM, Chevre JC, et al. A genome-wide scan in families with maturity-onset diabetes of the young: evidence for further genetic heterogeneity. Diabetes 2003;52(3):872–81.

[19] Kim SH, Ma X, Weremowicz S, et al. Identification of a locus for maturity-onset diabetes of the young on chromosome 8p23. Diabetes 2004;53(5):1375–84.

[20] Chevre JC, Hani EH, Boutin P, et al. Mutation screening in 18 Caucasian families suggest the existence of other MODY genes. Diabetologia 1998;41(9):1017–23.

[21] Costa A, Bescos M, Velho G, et al. Genetic and clinical characterisation of maturity-onset diabetes of the young in Spanish families. Eur J Endocrinol 2000;142(4):380–6.

[22] Frayling TM, Bulamn MP, Ellard S, et al. Mutations in the hepatocyte nuclear factor-1alpha gene are a common cause of maturity-onset diabetes of the young in the U.K. Diabetes 1997;46(4):720–5.

[23] Lindner TH, Cockburn BN, Bell GI. Molecular genetics of MODY in Germany. Diabetologia 1999;42(1):121–3.

[24] Fajans SS, Bell GI, Polonsky KS. Molecular mechanisms and clinical pathophysiology of maturity-onset diabetes of the young. N Engl J Med 2001;345(13):971–80.

[25] Sturis J, Kurland IJ, Byrne MM, et al. Compensation in pancreatic beta-cell function in subjects with glucokinase mutations. Diabetes 1994;43(5):718–23.

[26] Velho G, Froguel P, Clement K, et al. Primary pancreatic beta-cell secretory defect caused by mutations in glucokinase gene in kindreds of maturity onset diabetes of the young. Lancet 1992;340(8817):444–8.

[27] Byrne MM, Sturis J, Clement K, et al. Insulin secretory abnormalities in subjects with hyperglycemia due to glucokinase mutations. J Clin Invest 1994;93(3):1120–30.

[28] Velho G, Petersen KF, Perseghin G, et al. Impaired hepatic glycogen synthesis in glucokinase-deficient (MODY-2) subjects. J Clin Invest 1996;98(8):1755–61.

[29] Velho G, Vaxillaire M, Boccio V, et al. Diabetes complications in NIDDM kindreds linked to the MODY3 locus on chromosome 12q. Diabetes Care 1996;19(9):915–9.

[30] Hattersley AT, Beards F, Ballantyne E, et al. Mutations in the glucokinase gene of the fetus result in reduced birth weight. Nat Genet 1998;19(3):268–70.

[31] Velho G, Hattersley AT, Froguel P. Maternal diabetes alters birth weight in glucokinase-deficient (MODY2) kindred but has no influence on adult weight, height, insulin secretion or insulin sensitivity. Diabetologia 2000;43(8):1060–3.

[32] Weedon MN, Frayling TM, Shields B, et al. Genetic regulation of birth weight and fasting glucose by a common polymorphism in the islet cell promoter of the glucokinase gene. Diabetes 2005;54(2):576–81.

[33] Shih DQ, Stoffel M. Dissecting the transcriptional network of pancreatic islets during development and differentiation. Proc Natl Acad Sci U S A 2001;98(25):14189–91.

[34] Vaxillaire M, Pueyo ME, Clement K, et al. Insulin secretion and insulin sensitivity in diabetic and non-diabetic subjects with hepatic nuclear factor-1alpha (maturity-onset diabetes of the young-3) mutations. Eur J Endocrinol 1999;141(6):609–18.

[35] Isomaa B, Henricsson M, Lehto M, et al. Chronic diabetic complications in patients with MODY3 diabetes. Diabetologia 1998;41(4):467–73.

[36] Velho G, Benqué-Blanchet F, Vaxillaire M, et al. Renal proximal tubular defects associated to the MODY3 phenotype [abstract 108]. Diabetologia 1998;41(S1):418.

[37] Pontoglio M, Sreenan S, Roe M, et al. Defective insulin secretion in hepatocyte nuclear factor 1alpha-deficient mice. J Clin Invest 1998;101(10):2215–22.

[38] Vaxillaire M, Abderrahmani A, Boutin P, et al. Anatomy of a homeoprotein revealed by the analysis of human MODY3 mutations. J Biol Chem 1999;274(50):35639–46.

[39] Wang H, Maechler P, Hagenfeldt KA, et al. Dominant-negative suppression of HNF-1alpha function results in defective insulin gene transcription and impaired metabolism-secretion coupling in a pancreatic beta-cell line. EMBO J 1998;17(22):6701–13.

[40] Akpinar P, Kuwajima S, Krutzfeldt J, et al. Tmem27: A cleaved and shed plasma membrane protein that stimulates pancreatic beta cell proliferation. Cell Metab 2005;2(6):385–97.

[41] Hertz R, Magenheim J, Berman I, et al. Fatty acyl-CoA thioesters are ligands of hepatic nuclear factor-4alpha. Nature 1998;392(6675):512–6.

[42] Stoffel M, Duncan SA. The maturity-onset diabetes of the young (MODY1) transcription factor HNF4alpha regulates expression of genes required for glucose transport and metabolism. Proc Natl Acad Sci U S A 1997;94(24):13209–14.

[43] Gupta RK, Vatamaniuk MZ, Lee CS, et al. The MODY1 gene HNF-4alpha regulates selected genes involved in insulin secretion. J Clin Invest 2005;115(4):1006–15.

[44] Thomas H, Jaschkowitz K, Bulman M, et al. A distant upstream promoter of the HNF4α gene connects the transcription factors involved in maturity-onset diabetes of the young. Hum Mol Genet 2001;10(19):2089–97.

[45] Boj SF, Parrizas M, Maestro MA, et al. A transcription factor regulatory circuit in differentiated pancreatic cells. Proc Natl Acad Sci U S A 2001;98(25):14481–6.

[46] Lindner TH, Njolstad PR, Horikawa Y, et al. A novel syndrome of diabetes mellitus, renal dysfunction and genital malformation associated with a partial deletion of the pseudo-POU domain of hepatocyte nuclear factor-1beta. Hum Mol Genet 1999;8(11):2001–8.

[47] Bingham C, Bulman MP, Ellard S, et al. Mutations in the hepatocyte nuclear factor-1beta gene are associated with familial hypoplastic glomerulocystic kidney disease. Am J Hum Genet 2001;68(1):219–24.

[48] Bellanne-Chantelot C, Clauin S, Chauveau D, et al. Large genomic rearrangements in the hepatocyte nuclear factor-1{beta} (TCF2) gene are the most frequent cause of maturity-onset diabetes of the young type 5. Diabetes 2005;54(11):3126–32.

[49] Pearson ER, Starkey BJ, Powell RJ, et al. Genetic cause of hyperglycaemia and response to treatment in diabetes. Lancet 2003;362(9392):1275–81.

[50] Waeber G, Delplanque J, Bonny C, et al. The gene MAPK8IP1, encoding islet-brain-1, is a candidate for type 2 diabetes. Nat Genet 2000;24(3):291–5.

[51] Shimomura H, Sanke T, Hanabusa T, et al. Nonsense mutation of islet-1 gene (Q310X) found in a type 2 diabetic patient with a strong family history. Diabetes 2000;49(9):1597–600.

[52] Ashcroft FM. ATP-sensitive potassium channelopathies: focus on insulin secretion. J Clin Invest 2005;115(8):2047–58.

[53] Gloyn AL, Pearson ER, Antcliff JF, et al. Activating mutations in the gene encoding the ATP-sensitive potassium-channel subunit Kir6.2 and permanent neonatal diabetes. N Engl J Med 2004;350(18):1838–49.

[54] Vaxillaire M, Populaire C, Busiah K, et al. Kir6.2 mutations are a common cause of permanent neonatal diabetes in a large cohort of French patients. Diabetes 2004;53(10):2719–22.

[55] Huopio H, Otonkoski T, Vauhkonen I, et al. A new subtype of autosomal dominant diabetes attributable to a mutation in the gene for sulfonylurea receptor 1. Lancet 2003;361(9354): 301–7.

[56] Bernassola F, Federici M, Corazzari M, et al. Role of transglutaminase 2 in glucose tolerance: knockout mice studies and a putative mutation in a MODY patient. FASEB J 2002; 16(11):1371–8.

[57] Winckler W, Burtt NP, Holmkvist J, et al. Association of common variation in the HNF1alpha gene region with risk of type 2 diabetes. Diabetes 2005;54(8):2336–42.

[58] Love-Gregory LD, Wasson J, Ma J, et al. A common polymorphism in the upstream promoter region of the Hepatocyte Nuclear Factor-4α gene on chromosome 20q is associated with type 2 diabetes and appears to contribute to the evidence for linkage in an Ashkenazi Jewish population. Diabetes 2004;53(4):1134–40.

[59] Urhammer SA, Rasmussen SK, Kaisaki PJ, et al. Genetic variation in the hepatocyte nuclear factor-1 alpha gene in Danish Caucasians with late-onset NIDDM. Diabetologia 1997;40(4): 473–5.

[60] Vaxillaire M, Dina C, Lobbens S, et al. Effect of common polymorphisms in the HNF4α promoter on Type 2 diabetes susceptibility in the French Caucasian population. Diabetologia 2005;48(3):440–4.

[61] Neve B, Fernandez-Zapico ME, Ashkenazi-Katalan V, et al. Role of transcription factor KLF11 and its diabetes-associated gene variants in pancreatic beta cell function. Proc Natl Acad Sci U S A 2005;102(13):4807–12.

[62] Gloyn AL, Weedon MN, Owen KR, et al. Large scale association studies of variants in genes encoding the pancreatic beta-cell K-ATP channel subunits Kir6.2 (KCNJ11) and SUR1 (ABCC8) confirm that the KCNJ11 E23K variant is associated with increased risk of Type 2. Diabetes 2003;52(2):568–72.

[63] Love-Gregory L, Wasson K, Lin J, et al. An E23K single nucleotide polymorphism in the islet ATP-sensitive potassium channel gene (Kir6.2) contributes as much to the risk of type II diabetes in Caucasians as the PPARgamma. Diabetologia 2003;46(1):136–7.

[64] Florez JC, Burtt N, de Bakker PI, et al. Haplotype structure and genotype-phenotype correlations of the sulfonylurea receptor and the islet ATP-sensitive potassium channel gene region. Diabetes 2004;53(5):1360–8.

[65] Boutin P, Gresh L, Cisse A, et al. Missense mutation Gly574Ser in the transcription factor HNF-1alpha is a marker of atypical diabetes mellitus in African-American children. Diabetologia 1999;42(3):380–1.

[66] Iwasaki N, Oda N, Ogata M, et al. Mutations in the hepatocyte nuclear factor-1alpha/MODY3 gene in Japanese subjects with early- and late-onset NIDDM. Diabetes 1997; 46(9):1504–8.

[67] Triggs-Raine BL, Kirkpatrick RD, Kelly SL, et al. HNF-1alpha G319S, a transactivation-deficient mutant, is associated with altered dynamics of diabetes onset in an Oji-Cree community. Proc Natl Acad Sci U S A 2002;99(7):4614–9.

[68] Silander K, Mohlke KL, Scott LJ, et al. Genetic variation near the hepatocyte nuclear factor-4alpha gene predicts susceptibility to type 2 diabetes. Diabetes 2004;53(4):1141–9.

[69] Hani EH, Stoffers DA, Chevre JC, et al. Defective mutations in the insulin promoter factor-1 (IPF-1) gene in late-onset type 2 diabetes mellitus. J Clin Invest 1999;104(9):R41–8.

ELSEVIER
SAUNDERS

Endocrinol Metab Clin N Am
35 (2006) 385–396

ENDOCRINOLOGY
AND METABOLISM
CLINICS
OF NORTH AMERICA

New Insights in the Molecular Pathogenesis of the Maternally Inherited Diabetes and Deafness Syndrome

Johannes A. Maassen, PhD[a],*,
Roshan S. Jahangir Tafrechi, PhD[a],
George M.C. Janssen, PhD[a], Anton K. Raap, PhD[a],
Herman H. Lemkes, MD[b], Leen M. 't Hart, PhD[a]

[a]Department of Molecular Cell Biology, Leiden University Medical Centre,
Albinusdreef 2, 2333ZA Leiden, The Netherlands
[b]Department of Endocrinology and Metabolic Diseases, Leiden University Medical Centre,
Albinusdreef 2, 2333ZA Leiden, The Netherlands

A mutation at position 3243 in the mtDNA-encoded tRNA(Leu,UUR) gene has been found to be associated with the syndrome of maternally inherited diabetes and deafness syndrome (MIDD) [1]. This review addresses the molecular and physiologic processes by which this mutation leads to a disease state. Furthermore, it briefly summarizes some major clinical characteristics of this subtype of diabetes.

Mitochondrial function and genetics

Mitochondria are distinct organelles within eukaryotic cells. From an evolutionary point of view, it is assumed that mitochondria originated from bacteria by endosymbiotic mechanisms with proeukaryotic cells [2]. Mitochondria carry their own genetic material. In human beings, mtDNA is a circular molecule comprising 16,569 base pairs [3]. Several copies of circular DNA are present per mitochondrion. Furthermore, most cells contain hundreds of mitochondria that can undergo fusion and fission. Thus, in an average cell approximately 100 to 1000 mtDNA copies are present per nuclear genome. Human mtDNA encodes for only 13 proteins involved in

---

Funding was obtained through the Diabetes Fonds Nederland and Medische Wetenschappen-Nederlands Wetenschappelijk Onderzoek (MW-NWO).
* Corresponding author.
E-mail address: j.a.maassen@lumc.nl (J.A. Maassen).

0889-8529/06/$ - see front matter © 2006 Elsevier Inc. All rights reserved.
doi:10.1016/j.ecl.2006.02.014

endo.theclinics.com

oxidative phosphorylation and for the ribosomal and tRNA genes involved in mitochondrial protein synthesis. There are two tRNA genes for leucine with different codon use; tRNA(Leu,UUR) is one. Most mitochondrial components are encoded by nuclear DNA [4].

A large number of metabolic processes occur within the mitochondrion. Pyruvate, a product of the glycolytic flux, enters the mitochondrion and is further metabolized by the citric acid (Krebs) cycle. The resulting NADH and reduced flavin adenine dinucleotide ($FADH_2$) are reoxidized via the respiratory chain, and ATP is generated by oxidative phosphorylation of ADP. The transfer of electrons through the respiratory chain also contributes to the generation of oxygen-derived radicals [2], which have a strong effect on signaling pathways and gene expression. Furthermore, mitochondria are involved in fatty acid oxidation, the metabolism of some amino acids, and the regulation of cytosolic calcium concentrations [5]. Mitochondria are also major players in the regulation of apoptosis of cells. Under conditions that favor the release of cytochrome C from mitochondria to the cytosol, caspases that ultimately trigger the apoptotic process become activated. These processes are summarized in Fig. 1. We should thus consider the possibility that the pathogenesis of mitochondrial diseases resulting from mutations in mtDNA involves not only the impaired production of ATP but the possible deregulation of various other cellular processes.

The mtDNA in human beings shows a strict maternal inheritance, because during fertilization of the oocyte, the paternal mitochondria are not retained within the fertilized oocyte. Furthermore, mtDNA has a low recombination rate as well as a high mutation rate [6]. When a mutation is generated, it initially affects only one mtDNA molecule within a cell. During multiple cell divisions in which mitochondria are randomly divided over daughter cells, there is a gradual drift toward a state in which cells have predominantly wild-type (WT) or predominantly mutant mitochondria. The latter situation is called homoplasmy [2]. In the case in which a mutation has no or little effect on the function of the mitochondrion, a homoplasmic state is a stable end condition for cells, because the cell division rate and

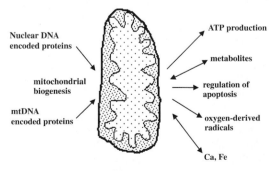

Fig. 1. Mitochondrial biogenesis and involvement in various metabolic processes. Ca, calcium; Fe, iron.

cellular lifespan are not or little affected. In the case of mutations that do impair the function of the mitochondrion, a situation in which all mitochondria carry mutated DNA is incompatible with proper cellular function and viability. Therefore, in vivo, these mutations generally do not progress to a homoplasmic state. Rather, one observes cells with a mixed population of WT and mutant mtDNA, a situation designated heteroplasmy. Thus, most pathogenic mtDNA mutations are found in a heteroplasmic state in patients.

Because mtDNA is not accessible for in situ manipulations, it is difficult to demonstrate a direct relation between a particular mtDNA mutation and altered mitochondrial function. King and Attardi [7] have developed a cybrid methodology in which mitochondria from patients' cells with a heteroplasmic mutation are introduced into recipient cells lacking mtDNA by cell fusion. Subsequent clonal selection allows the isolation of cells containing predominantly mutant mtDNA, which allows identification of the biochemical consequences of the mutation. Remarkably, the degree of heteroplasmy within an individual shows large variations when biopsies from different tissues are considered. Furthermore, even individual cells within a given tissue show differences in heteroplasmy levels [8]. Generally, there is a trend toward lower levels of heteroplasmy in rapidly dividing cells, such as leukocytes, when compared with slowly dividing tissues, such as muscle.

Point mutations show a strict maternal inheritance, and a carrier mother transmits the mutation to almost all her children. Aging is also associated with the accumulation of somatic point mutations and deletions in mtDNA. Especially under conditions that favor the induction of oxidative stress, such as hyperglycemia, somatic mutations in mtDNA are generated, including the appearance of the diabetogenic $3243A > G$ mutation [9]. Whether the latter mutation is a hot spot in mtDNA for mutation is unclear at this time. Generally, the heteroplasmy levels of somatic mutations remain low and are unlikely to affect the generation of ATP. One cannot exclude the possibility that these low-heteroplasmy levels of somatic mutations contribute to deregulation of particular cellular processes, however [10].

Physiology of glucose homeostasis

In the diabetic state, the complex interplay between the rates of glucose appearance and glucose disappearance in the circulation is deregulated and a state of persistent hyperglycemia develops. Glucose homeostasis in vivo is maintained by a balanced interaction between glucose disposal and glucose appearance. The rate of glucose disposal to most tissues is largely insulin independent and mediated by glucose-1 (Glut1) transporters. The flux of glucose to tissues through these transporters is determined by the actual glucose concentration in the blood. The excess glucose taken up by cells that is not metabolized by mitochondria or stored as glycogen or fat can be shuttled back to the liver in form of carbon-3 compounds, such as lactate or alanine. In the liver, these carbon-3 compounds have the ability to fuel gluconeogenesis. Only muscle and adipose tissue are regulated by insulin, with respect to glucose uptake, because these tissues express the insulin-sensitive Glut4 transporter. The number of Glut4 transporters on the cell surface of these tissues is increased by an increase in serum insulin. As a result, insulin enhances glucose disposal in muscle and fat and thus contributes to lowering of circulating glucose levels [11].

The liver is also regulated by insulin. At elevated insulin levels, the production of hepatic glucose is suppressed by inhibition of glycogenolysis and gluconeogenesis [12]. The combined action of insulin on muscle, fat, and liver results in a lowering of blood glucose.

Insulin secretion by pancreatic β-cells is regulated by circulating glucose concentrations. Glucose is taken up by the insulin-independent Glut2 transporter and is phosphorylated to glucose-6-phosphate by glucokinase, which is a high Michaelis-Menten reaction constant K (K_M) enzyme and seems to be rate limiting for glucose entering the glycolytic pathway [13]. Because β-cells have low lactate dehydrogenase levels, almost all the glucose taken up ends up in mitochondria and leads to ATP production. A high ATP/ADP ratio leads to a predominantly closed state of the potassium (K)-channel on the plasma membrane. The resulting membrane depolarization opens a voltage-gated calcium channel, and the increase in cytosolic calcium triggers the release of insulin. This sensing mechanism is schematically illustrated in Fig. 2.

A number of pathophysiologic mechanisms can lead to a state of persistent hyperglycemia. These include secretion of an inappropriate amount of insulin by the pancreas or inappropriate action of insulin on hepatic or peripheral tissues. A number of observations suggest that a major pathway

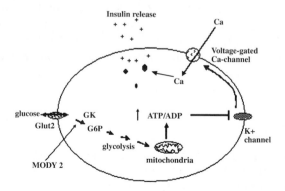

Fig. 2. Steps that contribute to the process of glucose-induced insulin secretion by pancreatic β-cells. Glucose enters the cells via Glut2 and undergoes subsequent phosphorylation by glucokinase (GK) to form glucose-6-phosphate (G6P). Subsequent metabolic conversions via glycolysis and mitochondria result in an increase in the ATP/ADP ratio, which closes the K+-channel. The resulting membrane depolarization opens a voltage-gated calcium (Ca) channel, and the increase in cytosolic Ca stimulates exocytosis of insulin-containing vesicles.

by which the 3243A > G mutation in mtDNA contributes to glucose intolerance involves impaired insulin secretion by the pancreas.

Clinical aspects of maternally inherited diabetes and deafness syndrome

The clinical appearance of MIDD has been discussed previously in several reviews [14–17]. Therefore, only some major hallmarks of the disease are given in the current review. These are summarized in Box 1.

For the most part, MIDD is a clinically unremarkable form of diabetes, with some patients becoming rapidly dependent on insulin treatment; before genetic testing, they are often diagnosed as having type 1 diabetes. Other patients can be managed by diet or oral hypoglycemic agents for a short time, and they are often diagnosed as having type 2 diabetes. Obesity is not seen as a major additional risk factor, as in common type 2 diabetes. After having diabetes for several years, all carriers tend to become dependent on insulin treatment.

The frequency of mitochondrial diabetes in the diabetes population depends on ethnic background and ranges between 0.2% and 2%, with the highest frequencies in Japan. Impaired hearing attributable to decreased perception of high tone frequencies is a characteristic comorbidity in most carriers of the 3243A > G mutation. This helps clinicians to recognize potential patients with MIDD, as does the strong familiar clustering with maternal inheritance.

In addition to diabetes and impaired hearing, a number of other comorbidities are sometimes seen to be associated with the 3243A > G mutation. These have been reviewed recently [17]. Why the 3243A > G mutation exhibits such a wide variability in clinical expression is unknown. The

---

Box 1. Major clinical characteristics of the MIDD syndrome

Clinical presentation of type 1–like and type 2–like diabetes with similar frequencies

Maternal mode of inheritance; all children from affected mother are carriers of the 3243A>G mutation

Average age of onset of diabetes is 38 years (age range: 8–69 years)

Impaired hearing and decreased perception of frequencies greater than 5 kHz, which are present in most carriers

Antibodies against β-cells are generally absent

Insulin resistance is generally absent

Other comorbidities, such as cardiomyopathy, may be severe; progressive kidney failure, muscular weakness (ptosis), and gastrointestinal complaints are seen at lower frequencies

distribution of the mutation load over individual tissues and the degree of the mutation load (heteroplasmy) may be factors that contribute to the phenotype. Only a few postmortem studies have been conducted to examine this aspect, and the results are not conclusive [18–20]. The mtDNA haplotype does not seem to contribute to the clinical phenotype [21]. Also, the lack of a suitable animal model system for the 3243A>G mutation is a major drawback in understanding the pathophysiology of this mutation.

A number of clinical studies have shown that insulin resistance of muscle and fat is not a characteristic phenomenon in most carriers of the 3243A>G mutation, at least when judged from the insulin/glucose ratio. Although insulin resistance has been reported in some carriers, this may be attributable to the fact that insulin resistance itself, independent of mtDNA mutations, is a common phenomenon in the general population. Another possibility to explain the diabetic state is that hepatic glucose output is enhanced and poorly suppressed by insulin in carriers of the 3243A>G mutation. This possibility is particularly relevant in view of enhanced peripheral lactate production in the case of mitochondrial dysfunction, which can fuel gluconeogenesis. To date, no clinical data are available regarding this possibility. The predominant process of glucose homeostasis that is affected by the 3243A>G mutation seems to be glucose-induced insulin secretion by pancreatic β-cells.

In nondiabetic carriers of the 3243A>G mutation, no abnormalities in insulin and glucose profiles are seen during oral glucose tolerance tests, suggesting normal β-cell function. When impaired glucose tolerance develops, however, a pronounced insulin secretory defect is seen in response to glucose stimulation of the pancreas in carriers of the 3243A>G mutation compared with noncarriers [15,22].

Mitochondrial myopathy, encephalopathy, lactic acidosis, and stroke-like episodes (MELAS) is another distinct syndrome that was originally found be associated with the 3243A>G mutation [23]. Its clinical phenotype has some resemblance to other neuromuscular diseases that are associated with mutations in mtDNA. The clinical characteristics of MELAS are compatible by suboptimal ATP production in muscular and neuronal tissues. Heteroplasmy levels tend to be high in MELAS, especially in muscle, although it should be kept in mind that no large-scale data exist on heteroplasmy values in the muscle of patients with MIDD because of the absence of clinically manifest muscular problems and the invasive nature of muscle biopsies.

Mechanisms leading to pancreatic dysfunction in 3243A>G carriers

Mitochondria carrying the 3243A>G mutation show reduced synthesis of mitochondrial proteins encoded by mtDNA in cybrid cell lines. In contrast, mitochondrial proteins encoded by nuclear DNA are synthesized in normal amounts. The resulting imbalance in mitochondrial proteins encoded by the two genomes results in the assembly of mitochondria with reduced activity of the respiratory chain and a reduced capacity to synthesize ATP [24]. In cybrid cell lines expressing variable ratios of WT versus 3243A > G mutant mitochondria, oxygen consumption only collapses at heteroplasmy values greater than 70% to 80%, suggesting a large spare capacity of the mitochondrial respiratory chain to maintain adequate ATP levels [25]. Nevertheless, patients with the 3243A > G mutation have heteroplasmy levels that are quite variable and mostly below the threshold for impairment of respiratory chain function [25]. Furthermore, the limited data on other tissues rarely show heteroplasmy levels that could interfere with the maintenance of adequate respiratory chain activity. Yet, these low heteroplasmy levels for the 3243A > G mutation are associated with a near 100% risk of developing glucose intolerance during life, and no major effect of high heteroplasmy levels in leukocytes is seen on the age of onset of diabetes [26].

This consistent observation in multiple ethnic backgrounds suggests that a simple decline in ATP production is unlikely to be the main pathogenic factor in the development of diabetes. In addition, tissues known to be dependent on high ATP production, such as muscle, are rarely clinically affected in most diabetic patients with the 3243A > G mutation. Furthermore, in the case of neuromuscular diseases attributable to other mutations in mtDNA, in which the phenotype seems to be determined by reduced ATP synthesis, diabetes is not seen in a substantial portion of the carriers. These considerations suggest that other or additional mechanisms rather than merely reduced ATP synthesis contribute to the high risk for diabetes in carriers of the 3243A > G mutation.

Reduced glucose-induced insulin secretion in 3243A > G carriers can, in theory, be explained by reduced ATP synthesizing activity of mutant mitochondria and, as a result, a change in the setting of the glucose sensor in pancreatic β-cells, as outlined in Fig. 2. The presence of mitochondria with the 3243A > G mutation within β-cells may alter the ATP/ADP ratio within these cells, thereby affecting the open-close probability of the K-channel and, as a result, the amount of insulin secreted. If this is the mechanism by which the 3243A > G mutation acts, one would expect to see glucose intolerance immediately after birth. A related situation occurs in newborns with inherited mutations in subunits of the K-channel (see Fig. 2), who do exhibit hyper- or hypoinsulinemia in the neonatal state, depending on the nature of the mutation [27]. Similarly, in the case of mutations in the glucokinase gene (which regulates the glucose flux through glycolysis and mitochondria, and thereby the ATP/ADP ratio), hyperglycemia or, more rarely, hypoglycemia is an early event in childhood [28,29]. Carriers of the 3243A > G mutation develop glucose intolerance at an average age of 38 years, however, indicating the contribution of age-dependent processes in the development of glucose intolerance rather than a genetically determined resetting of the glucose sensor. Carriers of the 3243A > G mutation also develop a decreased perception of high tone frequencies at an accelerated rate, which becomes manifest 10 to 20 years before glucose intolerance develops. Age-related hearing loss of high-frequency tones (presbyacusis) is a normal aging process in healthy individuals. In 3243A > G carriers, presbyacusis becomes clinically manifest at a relatively young age. Thus, it seems that premature aging of their auditory machinery occurs, and it is plausible that similar enhanced aging of pancreatic β-cells also takes place, leading to the gradual development of an insulinopenic state. There is a remarkable similarity in the biochemical mechanisms coupling mitochondrial function through the ATP/ADP ratio and the open probability of the K-channel in β-cells as well as cochlear hair cells of the ear. In the latter, a similar coupling occurs with K-channels of the KCNQ4 type [30]. The mechanism by which premature aging of cells carrying the A3243G mutation occurs seems to involve the enhanced production of radicals, as recently observed (Maechler et al submitted for publication, 2006).

The concept that mitochondrial mutations contribute to enhanced aging has been underscored recently by a transgenic mouse model with a proofreading defect in mtDNA polymerase γ. These mice accumulate mutations in mtDNA at an enhanced rate and, remarkably, exhibit a phenotype of enhanced aging with accelerated hearing loss [31,32].

An additional factor that may contribute to a state of impaired insulin secretion in diabetic patients having the 3243A > G mutation emerged from our studies in which we examined the consequences of the presence of the 3243A > G mutation on nuclear gene expression by whole-genome microarray studies. We observed that the presence of mitochondria with the 3243A > G mutation in cells leads to a coordinate reduction in the expression of the gene cluster encoding cytosolic ribosomal proteins. This coordinate reduction resulted in a 40% to 50% reduction in the rate of cytosolic protein synthesis [33]. Because the amount of insulin synthesis by pancreatic β-cells puts a great demand on the capacity of the protein synthesizing machinery, a reduction of cytosolic ribosomal protein synthesis by 40% to 50% could result in a decline in insulin secretion beyond the threshold needed to maintain normoglycemia. We would like to emphasize that the microarray studies were performed using a human osteosarcoma cell line as the model cell, because it is impossible to obtain viable pancreatic β-cells with mitochondria carrying the 3243A > G mutation. An additional factor that may contribute to reduced insulin synthesis and secretion in β-cells carrying 3243A > G mutants involves activation of AMP kinase. When ATP levels decline and ADP levels increase, ADP is converted into AMP and ATP. The appearance of AMP activates AMP-kinase, which switches off the initiation of ribosomal protein synthesis via a pathway involving mammalian target of rapamycin (mTOR) and p70S6 kinase [34]. Thus, the presence of mutant mitochondria may reduce the insulin production and secretion capacity of pancreatic β-cells by interfering at multiple steps in the process of protein synthesis (Fig. 3).

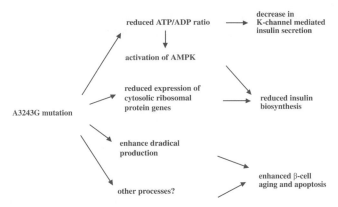

Fig. 3. Processes that are potentially affected in pancreatic β-cells by the 3243A > G mutation in mtDNA. AMPK, adenosine monophosphate–activated protein kinase.

Other genetic factors in mitochondrial diabetes

In addition to the 3243A > G mutation, many other point mutations, mostly in tRNA genes, have been identified as representing a risk factor for diabetes as well as for various other comorbidities. They have been discussed previously [15]. Their frequency is much lower compared with the 3243A > G mutation. Deletions in mtDNA are also associated with diabetes, mostly with juvenile-onset type 1–like diabetes (eg, Pearson syndrome, Kearns-Sayre syndrome) [35–37]. These diseases are extremely rare. Affected children often die before adulthood. In most cases, these deletions are sporadic, with little risk for other siblings. Recently, a nuclear gene involved in mitochondrial function has also been implicated in the risk for diabetes, probably by changing mitochondrial protein synthesis in a similar way as the mtDNA-encoded tRNA (Leu,UUR) mutation. This gene is the LARS2 gene, which encodes for mitochondrial Leu-tRNA synthase. This enzyme, synthesized in the cytosol, is imported by mitochondria, where it charges mtDNA-encoded tRNA (Leu) with leucine. Thus, this enzyme participates in the same biochemical pathway as tRNA(Leu,UUR). A genetic variant present within this gene has recently been found to be associated with an enhanced risk for developing type 2 diabetes mellitus [38]. The pathophysiologic mechanisms associated with this form of diabetes remain to be clarified, although carriers of this variant tend to have lower glucose-induced insulin secretion similar to the 3243A > G carriers.

Variants in the frataxin gene also modulate glucose-induced insulin secretion. Frataxin is a nuclear DNA–encoded protein involved in iron homeostasis within mitochondria. Certain severe mutations are involved in Friedreich ataxia, a disease characterized by neurologic abnormalities, with diabetes as a comorbid condition. Nonpathogenic variants in the gene have been shown to affect the insulin secretory response during glucose stimulation of the pancreas in vivo in human beings, supporting a critical role for mitochondrial iron metabolism in insulin secretion [39,40].

Summary

The 3243A > G mutation in mtDNA is associated with an almost 100% risk of developing diabetes during life. The mechanism by which this mutation contributes to the pathogenesis of diabetes is complex, and it is unlikely that this mechanism simply involves insufficient ATP production as the sole pathogenic factor. Rather, accelerated aging of β-cells, in conjunction with reduced insulin synthesis and changes in the ATP/ADP-mediated setting of insulin secretion by the β-cell, seems to be the factor that makes the organism vulnerable to the development of diabetes.

References

[1] van Den Ouweland JM, Lemkes HH, Ruitenbeek W, et al. Mutation in mitochondrial tRNA(Leu)(UUR) gene in a large pedigree with maternally transmitted type II diabetes mellitus and deafness. Nat Genet 1992;1(5):368–71.

[2] Wallace DC. Mitochondrial diseases in man and mouse. Science 1999;283(5407):1482–8.

[3] Anderson S, Bankier AT, Barrell BG, et al. Sequence and organization of the human mitochondrial genome. Nature 2000;290:457–65.

[4] Brown MD, Wallace DC. Molecular basis of mitochondrial DNA disease. J Bioenerg Biomembr 1994;26(3):273–89.

[5] Brini M, Pinton P, King MP, et al. A calcium signaling defect in the pathogenesis of a mitochondrial DNA inherited oxidative phosphorylation deficiency. Nat Med 1999;5(8):951–4.

[6] Hagelberg E, Goldman N, Lio P, et al. Evidence for mitochondrial DNA recombination in a human population of island Melanesia. Proc R Soc Lond B Biol Sci 1999;266(1418): 485–92.

[7] King MP, Attardi G. Human cells lacking mtDNA: repopulation with exogenous mitochondria by complementation. Science 1989;246(4929):500–3.

[8] van de Corput MP, van Den Ouweland JM, Dirks RW, et al. Detection of mitochondrial DNA deletions in human skin fibroblasts of patients with Pearson's syndrome by two-color fluorescence in situ hybridization. J Histochem Cytochem 1997;45(1):55–61.

[9] Nomiyama T, Tanaka Y, Hattori N, et al. Accumulation of somatic mutation in mitochondrial DNA extracted from peripheral blood cells in diabetic patients. Diabetologia 2002; 45(11):1577–83.

[10] Lenaz G. Role of mitochondria in oxidative stress and ageing. Biochim Biophys Acta 1998; 1366(1–2):53–67.

[11] Khan AH, Pessin JE. Insulin regulation of glucose uptake: a complex interplay of intracellular signalling pathways. Diabetologia 2002;45(11):1475–83.

[12] Roden M, Petersen KF, Shulman GI. Nuclear magnetic resonance studies of hepatic glucose metabolism in humans. Recent Prog Horm Res 2001;56:219–37.

[13] Matschinsky F, Liang Y, Kesavan P, et al. Glucokinase as pancreatic beta cell glucose sensor and diabetes gene. J Clin Invest 1993;92(5):2092–8.

[14] Guillausseau PJ, Massin P, Dubois-LaForgue D, et al. Maternally inherited diabetes and deafness: a multicenter study. Ann Intern Med 2001;134(9 Pt 1):721–8.

[15] Maassen JA, Janssen GM, 't Hart LM. Molecular mechanisms of mitochondrial diabetes (MIDD). Ann Med 2005;37(3):213–21.

[16] Maassen JA, 't Hart LM, van Essen E, et al. Mitochondrial diabetes: molecular mechanisms and clinical presentation. Diabetes 2004;53(Suppl 1):S103–9.

[17] Guillausseau PJ, Dubais-Laforgue D, Massin P, et al. Heterogenity of diabetes phenotype in patients with 3243 bp mutation of mitochondrial DNA (maternally inherited diabetes and deafness or MIDD). Diabetes Metab 2004;30(2):181–6.

[18] Kobayashi T, Nakanishi K, Nakase H, et al. In situ characterization of islets in diabetes with a mitochondrial DNA mutation at nucleotide position 3243. Diabetes 1997;46(10): 1567–71.

[19] Hamazaki S, Koshiba M, Sugiyama T. Organ distribution of mutant mitochondrial tRNA (leu(UUR)) gene in a MELAS patient. Acta Pathol Jpn 1993;43(4):187–91.

[20] Lynn S, Borthwick GM, Charnley RM, et al. Heteroplasmic ratio of the 3243A > G mitochondrial DNA mutation in single pancreatic beta cells. Diabetologia 2003;46(2):296–9.

[21] Torroni A, Campos Y, Rengo C, et al. Mitochondrial DNA haplogroups do not play a role in the variable phenotypic presentation of the 3243A > G mutation. Am J Hum Genet 2003; 72(4):1005–12.

[22] Velho G, Byrne MM, Clement K, et al. Clinical phenotypes, insulin secretion, and insulin sensitivity in kindreds with maternally inherited diabetes and deafness due to mitochondrial tRNALeu(UUR) gene mutation. Diabetes 1996;45(4):478–87.

[23] Goto Y, Nonaka I, Horai S. A mutation in the tRNA(Leu)(UUR) gene associated with the MELAS subgroup of mitochondrial encephalomyopathies [see comments]. Nature 1990; 348(6302):651–3.

[24] Janssen GM, Maassen JA, van Den Ouweland JM. The diabetes-associated 3243 mutation in the mitochondrial tRNA(Leu(UUR)) gene causes severe mitochondrial dysfunction without a strong decrease in protein synthesis rate. J Biol Chem 1999;274(42):29744–8.

[25] van Den Ouweland JM, Maechler P, Wollheim CB, et al. Functional and morphological abnormalities of mitochondria harbouring the tRNA(Leu)(UUR) mutation in mitochondrial DNA derived from patients with maternally inherited diabetes and deafness (MIDD) and progressive kidney disease. Diabetologia 1999;42(4):485–92.

[26] 't Hart LM, Jansen JJ, Lemkes HH, et al. Heteroplasmy levels of a mitochondrial gene mutation associated with diabetes mellitus decrease in leucocyte DNA upon aging. Hum Mutat 1996;7(3):193–7.

[27] Gloyn AL, Pearson ER, Antcliff JF, et al. Activating mutations in the gene encoding the ATP-sensitive potassium-channel subunit Kir6.2 and permanent neonatal diabetes. N Engl J Med 2004;350(18):1838–49.

[28] Cuesta-Munoz AL, Huopio H, Otonkoski T, et al. Severe persistent hyperinsulinemic hypoglycemia due to a de novo glucokinase mutation. Diabetes 2004;53(8):2164–8.

[29] Gloyn AL. Glucokinase (GCK) mutations in hyper- and hypoglycemia: maturity-onset diabetes of the young, permanent neonatal diabetes, and hyperinsulinemia of infancy. Hum Mutat 2003;22(5):353–62.

[30] Steel KP, Kros CJ. A genetic approach to understanding auditory function. Nat Genet 2001; 27(2):143–9.

[31] Kujoth GC, Hiona A, Pugh TD, et al. Mitochondrial DNA mutations, oxidative stress, and apoptosis in mammalian aging. Science 2005;309(5733):481–4.

[32] Trifunovic A, Wredenberg A, Falkenberg M, et al. Premature ageing in mice expressing defective mitochondrial DNA polymerase. Nature 2004;429(6990):417–23.

[33] Roshan S, Jahangir Tafrechi RS, Svensson P, et al. Distinct nuclear gene expression profiles in cells with mtDNA depletion and homoplasmic 3243A > G mutation. Mutat Res 2005;578: 43–52.

[34] Hardie DG. New roles for the LKB1 → AMPK pathway. Curr Opin Cell Biol 2005;17(2): 167–73.

[35] De Block CE, De Leeuw IH, Maassen JA, et al. A novel 7301-bp deletion in mitochondrial DNA in a patient with Kearns-Sayre syndrome, diabetes mellitus, and primary amenorrhoea. Exp Clin Endocrinol Diabetes 2004;112(2):80–3.

[36] Ballinger SW, Shoffner JM, Hedaya EV, et al. Maternally transmitted diabetes and deafness associated with a 10.4 kb mitochondrial DNA deletion. Nat Genet 1992;1(1):11–5.

[37] Wallace DC, Lott MT, Shoffner JM, et al. Diseases resulting from mitochondrial DNA point mutations. J Inherit Metab Dis 1992;15(4):472–9.

[38] 't Hart LM, Hansen T, Rietveld I, et al. Evidence that the mitochondrial leucyl tRNA synthetase (LARS2) gene represents a novel type 2 diabetes susceptibility gene. Diabetes 2005; 54(6):1892–5.

[39] Pandolfo M. Friedreich ataxia. Semin Pediatr Neurol 2003;10(3):163–72.

[40] Hart LM, Ruige JB, Dekker JM, et al. Altered beta-cell characteristics in impaired glucose tolerant carriers of a GAA trinucleotide repeat polymorphism in the frataxin gene. Diabetes 1999;48(4):924–6.

ELSEVIER
SAUNDERS

Endocrinol Metab Clin N Am
35 (2006) 397–404

ENDOCRINOLOGY
AND METABOLISM
CLINICS
OF NORTH AMERICA

Development of the Pancreas and Pancreatic Cancer

Brian C. Lewis, PhD[a,b,c]

[a]*Program in Gene Function and Expression, University of Massachusetts Medical School, 364 Plantation Street, LRB 521, Worcester, MA 01605 USA*
[b]*Program in Molecular Medicine, University of Massachusetts Medical School, 364 Plantation Street, LRB 521, Worcester, MA 01605 USA*
[c]*Cancer Center, University of Massachusetts Medical School, 364 Plantation Street, LRB 521, Worcester, MA 01605 USA*

The pancreas is specified during embryonic development from the gut endoderm. Among the signaling pathways required for the proper development of the organ are the notch and hedgehog signaling pathways. Both of these pathways are reactivated in pancreatic cancers, and sustained hedgehog signaling is required for the viability of most pancreatic cancer cell lines. Further, mouse models of the disease show activation of these pathways, and expression of pancreas progenitor markers. These findings indicate that developmentally regulated gene expression programs are important in the pathogenesis of pancreatic cancer.

Development of the pancreas

The pancreas is composed of three main cell types: (1) the acinar cells, which produce digestive enzymes; (2) the duct cells, which conduct these enzymes to the gut; and (3) the endocrine cells found in the islets of Langerhans, which produce hormones involved in the regulation of glucose homeostasis. The bulk of the pancreas, greater than 95%, is composed of the exocrine pancreas, which consists of the acinar cells and pancreatic ducts, whereas the endocrine cells are found in the discrete and morphologically distinct islets. Genetic studies in the mouse have demonstrated that these cell types are all derived from a common pancreatic progenitor [1]. In the mouse, the pancreas is specified at embryonic day 8.5 with the formation of the ventral and dorsal pancreatic buds from the primitive gut

E-mail address: brian.lewis@umassmed.edu

endoderm. Under the influence of extrinsic and intrinsic cues, these pancreatic buds develop to form the mature organ.

Intercellular signaling pathways regulating pancreatic development

The anatomic location of the developing pancreas is specified by many extrinsic signals including those provided by the hedgehog, notch, and transforming growth factor-β pathways [2]. Each of these signaling pathways plays a unique role in specifying pancreatic cell fate and location, and the correct integration of these signals is required for the proper development of the organ [2].

The expression of sonic hedgehog defines the boundary of the pancreas during embryonic development; sonic hedgehog–positive cells form the gut, whereas sonic hedgehog–negative cells develop into the pancreas [2]. The notch signaling pathway is also important during pancreatic development. Notch signaling promotes pancreatic progenitor self-renewal or exocrine lineage commitment and inhibits endocrine cell differentiation [3,4]. Indeed, enforced activation of the notch signaling pathway in pancreatic progenitors impairs their differentiation into the various pancreas cell lineages, whereas inactivation of notch signaling leads to premature differentiation of the endocrine pancreas [3–5]. Importantly, whereas the notch and hedgehog signaling pathways are inactive in the mature pancreas, both signaling pathways are reactivated in a large fraction of pancreatic cancers [6–8]. This finding suggests that, as in other cancers, developmentally regulated signaling pathways play critical roles in the genesis of pancreatic neoplasms.

Transcription factors involved in pancreatic development

The early pancreatic rudiments are marked by the expression of the homeobox transcription factor Pdx1. Lineage tracing and gene knockout studies demonstrated that Pdx1-positive cells give rise to all pancreatic cell types [9,10]. Indeed, deletion of Pdx1 in the mouse results in the absence of a mature pancreas; although the pancreatic buds form, they fail to expand and differentiate into a functional organ. These findings indicate that other intrinsic factors identify the earliest pancreatic precursors; however, the identity of these factors remains unknown. In addition to being a marker of early pancreatic progenitor cells, Pdx1 is also expressed in the β-cells of the mature pancreas and is important for the induction of insulin gene expression. In fact, mutations in Pdx1 are associated with one form of maturity-onset diabetes of the young [11]. Other transcription factors have been identified that play important roles in the development and differentiation of the pancreas, and gene knockout studies performed in mice have identified the roles of these transcription factors and the developmental defects that occur when they are inactivated [1,12]. Significantly, lineage-tracing studies have shown that the basic-helix-loop-helix transcription factor p48, whose expression in the mature organ is restricted to acinar cells, is expressed in pancreatic progenitors that give rise to all cell types within pancreas [12]. Expression of p48 is required for the formation of the exocrine pancreas, because this tissue fails to develop in p48-deficient mice [13]. Interestingly, in the absence of p48, pancreatic endocrine cells form, but the cells home to the spleen where they fail to form discrete clusters but rather exist as individual cells [13]. Collectively, these studies indicate that p48-positive cells give rise to all cell types within the pancreas, but that a p48-independent pathway exists for endocrine lineage development. Additional studies demonstrated that all of the endocrine cells within the pancreas are derived from an endocrine progenitor that expresses neurogenin3, because neurogenin3 null mice lack all pancreatic endocrine cells [14,15]. Additional transcription factors that are expressed at different times also regulate pancreatic development, and their inactivation leads to various perturbations of normal pancreatic development [1,16,17]. Therefore, a complex network of transcription factors regulates pancreatic development.

Pancreatic cancer

Pancreatic cancer is the fourth leading cause of cancer-related deaths in the western world. Consistent with this, the mean survival time after diagnosis of pancreatic ductal adenocarcinoma (PDAC) is approximately 6 months [18]. The poor prognosis for PDAC patients stems from multiple factors, including the late stage of presentation of the disease, the anatomic location of many tumors, the dissemination of the tumor to other organs by the time of diagnosis, and the profound resistance of this tumor type to currently used chemotherapy regimens.

Pancreatic tumors with the histologic features of each of the major cell types within the organ (acinar, ductal, and endocrine cells) occur in human patients. These tumors are believed to be derived from the transformation of their normal cellular counterparts. Another potential explanation is that these tumors arise from the transformation of pancreatic progenitor cells. Although tumors arise from each of the cellular compartments, greater than 85% of pancreatic tumors are PDAC [19].

Genetic alterations in pancreatic cancer

Studies of human tumor tissues have led to the identification of many common genetic alterations in PDAC, including activating mutations in the *KRAS2* oncogene; amplification of the *AKT2* oncogene; and loss, or inactivation, of the genes encoding the tumor-suppressor proteins p16, p53, and Smad4 [20]. The presence of these common genetic changes suggests that the pathways regulated by these molecules are critical for pancreatic cancer formation.

PDAC develops through the progression of precursor lesions called pancreatic intraductal neoplasms (PanIN) [21]. Each progressive stage displays increasing histologic and nuclear changes, and characteristic genetic alterations. Activating mutations in the *KRAS2* oncogene, present in approximately 90% of PDACs, are the earliest known genetic alteration in PDAC, and are commonly found in PanIN1 lesions [22]. Loss of the *INK4A* tumor-suppressor gene by allelic loss, inactivating point mutations, or gene silencing by DNA methylation is also present in PanIN1 lesions [23]. As the lesions progress to PanIN2 and 3, other commonly identified genetic alterations, such as loss of the tumor-suppressors genes *TP53* and *MADH4*, occur [24,25]. Interestingly, the genetic alterations commonly found in PDAC do not occur with appreciable frequency in acinar carcinomas or pancreatic endocrine neoplasms. Instead, acinar carcinomas commonly have mutations in *β-catenin* and *axin* that lead to stimulation of Wnt signaling; and endocrine tumors display inactivation of MEN1 [20,26].

Recently published studies have demonstrated that many pancreatic ductal tumors display activation of the hedgehog and notch signaling pathways, which are critical regulators of pancreatic development during embryogenesis [6–8]. The absence of active sonic hedgehog signaling in the adult pancreas, and its activation in most pancreatic cancer cell lines and tumors, suggests that this signaling pathway may play a critical role in the pathogenesis of this cancer. Indeed, the studies of Thayer and coworkers [7] and Berman and coworkers [6] showed that inhibition of the hedgehog signaling pathway by the antagonist cyclopamine led to growth arrest and apoptosis in many pancreatic cancer cell lines, and reduced tumor growth after subcutaneous transplantation [6,7]. Further, expression of sonic hedgehog under the control of a pancreas-specific promoter led to the formation of early pancreatic lesions that histologically resemble early PanIN lesions, and which bear activating mutations in *k-ras*, a hallmark lesion in PDAC [7].

Modeling pancreatic cancer in the mouse

Although analysis of human tumor material has led to the identification of the common genetic lesions in PDAC, it is difficult to analyze the molecular consequences of these changes in human tissue because of the presence of additional unidentified, and random, genetic changes, and the inherent genetic heterogeneity that defines the human population. In vivo model systems are therefore needed for the development of a clearer understanding of the consequences of specific genetic changes.

Several mouse models for pancreatic cancer have been generated over the past two decades [27]. Because of an inability specifically to target the pancreatic duct epithelium, these animal models have primarily modeled pancreatic acinar and endocrine neoplasms. Two recent mouse models have been described, however, that produce pancreatic lesions with many of the phenotypic and histologic characteristics of human PDAC [28–30]. In these models, the expression of an activated *k-ras* allele is induced specifically within the pancreas by means of cre-mediated excision of a transcriptional silencing element.

Importantly, the expression of the activated *k-ras* allele is under the control of its endogenous regulatory elements, a significant feature given that *k-ras* is activated, but not overexpressed, in human pancreatic tumors [20]. These animals develop progressive PanIN lesions with complete penetrance that infrequently progress to invasive carcinoma [28]. If these mice are crossed, however, with animals deleted for the *Ink4a/Arf* tumor-suppressor locus, or bearing mutant *p53* alleles, mice develop carcinomas that metastasize to the liver and other organs [29,30]. These models demonstrate that engineering of common genetic alterations found in PDAC leads to mouse models that recapitulate many of the salient features of the disease.

A novel somatic mouse model for pancreatic cancer

The previously mentioned mouse models are unlike human cancer development in one important aspect. In the models, expression of the activated *k-ras* allele occurs in every cell within the pancreas beginning during embryonic development. The current understanding in the field is that most carcinomas arise after the accumulation of a series of sporadic, somatically acquired genetic alterations. Other mouse models that model this aspect of the human disease will be of great value.

The author has recently published a mouse model for pancreatic cancer generated through the somatic delivery of oncogenes to the pancreata of mice that express TVA under the control of the elastase promoter (which is restricted to acinar cells in the adult pancreas) (elastase-*tv-a* mice) [31]. TVA is the receptor for avian leukosis sarcoma virus subgroup A (ALSV-A), and its presence on the cell surface is necessary and sufficient for infection by ALSV-A [32,33]. Mammalian cells do not express TVA, and tissue-specific infection by ALSV-A, or ALSV-A–based RCAS viruses, can be induced by using a tissue-specific promoter to direct expression of a transgene encoding the receptor. Delivery of RCAS viruses encoding markers, such as alkaline phosphatase, demonstrated that infection, and subsequent expression, occur in only a few cells. Further, it has been previously shown that there is no viral spread in mammalian cells after infection with RCAS viruses [34]. Infected pancreatic cells are surrounded by uninfected cells, more closely mimicking the scenario in human tumor development.

In this mouse model, delivery of RCAS viruses encoding different oncogenes into 2-day-old mice produced strikingly different effects. Delivery of chicken cells producing RCAS viruses encoding the mouse polyoma virus middle T antigen (RCAS-*PyMT*) to elastase-*tv-a* mice induced pancreatic lesions in approximately 25% of the animals sacrificed at 13 months of age. The induced lesions are microscopic and visible only after serial sectioning of the harvested pancreata. Histologically, the lesions most closely resemble early PanIN lesions with invaginated epithelium and the accumulation of mucin globules within the cytoplasm. Consistent with this, the lesions were positive for the ductal markers HNF1β and keratin 19. In addition, the lesions were all positive for the transcription factor Pdx1, a homeobox transcription factor that identifies beta cells in the mature pancreas, but also marks early pancreatic progenitors during the development of the organ [17]. In addition to expressing the progenitor marker Pdx1, the tumors were also positive for the neuroendocrine marker synaptophysin. Interestingly, no acinar cell pathology was seen in these mice, nor were there any signs of acinar-to-ductal metaplasia. These findings raised the possibility that the pancreatic lesions arose from the transformation of pancreas progenitor cells.

Delivery of RCAS viruses encoding PyMT to elastase-*tv-a* transgenic mice deficient for the *Ink4a/Arf* locus induced pancreatic tumors that were detectable as early as 4 months of age. Acinar carcinomas were identified in all tumor-bearing animals. Interestingly, in addition to the acinar carcinomas, most tumor-bearing animals also had ductal lesions. As was the case in the *Ink4a/Arf* wild-type mice, the tumors, irrespective of their histologic type, all expressed the progenitor marker Pdx1 and the neuroendocrine marker synaptophysin. Furthermore, the ductal tumors seem to arise de novo and not from the transdifferentiation of acinar cells as has been proposed in previously described transgenic mouse models, again suggestive of a pancreatic progenitor cell as the cell of origin [35].

In contrast to the induction of acinar and ductal lesions by RCAS-*PyMT*, introduction of RCAS–*c-myc* producer cells into elastase-*tv-a*, *Ink4a/Arf* null mice caused the formation of pancreatic endocrine neoplasms exclusively. The induced tumors are negative for all acinar-specific markers, and are positive for endocrine markers, such as synaptophysin, insulin, and the endocrine lineage-specific transcription factors Isl1, Nkx2.2, and Pax6. Interestingly, surveys of the pancreata of these mice failed to detect any acinar or ductal pathology. These findings support the hypothesis that the pancreatic tumors induced in this mouse model arise from the transformation of pancreatic progenitor cells that have the capacity to give rise to multiple cell lineages within the pancreas.

Collectively, the data from human pancreatic cancer cell lines and tissues, and from mouse models of the disease, demonstrate that pancreatic cancer initiation and progression involve the activation of signaling pathways and the expression of genes involved in pancreas development. They further raise the possibility that pancreatic tumors arise, at least in some instances, from the transformation of pancreas progenitor cells. Further studies are required to confirm the validity of this intriguing hypothesis.

References

[1] Edlund H. Pancreatic organogenesis: developmental mechanisms and implications for therapy. Nat Rev Genet 2002;3:524–32.

[2] Kim SK, Hebrok M. Intercellular signals regulating pancreas development and function. Genes Dev 2001;15:111–27.

[3] Jensen J, Pedersen EE, Galante P, et al. Control of endodermal endocrine development by Hes-1. Nat Genet 2000;24:36–44.

[4] Apelqvist A, Li H, Sommer L, et al. Notch signalling controls pancreatic cell differentiation. Nature 1999;400:877–81.

[5] Murtaugh LC, Stanger BZ, Kwan KM, et al. Notch signaling controls multiple steps of pancreatic differentiation. Proc Natl Acad Sci U S A 2003;100:14920–5.

[6] Berman DM, Karhadkar SS, Maitra A, et al. Widespread requirement for hedgehog ligand stimulation in growth of digestive tract tumours. Nature 2003;425:846–51.

[7] Thayer SP, di Magliano MP, Heiser PW, et al. Hedgehog is an early and late mediator of pancreatic cancer tumorigenesis. Nature 2003;425:851–6.

[8] Miyamoto Y, Maitra A, Ghosh B, et al. Notch mediates TGF alpha-induced changes in epithelial differentiation during pancreatic tumorigenesis. Cancer Cell 2003;3:565–76.

[9] Jonsson J, Carlsson L, Edlund T, et al. Insulin-promoter-factor 1 is required for pancreas development in mice. Nature 1994;371:606–9.

[10] Offield MF, Jetton TL, Labosky PA, et al. PDX-1 is required for pancreatic outgrowth and differentiation of the rostral duodenum. Development 1996;122:983–95.

[11] Stoffers DA, Ferrer J, Clarke WL, et al. Early-onset type-II diabetes mellitus (MODY4) linked to IPF1. Nat Genet 1997;17:138–9.

[12] Kawaguchi Y, Cooper B, Gannon M, et al. The role of the transcriptional regulator Ptf1a in converting intestinal to pancreatic progenitors. Nat Genet 2002;32:128–34.

[13] Krapp A, Knofler M, Ledermann B, et al. The bHLH protein PTF1-p48 is essential for the formation of the exocrine and the correct spatial organization of the endocrine pancreas. Genes Dev 1998;12:3752–63.

[14] Gradwohl G, Dierich A, LeMeur M, et al. Neurogenin3 is required for the development of the four endocrine cell lineages of the pancreas. Proc Natl Acad Sci U S A 2000;97:1607–11.

[15] Gu G, Dubauskaite J, Melton DA. Direct evidence for the pancreatic lineage: NGN3 + cells are islet progenitors and are distinct from duct progenitors. Development 2002;129:2447–57.

[16] Edlund H. Developmental biology of the pancreas. Diabetes 2001;50(Suppl 1):S5–9.

[17] Edlund H. Transcribing pancreas. Diabetes 1998;47:1817–23.

[18] Warshaw AL, Fernandez-del Castillo C. Pancreatic carcinoma. N Engl J Med 1992;326: 455–65.

[19] Moskaluk CA, Kern SE. Molecular genetics of pancreatic cancer. In: Reber HA, editor. Pancreatic cancer. Totowa (NJ): Humana Press; 1998. p. 3–20.

[20] Bardeesy N, DePinho RA. Pancreatic cancer biology and genetics. Nat Rev Cancer 2002;2: 897–909.

[21] Hruban RH, Goggins M, Parsons J, et al. Progression model for pancreatic cancer. Clin Cancer Res 2000;6:2969–72.

[22] Caldas C, Hahn SA, Hruban RH, et al. Detection of K-ras mutations in the stool of patients with pancreatic adenocarcinoma and pancreatic ductal hyperplasia. Cancer Res 1994;54: 3568–73.

[23] Wilentz RE, Geradts J, Maynard R, et al. Inactivation of the p16 (INK4A) tumor-suppressor gene in pancreatic duct lesions: loss of intranuclear expression. Cancer Res 1998;58: 4740–4.

[24] Wilentz RE, Iacobuzio-Donahue CA, Argani P, et al. Loss of expression of Dpc4 in pancreatic intraepithelial neoplasia: evidence that DPC4 inactivation occurs late in neoplastic progression. Cancer Res 2000;60:2002–6.

[25] DiGiuseppe JA, Hruban RH, Goodman SN, et al. Overexpression of p53 protein in adenocarcinoma of the pancreas. Am J Clin Pathol 1994;101:684–8.

[26] Abraham SC, Wu TT, Hruban RH, et al. Genetic and immunohistochemical analysis of pancreatic acinar cell carcinoma: frequent allelic loss on chromosome 11p and alterations in the APC/beta-catenin pathway. Am J Pathol 2002;160:953–62.

[27] Leach SD. Mouse models of pancreatic cancer: the fur is finally flying!. Cancer Cell 2004;5: 7–11.

[28] Hingorani SR, Petricoin EF, Maitra A, et al. Preinvasive and invasive ductal pancreatic cancer and its early detection in the mouse. Cancer Cell 2003;4:437–50.

[29] Hingorani SR, Wang L, Multani AS, et al. Trp53(R172H) and Kras(G12D) cooperate to promote chromosomal instability and widely metastatic pancreatic ductal adenocarcinoma in mice. Cancer Cell 2005;7:469–83.

[30] Aguirre AJ, Bardeesy N, Sinha M, et al. Activated Kras and Ink4a/Arf deficiency cooperate to produce metastatic pancreatic ductal adenocarcinoma. Genes Dev 2003;17:3112–26.

[31] Lewis BC, Klimstra DS, Varmus HE. The *c-myc* and *PyMT* oncogenes induce different tumor types in a somatic mouse model for pancreatic cancer. Genes Dev 2003;17:3127–38.

[32] Bates P, Young JA, Varmus HE. A receptor for subgroup A Rous sarcoma virus is related to the low density lipoprotein receptor. Cell 1993;74:1043–51.

[33] Young JA, Bates P, Varmus HE. Isolation of a chicken gene that confers susceptibility to infection by subgroup A avian leukosis and sarcoma viruses. J Virol 1993;67:1811–6.

[34] Fisher GH, Orsulic S, Holland E, et al. Development of a flexible and specific gene delivery system for production of murine tumor models. Oncogene 1999;18:5253–60.

[35] Wagner M, Luhrs H, Kloppel G, et al. Malignant transformation of duct-like cells originating from acini in transforming growth factor transgenic mice. Gastroenterology 1998;115: 1254–62.

ELSEVIER
SAUNDERS

Endocrinol Metab Clin N Am
35 (2006) 405–415

ENDOCRINOLOGY
AND METABOLISM
CLINICS
OF NORTH AMERICA

Genotype/Phenotype of Familial Pancreatic Cancer

Randall E. Brand, MD[a,b,*], Henry T. Lynch, MD[c]

[a]Department of Medicine, Northwestern University, Feinberg School of Medicine,
Chicago, IL 60611, USA
[b]Section of Gastroenterology, Evanston Northwestern Healthcare,
2100 Pfingsten Road, Glenview, IL 60026, USA
[c]Department of Preventive Medicine/Public Health, Creighton University School of Medicine,
2300 California Plaza, Omaha, NE 68178, USA

Despite our growing understanding regarding the genetic alterations of pancreatic adenocarcinoma, it continues to have the worst prognosis of any major cancer, with an overall 5-year survival rate of less than 5% [1]. In the year 2005, 32,180 new cases of pancreatic cancer and 31,800 deaths were expected [1]. It is estimated that hereditary factors may play a significant role in the development of pancreatic cancer in approximately 5% to 10% of cases [2,3]. Most of these familial aggregations have an autosomal dominant pattern of inheritance [4], whereas other families develop pancreatic cancer associated with known cancer syndromes [5,6]. For most pancreatic cancer kindreds, the responsible germline mutation has not been identified. The goal of this article is to review the challenges in identifying pancreatic cancer–prone families and how environmental factors interact with genetic factors in these families.

Recognition of familial pancreatic cancer

It was first recognized approximately 40 years ago that a subset of pancreatic adenocarcinoma cases had a hereditary component. Lynch [7] first reported in 1967 on the occurrence of pancreatic cancer in the setting of cancer-prone families with a high incidence of adenocarcinoma of multiple anatomic sites. In the early 1970s, there were a few reports of families with a predisposition for developing pancreatic cancer [8,9]. An initial study in 1972 reported an apparent association between hereditary pancreatitis and

---

* Corresponding author. Section of Gastroenterology, Evanston Northwestern Healthcare, 2100 Pfingsten Road, Glenview, IL 60026.
   E-mail address: rbrand@enh.org (R.E. Brand).

0889-8529/06/$ - see front matter © 2006 Elsevier Inc. All rights reserved.
doi:10.1016/j.ecl.2006.02.015 *endo.theclinics.com*

pancreatic adenocarcinoma [8]. In 1973, a family was described in whom four of six siblings developed adenocarcinoma of the pancreas in a setting without a history of any other types of cancer or hereditary pancreatitis [9].

In addition to these and other anecdotal reports of familial aggregation [10–12], further support for the concept of hereditary susceptibility to pancreatic cancer comes from case-control studies. A case-control study performed by Falk and colleagues [13] in Louisiana of 363 subjects with pancreatic cancer and 1234 controls found a more than fivefold risk (odds ratio [OR] = 5.25, 95% confidence interval [CI]: 2.08–13.21) in those individuals with a family history of pancreatic cancer. Furthermore, having a history of any cancer in a first-degree relative also increased one's risk approximately twofold for developing pancreatic cancer (OR = 1.86, 95% CI: 1.42–2.44). A population-based case-control study of pancreatic cancer in French Canadians from Montreal reported a 13-fold difference in the frequency of family history for pancreatic cancer between cases and their controls ($P < .001$) [14]. Among the 179 patients with pancreatic cancer, 14 (7.8%) had a histologically confirmed positive family history of pancreatic cancer as compared with only 1 (0.6%) of 179 controls. In a large population-based case-control study, 484 cases of pancreatic cancer from Detroit, Atlanta, and New Jersey identified through cancer registries were compared with 2099 controls from the general population of these study areas [15]. Similar to previous studies, there was a threefold increased risk (OR = 3.2, 95% CI: 1.8–5.6) associated with a family history of pancreatic cancer. This study also found that a family history of any cancer among first-degree relatives was associated with a significant 30% (OR = 1.3, 95% CI: 1.1–1.6) increased risk of pancreatic cancer.

Hereditary pancreatic cancer syndromes

For most pancreatic cancer–prone families, the responsible germline mutation has not been identified. In a small subset of families, however, pancreatic cancer may also be an integral tumor of recognized inherited syndromes. These hereditary syndromes (and their risk for developing pancreatic adenocarcinoma) include (1) hereditary breast-ovarian cancer (HBOC) syndrome in families with the *BRCA1* and *BRCA2* mutations (three- to fourfold) [16,17], (2) hereditary pancreatitis caused by mutation of the cationic trypsinogen gene (54-fold) [18], (3) Peutz-Jeghers polyposis (> 100-fold) [19], and (4) the subset of familial atypical multiple mole melanoma (FAMMM) syndrome attributable to the *CDKN2A* (*p16*) germline mutation (13–52-fold) [20,21]. For most pancreatic cancer kindreds, the responsible germline mutation has not been identified.

Identifying familial pancreatic cancer families

Unlike many cancers, there is no widely accepted formal definition of hereditary pancreatic adenocarcinoma. Furthermore, there are no standardized clinical criteria that can be used to identify families at high risk for pancreatic cancer. As discussed elsewhere in this article, this is partially attributable to our inability to differentiate a hereditary pancreatic cancer from a sporadic cancer on the basis of the clinical presentation or histologic findings. Many centers define familial pancreatic cancer narrowly as two or more first-degree relatives with pancreatic cancer. It is our belief, however, that the definition must be broad enough to allow identification of the aforementioned syndromes that include pancreatic cancer. Although it is often necessary in research settings to be stricter in defining familial pancreatic cancer, it is the authors' belief that many pancreatic cancer cases are genetic in etiology, based not on a classic autosomal inherited pattern but rather on inherited susceptibility factors. Further, one must always search for cancer of all anatomic sites when assessing a pedigree's significance or demonstrating a hereditary phenomenon.

As shown in Fig. 1, we hypothesize that there is a spectrum of cases that are genetically based. It is easy to accept the genetic basis in those individuals having one, two, or three or more first-degree relatives affected with pancreatic cancer, based on a study from the Johns Hopkins National Familial Pancreas Tumor Registry [22]. This important study, which defined pancreatic cancer–prone families as having at least two first-degree relatives with pancreatic cancer, found that among unaffected first-degree relatives, there was a ninefold risk for developing pancreatic cancer. As expected, the number of affected individuals in the family factored into the magnitude of this increased risk, with those individuals with three or more first-degree relatives having a 32-fold increased risk for developing pancreatic cancer, whereas a 6.4-fold risk and a 4.6-fold risk were observed for individuals with two or one first-degree relatives, respectively.

Genotypic and phenotypic variation in hereditary cancer syndromes must be given consideration when evaluating pancreatic cancer–prone syndrome pedigrees. As mentioned in the previous section, the risk for developing pancreatic cancer is variable, ranging from greater than 100-fold for Peutz-Jeghers syndrome to a modest 1.5-fold in Lynch syndrome [19,23]. The diagnosis of familial pancreatic cancer in a variety of syndromes requires knowledge of its heterogeneity; each with multiple organ sites that are integral for

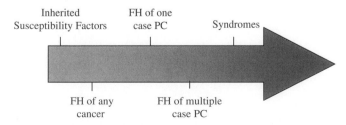

Fig. 1. How many cases are actually of genetic etiology? FH, family history; PC, pancreatic cancer.

pancreatic cancer association must be considered. The challenge is the fact that pancreatic cancer may occur only infrequently in each of these hereditary cancer syndromes in accord with reduced penetrance of the deleterious mutations. Nevertheless, their presence in these disorders is clearly integral in that they significantly exceed population expectations.

The review of the following pedigrees demonstrates the importance of obtaining a complete medical history. Fig. 2 shows a pedigree from a FAMMM family found to have a p16 germline mutation. If one only looked at the subset of the kindred (II-2 and her progeny), he or she would not appreciate the occurrence of pancreatic cancer (II-5, III-15) or earlier age melanoma (III-15, III-16). Fig. 3 shows an example of a BRCA2 family. This pedigree reveals cases of pancreatic cancer and early age onset breast cancer extended over multiple generations. The last pedigree from Fig. 4 shows multiple cases of pancreatic cancer that do not seem to be part of a known hereditary syndrome.

It has been suggested that cancer susceptibility is a polygenic trait [24]. The occurrences of the previously mentioned high-risk alleles (a highly penetrant allele that is associated with a high likelihood of disease) are rare and are estimated to account for approximately 5% of cancer cases in the general population [24]. Even in the presence of high-risk alleles, it seems that the presence of additional genetic modifiers influences the penetrance of these high-risk alleles. For example, the FAMMM syndrome is an autosomal dominantly inherited disorder with incomplete penetrance. It is characterized by multiple nevi (usually in the hundreds), multiple atypical nevi, and multiple melanomas. In 1990, Bergman and coworkers [25] reported a significantly increased risk of pancreatic cancer in a subset of FAMMM kindreds. Pancreatic adenocarcinoma showed a standard incidence ratio of 13.4 in 200 individuals from nine Dutch families. Other types of gastrointestinal tract

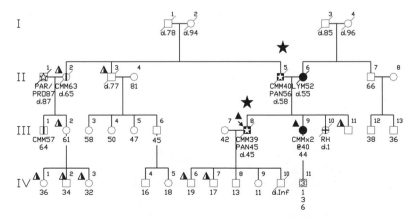

Fig. 2. Pedigree of a FAMMM kindred. Arrow, proband; slashed line, dead; □, male; ○, female; ■, verified cancer; ▲, individual also has melanoma; ★, pancreatic cancer case; ▨, cancer verified by review of medical records or death certificates; ▲, individuals have multiple nevi.

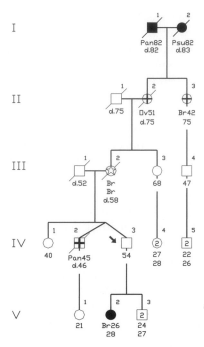

Fig. 3. Pedigree of a BRCA2 family. Arrow, proband; slashed line, dead; □, male; ○, female; ■, verified cancer; ▲, individual also has melanoma; ★, pancreatic cancer case; ⊠, cancer verified by review of medical records or death certificates; ▲, individuals have multiple nevi.

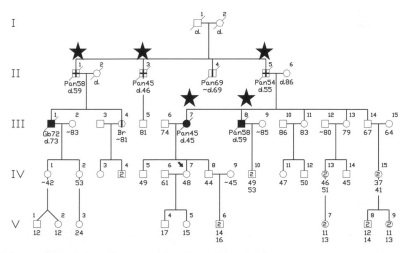

Fig. 4. Pedigree shows multiple cases with pancreatic adenocarcinoma. Arrow, proband; slashed line, dead; □, male; ○, female; ■, verified cancer; ▲, individual also has melanoma; ★, pancreatic cancer case; ⊠, cancer verified by review of medical records or death certificates; ▲, individuals have multiple nevi.

cancer were also found in excess in these nine families, with a standard incidence ratio of 3.3. Further analysis of the kindreds showed that all cases of pancreatic carcinoma occurred in just three of the nine families.

After identification of mutations in the *CDKN2* gene that impaired the function of the p16 protein in FAMMM kindreds, a subsequent study of these same Dutch kindreds [26] demonstrated that those three families with pancreatic cancer had a 19–base pair (bp) germline deletion in the *CDKN2* gene. The importance of the *CDKN2* mutation in the development of pancreatic cancer in these families was confirmed by the finding of a mutated allele and the loss of the wild-type allele in the primary pancreatic tumor tissue from an individual who was a carrier of the *CDKN2* mutation. It was noteworthy that in three of the nine families with FAMMM that were sufficiently large to express the gastrointestinal cancer trait, the same 19-bp deletion in the *CDKN2* gene was identified in the absence of any excess incidence of systemic cancers. Another study suggests that only approximately one third of families with a mutation in the *CDKN2* gene are observed to have cases of pancreatic cancer [27]. These observations indicate that in addition to the type of *p16* mutation, other factors or genes likely influence the development of pancreatic cancer in these families. Similar findings have been seen in other cancers, such as breast cancer [28], supporting the finding that even in individuals with high-risk alleles, cancer susceptibility is a polygenic trait [24].

Further evidence for the presence of cancer susceptibility genes comes from the aforementioned case-control studies, which have demonstrated a modest (approximately twofold) increased risk for pancreatic cancer in those individuals with a family history of any cancer and the association of genetic polymorphisms with a risk of pancreatic cancer. Recent evidence suggests that 5,10-methylenetetrahydrofolate reductase (*MTHFR*) polymorphisms modify the risk of developing pancreatic cancer [29]. Specifically, the 667TT genotype was found to confer an approximately twofold statistically significant increased risk for pancreatic cancer as compared with the CC/CT genotypes. Additionally, certain polymorphisms in the phase II detoxifying enzymes, uridine 5′-diphosphate glucuronosyltransferases (UGTs), have been associated with a higher risk for pancreatic cancer development [30]. Ockenga and colleagues [30] have shown a twofold increased risk for pancreatic adenocarcinoma in individuals with the polymorphism UGT1A7*3, which encodes for a protein that has a significant decrease in detoxification activity.

Our inability to identify familial pancreatic cancer cases based on the clinical presentation and histologic findings has been suggested on the basis of studies from several pancreatic cancer–prone registries. Lynch and coworkers [4] first reported in 1990 on 18 families in which pancreatic cancer occurred in two or more first-degree relatives. No differences in the observed sex ratio (43% female, 57% male), age of onset (median = 70 years, range: 46–94 years), histologic type, or length of survival in the hereditary pancreatic cancer cases were found when they were compared with a large nonfamilial series. Limitations of this study were its small numbers and lack of a population-based case-control design. Results comparable to those of this study by Lynch and coworkers [4] regarding age of onset were reported by Hruban and colleagues [6] when they examined data from the index cases of 212 kindreds enrolled in their National Familial Pancreas Tumor Registry. They defined familial pancreatic cancer cases as those patients with pancreatic cancer and at least one first-degree relative with pancreatic cancer and sporadic pancreatic cancer cases as those patients with pancreatic cancer and no first-degree relatives with pancreatic cancer. Eighty patients met the criteria for familial pancreas cancer, and 132 patients met the criteria for sporadic pancreatic cancer. Similar to the study by Lynch and coworkers [4], no difference was observed in age of onset between the familial and sporadic cases, with both groups having a mean age of 65 years, with a range of 31 to 92 years and 32 to 85 years, respectively.

The age at diagnosis may suggest a genetic etiology in a subset of patients based on a literature review of ductal adenocarcinoma in patients younger than the age of 40 years, however [31]. This review of 63 publications involving more than 6 patients found that only 20 of a reported 71 cases of pancreatic carcinoma could be classified reliably as ductal adenocarcinoma. Of these 20 patients, 7 (35%) reportedly had an identifiable genetic risk factor. There were 3 patients with a hereditary pancreatic cancer syndrome, 2 with Peutz-Jeghers syndrome, 1 with hereditary nonpolyposis colorectal cancer (HNPCC), and 1 with juvenile polyposis. Limitations of this study, such as its small sample size and the potential bias on types of cases reported in the literature, make it difficult to draw a meaningful conclusion. Support for this last statement comes from the same study. The investigators reviewed their own files for pancreatic adenocarcinoma and only found 10 patients younger than 40 years of age from a total of 439 cases, for a relative frequency of 0.3%; importantly, after review of the family histories of these patients, they did not find an obvious hereditary background in any of these patients. A recent retrospective study from Roswell Park Cancer Institute in New York compared 30 patients in a familial cohort based on their having at least one first-degree relative with documented pancreatic cancer with 796 patients in a sporadic cohort [32]. A statistically significant difference was seen in the familial cohort in regard to age of diagnosis, with 36% of diagnoses occurring in patients less than 50 years old as compared with 18.3% in the sporadic cohort. One must recognize that there was a greater proportion of smokers in the familial cohort (87% versus 66%; $P = .06$), however. This fact is important, because Rulyak and colleagues [33] have demonstrated that pancreatic cancer developed approximately 10 years earlier in smokers as compared with nonsmokers in members of pancreatic cancer–prone families.

Because there are no specific clinical or pathologic criteria available to identify high-risk families reliably, the only means at the present time is by obtaining a complete family history. There is a spectrum of genetic factors ranging from high-risk mutations to genetic polymorphisms that predispose individuals to developing pancreatic cancer. Presently, with a good family history, it is possible to identify those families with an excess of pancreatic cancer and those with syndromes associated with an increased risk for developing pancreatic cancer. More challenging is the identification of those genetic polymorphisms in the general population that affect one's risk for developing pancreatic cancer and how to incorporate this information, analogous to breast cancer [34], into different models for assessing the genetic component of pancreatic cancer risk.

Factors having an impact on phenotype of familial pancreatic cancer

Phenotypic expression of pancreatic cancer in these high-risk families is dependent not only on the genetic variables but on nongenetic factors. The single nonhereditary risk factor consistently linked to pancreatic adenocarcinoma is cigarette smoking (1.5–5.5-fold) [35,36]. There is a need to recognize the interactions between nonhereditary factors and hereditary factors on pancreatic cancer development, including incidence and age of onset. For example, cigarette smoking enhances pancreatic cancer risk in individuals with hereditary pancreatitis from 54-fold to 154-fold as compared with the general population [37]. Moreover, in these patients, cancer developed, on average, 20 years earlier in smokers than in nonsmokers. The previously discussed nested case-control study of pancreatic cancer–prone families with two or more members with pancreatic cancer found the greatest risk for pancreatic cancer in smokers less than 50 years of age (OR = 7.6) or in male family members (OR = 5.2) [33].

Additionally, smoking seems to interact with the risk for developing pancreatic cancer in less well-defined genetic susceptibility situations. As stated previously, there is an association between the polymorphism UGT1A7*3 and pancreatic adenocarcinoma [30]. The UGT family of proteins is involved in cellular protection and the detoxification of a variety of compounds, including drugs, dietary byproducts, and tobacco-borne toxicants. The UGT1A7*3 polymorphism causes low detoxification activity. An allelic frequency of 0.34 was found for the UGT1A7*3 polymorphism in pancreatic cancer cases as compared with 0.21 in a normal control group, leading to an OR of 1.98 (95% CI: 1.24–3.14). It is worth mentioning that the association between UGT1A7*3 and smoking was particularly strong in younger patients. Five of the 52 patients with pancreatic adenocarcinoma were younger than 50 years of age, and another 5 patients (total of 10) were younger than 55 years of age. All 10 of these patients were smokers; 4 of the 5 patients younger than 50 years of age had the UGT1A7*3 polymorphism (OR = 5.8, 95% CI: 1.6–21.1), as did 7 of the 10 patients younger than 55 years of age (OR = 4.7, 95% CI: 1.9–11.8).

Similarly, environmental factors also enhanced the association for pancreatic adenocarcinoma with the previously described *MTHFR* 667TT polymorphism [29]. A multivariate analysis demonstrated that the effect of the 677TT genotype was present in ever alcohol drinkers (OR = 3.16, 95% CI: 1.30–7.69) and ever smokers (OR = 5.53, 95% CI: 2.0–15.3) but not in never alcohol drinkers (OR = 1.42, 95% CI: 0.56–3.62) or never smokers (OR = 0.82, 95% CI: 0.33–2.06). This association was even greater among heavy smokers or heavy alcohol consumers.

Other challenges in high-risk families include better understanding and recognition of the phenotypic variations of cancer presentations that are associated with these pancreatic cancer–prone syndromes. This is well illustrated in an article by Lynch and colleagues [38] describing eight extended *CDKN2A* FAMMM families that also manifested pancreatic cancer in their pedigrees. These families demonstrate the diversity of cancer presentation within and among kindreds. Some families had multiple cases of melanoma, whereas other extended pedigrees only had a single documented case. Age of onset varied, with half of the families having at least one case of pancreatic carcinoma diagnosed in a family member less than 50 years of age. Finally, this report illustrated the spectrum of cancers associated with this mutation, including sarcoma, esophageal carcinoma, and possibly an early-age endometrial carcinoma.

We have previously described points that need to be considered when identifying pancreatic cancer–prone families [39]. In the context of this article, it is warranted to repeat several of them:

1. With the exception of a few syndromes with cutaneous manifestations, such as the Peutz-Jeghers syndrome, FAMMM, and ataxia telangiectasia (all predisposing to pancreatic cancer and all with germline mutations), we are essentially unable to employ premorbid signs of hereditary cancer risk short of a meticulous family history; therein, we must include cancer of all anatomic sites, because variable tumor combinations may enable us to establish the hereditary pancreatic cancer syndrome of concern.

2. Hereditary pancreatitis is the only hereditary pancreatic cancer syndrome that predisposes exclusively to pancreatic cancer. The so-called "site-specific" pancreatic cancer families, in the absence of hereditary pancreatitis, require more medical genetic evaluation before these cases can be considered site specific.

3. Pattern recognition, defined as a more global view of the pedigree, giving due consideration to factors inclusive of early age of onset, multiple primary cancers, transmission of cancer in accord with a likely Mendelian inheritance pattern, and differences in gene penetrance, is particularly helpful in the diagnosis of hereditary forms of pancreatic carcinoma. Pattern recognition should thus embrace the known tumor spectrum for a particular pancreatic cancer–prone syndrome as well as extracancer phenotypic features. Examples of these extracancer phenotypic features include the mucocutaneous features of Peutz-Jeghers

syndrome and multiple cutaneous nevi, with a large size, irregular contours, and variegation in coloration, of the FAMMM syndrome.

Summary

The challenges in defining pancreatic cancer are great because of our recognition that even sporadic cancer cases are likely at the end of a spectrum, where the individual genetic etiologies are more difficult to identify [24]. A polygenic model that takes into account nongenetic risk factors, most notably smoking, seems to be most appropriate for pancreatic cancer. With few exceptions (eg, hereditary pancreatitis), Mendelian inherited pancreatic cancer–prone syndromes involve a variety of cancers of different anatomic sites, wherein their phenotypic and genotypic heterogeneity may be extant.

References

[1] American Cancer Society. Cancer facts and figures 2005. Atlanta (GA): American Cancer Society; 2005.

[2] Brand R, Lynch HT. Hereditary pancreatic adenocarcinoma: a clinical perspective. Med Clin North Am 2000;84(3):665–75.

[3] Lynch HT, Smyrk T, Kern SE, et al. Familial pancreatic cancer: a review. Semin Oncol 1996; 23:251–75.

[4] Lynch HT, Fitzsimmons ML, Smyrk TC, et al. Familial pancreatic cancer: clinicopathologic study of 18 nuclear families. Am J Gastroenterol 1990;85:54–60.

[5] Lynch HT. Genetics and pancreatic cancer. Arch Surg 1994;129(3):266–8.

[6] Hruban RH, Petersen GM, Ha PK, et al. Genetics of pancreatic cancer. From genes to families. Surg Oncol Clin N Am 1998;7(1):1–23.

[7] Lynch HT. "Cancer families": adenocarcinomas (endometrial and colon carcinomas) and multiple primary malignant neoplasms. Recent Results Cancer Res 1967;12:125–42.

[8] Castleman B, Scully RE, McNeely BU. Case records of the Massachusetts General Hospital. N Engl J Med 1972;286:1353–9.

[9] MacDermott RP, Kramer P. Adenocarcinoma of the pancreas in four siblings. Gastroenterology 1973;65:137–9.

[10] Reimer RR, Fraumeni JF Jr, Ozols RF, et al. Pancreatic cancer in father and son [letter]. Lancet 1977;1:911.

[11] Danes BS, Lynch HT. A familial aggregation of pancreatic cancer: an in vitro study. JAMA 1982;247:2798–802.

[12] Ehrenthal D, Haeger L, Griffin T, et al. Familial pancreatic adenocarcinoma in three generations: a case report and a review of the literature. Cancer 1987;59:1661–4.

[13] Falk T, Pickle LW, Fontham ET, et al. Life-style risk factors for pancreatic cancer in Louisiana: a case-control study. Am J Epidemiol 1988;18:324–36.

[14] Ghadirian P, Boyle P, Simard A, et al. Reported family aggregation of pancreatic cancer within a population-based case-control study in Francophone Community in Montreal, Canada. Int J Pancreatol 1991;10:183–96.

[15] Silverman DT, Schiffman M, Everhart J, et al. Diabetes mellitus, other medical conditions and familial history of cancer as risk factors for pancreatic cancer. Br J Cancer 1999;80: 1830–7.

[16] Brose MS, Rebbeck TR, Calzone KA, et al. Cancer risk estimates for BRCA1 mutation carriers identified in a risk evaluation program. J Natl Cancer Inst 2002;94:1365–72.

[17] Breast Cancer Linkage Consortium. Cancer risks in BRCA2 mutation carriers. The Breast Cancer Linkage Consortium. J Natl Cancer Inst 1999;91:1310–6.

[18] Lowenfels AB, Maisonneuve P, DiMagno EP, et al. Hereditary pancreatitis and the risk of pancreatic cancer. International Hereditary Pancreatitis Study Group. J Natl Cancer Inst 1997;89:442–6.

[19] Giardiello FM, Brensinger JD, Tersmette AC, et al. Very high risk of cancer in familial Peutz-Jeghers syndrome. Gastroenterology 2000;119:1447–53.

[20] Goldstein AM, Fraser MC, Struewing JP, et al. Increased risk of pancreatic cancer in melanoma-prone kindreds with p16INK4 mutations. N Engl J Med 1995;333:970–4.

[21] Goldstein AM, Struewing JP, Fraser MC, et al. Prospective risk of cancer in CDKN2A germline mutation carriers. J Med Genet 2004;41:421–4.

[22] Klein AP, Brune KA, Petersen GM, et al. Prospective risk of pancreatic cancer in familial pancreatic cancer kindreds. Cancer Res 2004;64:2634–8.

[23] Watson P, Lynch HT. Extracolonic cancer in hereditary nonpolyposis colorectal cancer. Cancer 1993;71:677–85.

[24] Mohrenweiser HW, Wilson DM, Jones IM. Challenges and complexities in estimating both the functional impact and the disease risk associated with the extensive genetic variation in human DNA repair genes. Mutat Res 2003;526:93–125.

[25] Bergman W, Watson P, de Jong J, et al. Systemic cancer and the FAMMM syndrome. Br J Cancer 1990;61:932–6.

[26] Gruis NA, Sandkuijl LA, van der Velden PA, et al. CDKN2 explains part of the clinical phenotype in Dutch familial atypical multiple-mole melanoma (FAMMM) syndrome families. Melanoma Res 1995;5:169–77.

[27] Vasen HF, Gruis NA, Frants RR, et al. Risk of developing pancreatic cancer in families with familial atypical multiple mole melanoma associated with a specific 19 deletion of *p16* (*p16-LEIDEN*). Int J Cancer 2000;87:809–11.

[28] Begg CB. On the use of familial aggregation in population-based case probands for calculating penetrance. J Natl Cancer Inst 2002;94:1221–6.

[29] Li D, Ahmed M, Li Y, et al. 5,10-Methylenetetrahydrofolate reductase polymorphisms and the risk of pancreatic cancer. Cancer Epidemiol Biomarkers Prev 2005;14(6):1470–6.

[30] Ockenga J, Vogel A, Teich N, et al. UDP glucuronosyltransferase (UGT1A7) gene polymorphisms increase the risk of chronic pancreatitis and pancreatic cancer. Gastroenterology 2003;124:1802–8.

[31] Luttges J, Stigge C, Pacena M, et al. Rare ductal adenocarcinoma of the pancreas in patients younger than age 40 years. Cancer 2004;100(1):173–82.

[32] James TA, Sheldon DG, Rajput A, et al. Risk factors associated with earlier age of onset in familial pancreatic carcinoma. Cancer 2004;101 2722–2.

[33] Rulyak SJ, Lowenfels AB, Maisonneuve P, et al. Risk factors for the development of pancreatic cancer in familial pancreatic cancer kindreds. Gastroenterology 2003;124:1292–9.

[34] Pharoah PD, Antoniou A, Bobrow M, et al. Polygenic susceptibility to breast cancer and implications for prevention. Nat Genet 2002;31:33–6.

[35] Fuchs CS, Colditz GA, Stamper MJ, et al. A prospective study of cigarette smoking and the risk of pancreatic cancer. Arch Intern Med 1996;156(19):2255–60.

[36] Gold EB, Goldin SB. Epidemiology of and risk factors for pancreatic cancer. Surg Oncol Clin N Am 1998;7:67–91.

[37] Lowenfels AB, Maisonneuve P, Whitcomb DC, et al. Cigarette smoking as a risk factor for pancreatic cancer in patients with hereditary pancreatitis. JAMA 2001;286:169–70.

[38] Lynch HT, Brand RE, Hogg D, et al. Phenotypic variation in eight extended *CDKN2A* germline mutation familial atypical multiple mole melanoma-pancreatic carcinoma-prone families. Cancer 2002;94:84–96.

[39] Brand RE, Lynch HT. Identification of high-risk pancreatic cancer-prone families. Gastroenterol Clin North Am 2004;33:907–18.

ELSEVIER
SAUNDERS

Endocrinol Metab Clin N Am
35 (2006) 417–430

ENDOCRINOLOGY
AND METABOLISM
CLINICS
OF NORTH AMERICA

Familial Pancreatic Cancer Syndromes

Nils Habbe, MD[a], Peter Langer, MD[a],
Mercedes Sina-Frey, MD[b], Detlef K. Bartsch, MD[c],*

[a]Department of Surgery, Philipps-University Marburg, Baldiger Strasse,
Marburg 35033, Germany
[b]Institute of Clinical Genetics, Philipps-University Marburg, Bahnhofstrasse 7,
Marburg 35037, Germany
[c]Department of Surgery, Städtische Kliniken Bielefeld-Mitte, Teutoburgerstrasse 50,
Bielefeld 33042, Germany

The existence of hereditary pancreatic cancer (PC) was initially suggested by several case reports of a familial aggregation of ductal pancreatic adenocarcinomas. Until the late 1980s, only case reports have suggested that PC aggregates in some families [1–3]. The first systematic study of a larger cohort of families with PC was published in 1989 [4]. Afterward, several registries for PC families were established in the United States [5] and Europe [6,7] to collect and analyze data on these rare families. Two prospective studies from Sweden and Germany demonstrated a familial aggregation of PC of only 2.7% and 1.9%, respectively, if the strict criteria of confirmation by histology and medical records were used [8,9].

There is much confusion in the literature regarding the use of the terms *familial pancreatic carcinoma* and *hereditary pancreatic carcinoma*, because there is a large phenotypic heterogeneity. The authors believe that a mostly syndrome-specific classification is the only way to separate the different forms of hereditary PC. An inherited predisposition to PC is believed to occur in three distinct clinical settings (Table 1). First, it occurs in hereditary tumor predisposition syndromes that are defined primarily by a clinical phenotype other than PC but are known to be associated with an increased risk of PC. The second setting is hereditary pancreatitis (HP) and cystic fibrosis (CF), in which genetically determined early age onset changes of the pancreas can predispose to the development of PC. In contrast, the term *familial pancreatic cancer* (FPC) is applied by most experts to families with two or

This work was supported by a grant of the Deutsche Krebshilfe (70-3085-Ba4).
* Corresponding author.
E-mail address: detlef.bartsch@sk-bielefeld.de (D.K. Bartsch).

endo.theclinics.com

Table 1
Different settings of hereditary pancreatic cancer

	Gene	Pancreatic cancer risk until 70 years
Tumor syndromes		
Peutz-Jeghers syndrome	LKB1	36%
FAMMM-PC/MPCS	CDKN2a	17%
HBOC	BRCA1/2	3.9–8
HNPCC	MLH1, MSH2	<5%
FAP	APC	<5%
Ataxia teleangiectasia	ATM	<5%
PC/BCC syndrome	?	?
Hereditary parcreatitis	PRSS1, SPINK1	40%
Cystic fibrosis	CFTR	<5%
EPC syndrome	BRCA2, ?	>50%?

Abbreviations: EAMMM-PC/MPCS, familial atypical multiple mole melanoma pancreatic carcinoma; MPCS, melanoma pancreatic carcinoma syndrome; HBOC, hereditary breast and ovarian cancer; FAP, familial adenomatous polyposis; PC/BC, pancreatic carcinoma/basal cell carcinoma syndrome; FPC, familial pancreatic cancer.

more first-degree relatives with PC without fulfilling the criteria of another inherited tumor syndrome.

Hereditary tumor syndromes associated with pancreatic cancer

Peutz-Jeghers syndrome

Peutz-Jeghers syndrome (PJS) is an autosomal dominant tumor syndrome with an incidence of 1 in 25,000. The clinical phenotype consists of multiple hamartomatous intestinal polyps in association with mucocutaneous pigmentations. This disease is caused by germline mutations of the serine/threonine kinase 11 (STK11/LKB1) gene. Patients with PJS have a 132-fold increased risk for developing PC and an estimated lifetime risk of 36% [10–12].

Familial atypical multiple mole melanoma

Familial atypical multiple mole melanoma (FAMMM) is characterized by 50 or more partly dysplastic nevi and malignant melanoma in two or more first- and second-degree relatives. PC is associated with approximately 25% of the FAMMM families. In approximately 50% of FAMMM families with PC, oncogenic germline mutations of the cyclin-dependent kinase 2A (CDKN2A) gene were identified. Conversely, no PC has yet been observed in melanoma-prone kindreds without CDKN2A germline mutations. The penetrance of CDKN2A mutations varies considerably. The metachronous occurrence of malignant melanoma and PC as well as melanoma or PC as the prevailing phenotype has been observed. In FAMMM families, CDKN2A mutation carriers have been shown to have a 13- to 22-fold increased risk for the development of PC [13]. In carriers of a distinct CDKN2A mutation (p16-Leiden), the cumulative risk for the development of PC by the age of 75 years was estimated at 17% [14]. PC has not yet been observed in melanoma-prone kindreds without CDKN2A germline mutations, however.

In 1995, a CDKN2a germline mutation was first identified in a kindred with PC and melanoma that did not exhibit the FAMMM phenotype [15]. Consequently, in other families with PC and melanoma, cosegregating CDKN2a mutations were detected [16–18]. In contrast, CDKN2a mutations have not yet been described in families with FPC [18]. Thus, the joint occurrence of melanoma and PC seems to be a distinct tumor predisposition syndrome and is now called melanoma–pancreatic cancer syndrome (MPCS; OMIM 606719; Fig. 1).

Hereditary breast and ovarian cancer

Hereditary breast and ovarian cancer (HBOC) is mainly caused by germline mutations in the BRCA 1 or BRCA 2 genes. Several reports have revealed evidence for an increased frequency of PC among BRCA1 and BRCA2 families [19–21]. An analysis of 11,847 individuals from 699 families segregating a BRCA1 mutation showed a significantly increased relative risk of 2.26 for the development of PC in BRCA1 mutation carriers [21]. Similar large studies are not available for BRCA2 families. One smaller study showed an estimated relative risk of PC among BRCA2 families of 2.2 [22]. This study also suggested that the elevated risk not only for PC but for colorectal, stomach, and prostate cancer was associated with mutations within the ovarian cancer cluster region (OCCR) of exon 11. In summary, current data from available retrospective studies suggest an increased relative risk for PC between 2 and 5 for BRCA1/BRCA2 mutation carriers from HBOC families [23,24].

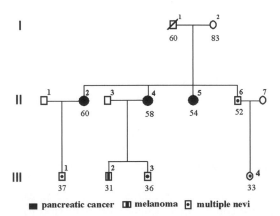

Fig. 1. Pedigree of MPCS family 25-9-0044 of the FaPaCa registry. □, male; ○, female.

Hereditary nonpolyposis colorectal cancer, familial adenomatous polyposis

Although PC is a rare cancer in patients with hereditary nonpolyposis colorectal cancer (HNPCC), HNPCC may predispose affected individuals to PC [25]. HNPCC is caused by germline mutations in one of the mismatch repair (MMR) genes, including hMSH2 and hMLH1 [25–27]. These genes code for proteins that correct the small errors normally occurring during DNA replication. In a Finnish study, 1% of MMR gene mutation carriers developed PC [28]. Furthermore, a few studies have shown that the prevalence of colon cancer is increased in some PC families [5,29]. Therefore, some cases of PC, especially those that develop in patients with a family history of colorectal cancer, may be associated with HNPCC. Overall, for HNPCC, the estimated cumulated risk of PC is thought to be less than 5%.

Familial adenomatous polyposis (FAP) is an autosomal dominant inherited disease in which affected individuals develop hundreds of adenomatous polyps during the second and third decades of life. The syndrome is caused by germline mutations of the APC gene, leading to accelerated tumor initiation. Occasional observations of an increased incidence of PC among FAP families have been reported [30,31]. Because the number of these cases is small, a definitive link between FAP and PC risk cannot be established [32].

Ataxia telangiectasia

Ataxia telangiectasia (AT) is an autosomal recessive inherited disease. The clinical phenotype consists of cerebellar ataxia in combination with oculocutaneous telangiectasia and cellular and humoral immune deficiencies. Germline mutations in the ATM gene are responsible for this syndrome. An increased risk for PC, albeit low, seems to be associated with this disease [33].

Pancreatic cancer and basal cell carcinoma

The joint occurrence of PC and basal cell carcinoma of the skin in three families has recently led to the suggestion that this might represent a rare new tumor syndrome [34]. Four of 70 FPC families of the German National Case Collection of Familial Pancreatic Cancer (FaPaCa) revealed this phenotype (Fig. 2). Further studies are warranted to confirm this potential tumor syndrome and to evaluate the underlying gene defect.

Hereditary pancreatitis and cystic fibrosis

Hereditary pancreatitis is characterized by recurring abdominal pain attacks attributable to acute pancreatitis and progression to chronic pancreatitis with an early onset, often in childhood. The disease is inherited in an

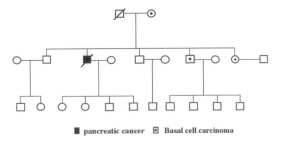

■ pancreatic cancer   ⊡ Basal cell carcinoma

Fig. 2. Pedigree of PC-basal cell carcinoma family 25-9-0032 of the FaPaCa registry. □, male; ○, female; slashed line, deceased.

autosomal dominant fashion, and mutations of the cationic trypsinogen gene (protease serine 1 [PRSS1]) were identified in 70% of cases [35]. The mutations prevent the autolytic inactivation of trypsin; as a result, untimely intra-acinous activation of the zymogene activation cascade occurs. This leads to autodigestion of the pancreas and chronic pancreatitis, which is the long-term stimulus for PC development [35]. In a few other families, germline mutations in the serine protease inhibitor, Kazal type 1 gene (SPINK1), have been found to be associated with HP but may only function as modifier genes [36]. Patients with HP have a relative risk of 100 and a lifetime risk of 40% for the development of PC until the age of 70 years. The risk seems to be further increased in individuals with paternal inheritance of the disease and by cigarette smoking [37–39].

Cystic fibrosis is one of the most common life-shortening inherited disorders. Mutations in the cystic fibrosis transmembrane regulator (CFTR) gene disrupt the localization and function of the cyclic adenosine monophosphate (cAMP)–mediated chloride channel. The CFTR is a cAMP-activated chlorine (Cl)-negative channel expressed in epithelial cells in the airways, pancreas, intestine, and other fluid-transporting tissues. The main pathologic changes of CF result from obstruction of ducts in several organs, including the pancreas, by mucous secretions. There have been a number of reports showing an increased risk for PC in CF patients [40,41]. Because of the overall low frequency of PC reported to date in CF families, it is difficult to estimate the actual contribution of CFTR mutations to the PC risk.

Familial pancreatic cancer syndrome

The previous sections summarize the hereditary syndromes that have a more or less unequivocal association with an increased risk for PC. This section focuses on the most likely heterogeneous group of families with at least two first-degree relatives with confirmed PC that do not fulfill the criteria of other cancer syndromes. These families are currently unified under the term *familial pancreatic carcinoma*. Of note, this definition of FPC has to be regarded as an operational definition, which was suggested by Hruban and colleagues [5], and it is currently used by most researchers in the field. Some groups also use the term *familial pancreatic carcinoma* for families with PC in three or more relatives of any degree [6,25]. A typical FPC family is shown in Fig. 3. Frequently, other tumor types, such as breast, colon, lung, and prostate cancer, can be associated with FPC, causing phenotypic heterogeneity of FPC families (Fig. 4). Clearly, in the future, it would be desirable to define FPC by the distinct genetic alterations responsible for the increased PC risk in these families.

The first systematic study of a larger cohort of FPC families was published by Lynch and coworkers [4] in 1989. Afterward, international and national tumor registries were established to collect data on families so as to determine the characteristics and underlying gene defect(s) of FPC. These include the North American National Familial Pancreatic Tumor Registry (NFPTR), the German National Case Collection of Familial Pancreatic Cancer (FaPaCa), and European Registry of Hereditary Pancreatitis and Familial Pancreatic Cancer (EUROPAC) [5–7]. The comprehensive clinical and genetic analysis of FPC families within these registries came up with some important data about FPC. The vertical pattern of cancer observed in most FPC families is consistent with an autosomal dominant trait. One prospective study of the NFPTR determined the risk for developing PC among first-degree relatives of a PC patient to be 18-fold in kindreds with two affected family members and as high as 57-fold in kindreds with three or more affected family members [42]. This relatively high risk was confirmed in a recent follow-up study of the same group [43]. A study of EUROPAC and FaPaCa registries on 106 FPC families, including 80 parent-child pairs, provides the first strong evidence for anticipation in FPC, because patients in younger generations died approximately 10 years earlier than their affected parent [44]. It has also been shown that resected pancreata of FPC patients often reveal multifocal dysplasias or carcinomas, which is consistent with an inherited disease.

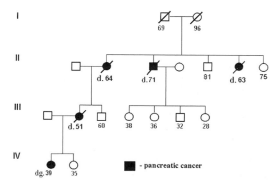

Fig. 3. Pedigree of FPC family 25-5-11 of the FaPaCa registry. D. number, age of death; dg. number, age of diagnosis (year); □, male; ○, female.

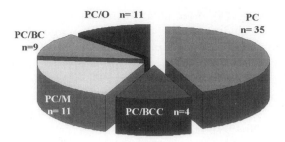

Fig. 4. Tumor spectrum of FPC families of the FaPaCa registry. PC, pancreatic cancer only; PC/BCC, pancreatic cancer and basal cell carcinoma; PC/BC, pancreatic cancer and breast cancer; PC/M, pancreatic cancer and melanoma; PC/O, pancreatic cancer and other cancers (eg, prostate, lung, colon).

Genetic studies in familial pancreatic cancer syndrome

In contrast to studies in other hereditary tumor syndromes, such as HNPCC and FAP, which were rewarded by identifying major tumor genes, similar success has not yet been granted to the researchers searching for the "major" FPC gene(s). One reason might be that FPC comprises a genetic rather heterogeneous group and large numbers of families with many affected family members over several generations are rare for the identification of chromosomal loci that may be linked to the disease using classic approaches, such as linkage analysis. Thus, the major underlying gene defect(s) is still unknown in FPC.

There has been one segregation analysis study suggesting that there is a rare major gene influencing the susceptibility to PC [45]. With respect to this study, it is of note that there has been a recent report of linkage to chromosome 4q32-34 of a younger onset PC and endocrine pancreatic insufficiency phenotype in a single kindred [46]. An allelotype analysis of 77 European FPC families could not confirm this potential linkage, suggesting that 4q32-34 does not contain a major locus for European FPC families (Detlef K. Bartsch, MD, unpublished data, 2006).

Studies testing the hypothesis that FPC may be caused by germline mutations in one of the major sporadic PC tumor suppressor genes (TP53, MADH4/DPC4, and CDKN2a) have so far failed to detect inactivating mutations in FPC patients [18,47,48]. In addition, none or only a few indeterminable germline alterations could be identified in other candidate genes, such as STK11/LKB1, RNASEL, and CHEK2 [49–51]. Similarly, the published mutation analyses of the so-called "minor" genes came up negative for the tested genes MAP2K4, ACVR1B/ALK4, and ACVR2 [48]. The significance of the NOD23020insC mutation remains unclear because it was detected in 2 (7%) of 31 FPC patients and in 3% of controls [52]. Mutations in the Fanconi genes FANCC and FANCG were identified in two cases of sporadic PC with an early onset of the disease (<50 years). In a further analysis of these genes in 38 FPC families, however, no germline mutations could be identified [53,54]. A recent study postulated an association between familial cancer, including a few cases of PC, and the polymorphism Trp149X of the ARLTS1 gene [55]. We could not identify this or other relevant ARLTS1 gene alterations in 15 FPC index patients, however, suggesting no important role of this gene for FPC (Detlef K. Bartsch, MD, unpublished data, 2006).

To date, the only exception to the rather disappointing outcome of these numerous mutation analyses is BRCA2. BRCA2 was initially considered to be a candidate pancreas tumor suppressor gene; before its discovery, a homozygous deletion at 13q12.3 was reported in PC by Schutte and coworkers [56], which aided in the cloning of the BRCA2 gene. There are now two available studies on a total of 55 families reporting BRCA2 germline mutations in the setting of FPC. The study by Murphy and colleagues [48] reported BRCA2 germ line mutations in 5 (17.2%) of 29 families with three or more relatives with PC. Of note, 3 of the 5 families reported to have BRCA2 germline mutations were of Ashkenazi Jewish descent and harbored the common 6174delT frameshift mutation previously found in "sporadic" PC cases. The study by Hahn and colleagues [57] included families with two or more first-degree relatives with histologically confirmed PC. This led to the discovery of a BRCA2 germline in 4 (15%) of 26 European families of non-Jewish descent, including one BRCA2 mutation-positive family with only two first-degree relatives with PC. The 6174delT mutation was not identified in the European families. In addition, a recent study has demonstrated that the BRCA2 K3326X alteration was significantly more prevalent in individuals with FPC (5.6%) than in controls (1.2%; $P < .01$) and therefore might contribute to the risk of PC [58]. These data make BRCA2 germline mutations the most frequent inherited genetic alteration yet identified in FPC.

Surveillance strategies and treatment options in hereditary pancreatic cancer

For several hereditary tumor syndromes, such as multiple endocrine neoplasia type 2 and FAP, the causative germline mutations have been identified, providing options for preventive screening and prophylactic treatment. Unfortunately, this is not yet the case for hereditary PC. For most settings of hereditary PC, the penetrance is not defined and the underlying gene defect(s) is unknown in most of the large group of FPC families. The appropriate classification of a family to a tumor syndrome predisposing to PC is prerequisite to the most realistic determination of the risk to family members and the consequences for their further medical care, however. The heterogeneity of tumor predisposition syndromes with a high risk of PC requires a thorough analysis of the family tree over at least three generations, including confirmation of the diagnoses by medical records and histology.

Based on the diagnosis of a hereditary disease, an approximate estimation of an individual's risk of PC can be made.

According to a consensus conference of experts, high-risk individuals should be recommended for participation in controlled screening programs [59]. Ideally, screening should be performed in expert centers within multidisciplinary institutional review board–approved protocols, allowing a precise evaluation of the screening program with special attention to outcome. High-risk individuals ($\geq$10-fold risk) for the development of PC include first-degree relatives of an affected patient of a FPC family as well as carriers of CDKN2a mutations of an MPCS kindred (Box 1). The screening should start at least 10 years before the youngest age of onset in the family or by the age of 40 years. Nevertheless, there are some strong limitations regarding PC screening. Reliable diagnostic markers or imaging procedures for the detection of a small PC or, even better, its precursor lesions are currently not available. In addition, it remains to be proven that the early detection of PC or its precursor lesions (PanIN2b and PanIN3) can prolong an individual's life expectancy. There are early reports recommending that high-risk family members of FPC families might benefit from close surveillance, however. In a recent study, 12 of 35 high-risk persons were thought to have manifested dysplasia of the pancreas on the basis of their clinical history, coupled with subtle abnormalities on imaging (CT, endoscopic ultrasound [EUS], and endoscopic retrograde cholangiopancreatography [ERCP]), and they underwent a total pancreatectomy. Histopathologic examination of all 12 specimens demonstrated pancreatic dysplasia (mostly PanIN2) but no PC. There has been no perioperative mortality, and none of these 12 patients developed PC during a follow-up period up to 48 months [60]. Using an EUS-based approach, Canto and coworkers [61] screened 38 high-risk individuals of 17 FPC families initially by EUS and CT, followed by ERCP in case of a detected suspicious lesion. Six of these patients had suspicious lesions on EUS with fine-needle aspiration (FNA) and ERCP; thus, limited pancreatic

---

Box 1. Definition of high-risk individuals who should be recommended for participation in controlled PC screening programs

- Individuals with at least two first-degree relatives with PC
- Individuals with at least three relatives with PC independent of degree
- BRCA2 mutation carriers with at least one PC case in a first- or second-degree relative
- CDKN2a mutation carriers of a family with MPCS
- Individuals with PJS
- Individuals with HP

resections were performed in these individuals. Histopathologic analysis revealed PC in 1 patient, benign serous cystadenoma in 2 patients, an intraductal papillary mucinous tumor (IPMT) in 1 patient, and nonneoplastic lesions in 2 patients. All specimens revealed PanIN1A and PanIN1b lesions. Hence, the diagnostic yield for detecting clinically significant pancreatic neoplasms was 5.3% (2 of 38 cases). The authors concluded that EUS-based screening of asymptomatic high-risk individuals can detect prevalent resectable pancreatic neoplasias but that false-positive diagnoses also occur. These results were confirmed by data of the FaPaCa registry [62]. The PC screening (Fig. 5) in 39 high-risk individuals (18 mutation carriers) with EUS and MRI revealed mostly single lesions in 13 (33%) of 39 persons. Therefore, limited pancreatic resection has not yet been performed in 4 individuals, whereas the other 9 persons are under close surveillance. Histopathologic examination showed pancreatic lipoma in 1 patient, focal fibrosis with PanIN1b lesions in 2 patients, and a ductal epithelial cyst with PanIN1b lesion in 1 patient.

It seems reasonable to proceed to surgery once dysplastic or tumorous lesions in the pancreas have been diagnosed by imaging in a high-risk individual. Previously, we and others stated that the multifocal nature of dysplastic lesions in the setting of FPC precludes any type of operation that would leave behind pancreatic tissue [7,8,60]. Based on the aforementioned data, we changed our strategy to avoid overtreatment and the significant drawbacks of a total pancreatectomy, including Briddles' diabetes. We now first resect the part of the pancreas that contains the suspicious lesion and perform testing on a frozen section. If examination of the frozen section leads to a diagnosis of PC or high-grade PanIN lesions, we then proceed to a total pancreatectomy (otherwise not). Currently, a prophylactic pancreatectomy cannot be recommended in asymptomatic high-risk patients given the

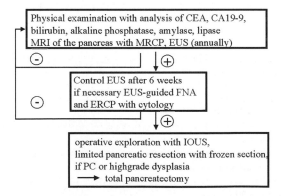

Fig. 5. Screening program of the FaPaCa registry for high-risk individuals of FPC kindreds. CEA, carcinoembryonic antigen; MRCP, magnetic resonance cholangiopancreatography; IOUS, intraoperative ultrasound.

significant morbidity of the procedure and the unknown penetrance of PC in the different settings of inherited PC.

Summary

Hereditary PC is rare and extremely heterogeneous, and it accounts for approximately 2% of all PC cases. The major component of hereditary PC is the FPC syndrome. Although up to 20% of hereditary PC cases are associated with germline mutations in the BRCA2, CDKN2A, PRSS1, STK11, or MMR gene, the major underlying gene defect(s) is still unknown.

Although hereditary PC is rare, the data on PC families that have been collected by various study groups worldwide provide a unique opportunity to evaluate the natural history, causative gene alterations, new diagnosis, and chemoprevention strategies as well as treatment modalities. More international collaboration may increase the chances of identifying one or more genes responsible for FPC. In addition, screening and treatment strategies could be assessed more reliably. High-risk individuals in FPC families would greatly benefit from new methods that enable the detection of PC at its earliest possible stage, thus providing a chance for cure. Such knowledge might also be useful in improving the diagnosis and prognosis of the much more common sporadic form of PC.

References

[1] Ehrenthal D, Haeger L, Griffin T, et al. Familial pancreatic adenocarcinoma in three generations. A case report and a review of the literature. Cancer 1987;59(9):1661–4.
[2] MacDermott RP, Kramer P. Adenocarcinoma of the pancreas in four siblings. Gastroenterology 1973;65(1):137–9.
[3] Reimer RR, Fraumeni JF Jr, Ozols RF, et al. Pancreatic cancer in father and son [letter]. Lancet 1977;1(8017):911.
[4] Lynch HT, Lanspa SJ, Fitzgibbons RJ Jr, et al. Familial pancreatic cancer (part 1): genetic pathology review. Nebr Med J 1989;74(5):109–12.
[5] Hruban RH, Petersen GM, Ha PK, et al. Genetics of pancreatic cancer. From genes to families. Surg Oncol Clin N Am 1998;7(1):1–23.
[6] Applebaum SE, Kant JA, Whitcomb DC, et al. Genetic testing. Counseling, laboratory, and regulatory issues and the EUROPAC protocol for ethical research in multicenter studies of inherited pancreatic diseases. Med Clin North Am 2000;84(3):575–88.
[7] Bartsch DK, Sina-Frey M, Ziegler A, et al. Update of familial pancreatic cancer in Germany. Pancreatology 2001;1(5):510–6.
[8] Bartsch DK, Kress R, Sina-Frey M, et al. Prevalence of familial pancreatic cancer in Germany. Int J Cancer 2004;110(6):902–6.
[9] Hemminki K, Li X. Familial and second primary pancreatic cancers: a nationwide epidemiologic study from Sweden. Int J Cancer 2003;103(4):525–30.
[10] Jenne DE, Reimann H, Nezu J, et al. Peutz-Jeghers syndrome is caused by mutations in a novel serine threonine kinase. Nat Genet 1998;18(1):38–43.
[11] Su GH, Hruban RH, Bansal RK, et al. Germline and somatic mutations of the STK11/LKB1 Peutz-Jeghers gene in pancreatic and biliary cancers. Am J Pathol 1999;154(6):1835–40.

[12] Giardiello FM, Welsh SB, Hamilton SR, et al. Increased risk of cancer in the Peutz-Jeghers syndrome. N Engl J Med 1987;316(24):1511–4.

[13] Goldstein AM, Fraser MC, Struewing JP, et al. Increased risk of pancreatic cancer in melanoma-prone kindreds with p16INK4 mutations. N Engl J Med 1995;333(15): 970–4.

[14] Vasen HF, Gruis NA, Frants RR, et al. Risk of developing pancreatic cancer in families with familial atypical multiple mole melanoma associated with a specific 19 deletion of p16 (p16-Leiden). Int J Cancer 2000;87(6):809–11.

[15] Whelan AJ, Bartsch D, Goodfellow PJ. Brief report: a familial syndrome of pancreatic cancer and melanoma with a mutation in the CDKN2 tumor-suppressor gene. N Engl J Med 1995;333(15):975–7.

[16] Moskaluk CA, Hruban H, Lietman A, et al. Novel germline p16(INK4) allele (Asp145Cys) in a family with multiple pancreatic carcinomas. Mutations in brief no. 148. Hum Mutat 1998;12(1):70.

[17] Lynch HT, Brand RE, Hogg D, et al. Phenotypic variation in eight extended CDKN2A germline mutation familial atypical multiple mole melanoma-pancreatic carcinoma-prone families: the familial atypical mole melanoma-pancreatic carcinoma syndrome. Cancer 2002;94(1):84–96.

[18] Bartsch DK, Sina-Frey M, Lang S, et al. CDKN2A germline mutations in familial pancreatic cancer. Ann Surg 2002;236(6):730–7.

[19] Tonin P, Ghadirian P, Phelan C, et al. A large multisite cancer family is linked to BRCA2. J Med Genet 1995;32(12):982–4.

[20] Simard J, Tonin P, Durocher F, et al. Common origins of BRCA1 mutations in Canadian breast and ovarian cancer families. Nat Genet 1994;8(4):392–8.

[21] Thompson D, Easton DF, for the Breast Cancer Linkage Consortium. Cancer incidence in BRCA1 mutation carriers. J Natl Cancer Inst 2002;94(18):1358–65.

[22] Risch HA, McLaughlin JR, Cole DE, et al. Prevalence and penetrance of germline BRCA1 and BRCA2 mutations in a population series of 649 women with ovarian cancer. Am J Hum Genet 2001;68(3):700–10.

[23] Ozcelik H, Schmocker B, Di Nicola N, et al. Germline BRCA2 6174delT mutations in Ashkenazi Jewish pancreatic cancer patients. Nat Genet 1997;16(1):17–8.

[24] The Breast Cancer Linkage Consortium. Cancer risks in BRCA2 mutation carriers. J Natl Cancer Inst 1999;91:1310–6.

[25] Lynch HT, Brand RE, Deters CA, et al. Hereditary pancreatic cancer. Pancreatology 2001; 1(5):466–71.

[26] Leach FS, Nicolaides NC, Papadopoulos N, et al. Mutations of a mutS homolog in hereditary nonpolyposis colorectal cancer. Cell 1993;75(6):1215–25.

[27] Fishel R, Lescoe MK, Rao MR, et al. The human mutator gene homolog MSH2 and its association with hereditary nonpolyposis colon cancer. Cell 1993;75:1027–8.

[28] Aarnio M, Sankila R, Pukkala E, et al. Cancer risk in mutation carriers of DNA-mismatch-repair genes. Int J Cancer 1999;81(2):214–8.

[29] Lynch HT, Voorhees GJ, Lanspa SJ, et al. Pancreatic carcinoma and hereditary nonpolyposis colorectal cancer: a family study. Br J Cancer 1985;52:271–3.

[30] Stewart CJ, Imrie CW, Foulis AK. Pancreatic islet cell tumour in a patient with familial adenomatous polyposis. J Clin Pathol 1994;47(9):860–1.

[31] Maire F, Hammel P, Terris B, et al. Intraductal papillary and mucinous pancreatic tumour: a new extracolonic tumour in familial adenomatous polyposis. Gut 2002;51(3):446–9.

[32] Yashima K, Nakamori S, Murakami Y, et al. Mutations of the adenomatous polyposis coli gene in the mutation cluster region: comparison of human pancreatic and colorectal cancers. Int J Cancer 1994;59(1):43–7.

[33] Lynch HT. Genetics and pancreatic cancer. Arch Surg 1994;129(3):266–8.

[34] Sina-Frey M, Bartsch DK, Grundei T, et al. Pancreatic cancer and basal-cell carcinoma [letter]. Lancet 2003;361(9352):180.

[35] Whitcomb DC, Gorry MC, Preston RA, et al. Hereditary pancreatitis is caused by a mutation in the cationic trypsinogen gene. Nat Genet 1996;14(2):141–5.

[36] Witt H, Luck W, Hennies HC, et al. Mutations in the gene encoding the serine protease inhibitor, Kazal type 1 are associated with chronic pancreatitis. Nat Genet 2000;25(2): 213–6.

[37] Lowenfels AB, Maisonneuve P, Whitcomb DC. Risk factors for cancer in hereditary pancreatitis. International Hereditary Pancreatitis Study Group. Med Clin North Am 2000;84(3): 565–73.

[38] Lowenfels AB, Maisonneuve P, Whitcomb DC, et al. Cigarette smoking as a risk factor for pancreatic cancer in patients with hereditary pancreatitis. JAMA 2001;286(2):169–70.

[39] Lowenfels AB, Maisonneuve P. Risk factors for pancreatic cancer. J Cell Biochem 2005; 95(4):649–56.

[40] Tedesco FJ, Brown R, Schuman BM. Pancreatic carcinoma in a patient with cystic fibrosis. Gastrointest Endosc 1986;32(1):25–6.

[41] Tsongalis GJ, Faber G, Dalldorf FG, et al. Association of pancreatic adenocarcinoma, mild lung disease, and delta F508 mutation in a cystic fibrosis patient. Clin Chem 1994;40(10): 1972–4.

[42] Tersmette AC, Petersen GM, Offerhaus GJ, et al. Increased risk of incident pancreatic cancer among first-degree relatives of patients with familial pancreatic cancer. Clin Cancer Res 2001;7:738–44.

[43] Klein AP, Brune KA, Petersen GM, et al. Prospective risk of pancreatic cancer in familial pancreatic cancer kindreds. Cancer Res 2004;64(7):2634–8.

[44] McFaul C, Greenhalf W, Earl J, et al. Anticipation in familial pancreatic cancer. Gut 2006; 55:252–8.

[45] Klein AP, Beaty TH, Bailey-Wilson JE, et al. Evidence for a major gene influencing risk of pancreatic cancer. Genet Epidemiol 2002;23(2):133.

[46] Eberle MA, Pfutzer R, Pogue-Geile KL, et al. A new susceptibility locus for autosomal dominant pancreatic cancer maps to chromosome 4q32-34. Am J Hum Genet 2002; 70(4):1044–8.

[47] Hruban RH, Petersen GM, Goggins M, et al. Familial pancreatic cancer. Ann Oncol 1999; 10(Suppl 4):69–73.

[48] Murphy KM, Brune KA, Griffin C, et al. Evaluation of candidate genes MAP2K4, MADH4, ACVR1B, and BRCA2 in familial pancreatic cancer: deleterious BRCA2 mutations in 17%. Cancer Res 2002;62(13):3789–93.

[49] Grützmann R, McFaul C, Bartsch DK, et al. No evidence for germline mutations of the LKB1/STK11 gene in familial pancreatic carcinoma. Cancer Lett 2004;214(1):63–8.

[50] Bartsch DK, Fendrich V, Slater EP, et al. RNASEL germline variants are associated with pancreatic cancer. Int J Cancer 2005;117(5):718–22.

[51] Bartsch DK, Krjusewski K, Sina-Frey M, et al. Low frequency of CHEK2 mutations in familial pancreatic cancer. Fam Cancer, in press.

[52] Nej K, Bartsch DK, Sina-Frey M, et al. The NOD3020insC mutation and the risk of familial pancreatic cancer. Hered Cancer Clin Pract 2004;2:149–50.

[53] van der Heijden MS, Yeo CJ, Hruban RH, et al. Fanconi anemia gene mutations in young-onset pancreatic cancer. Cancer Res 2003;63(10):2585–8.

[54] Rogers CD, van der Heijden MS, Brune K, et al. The genetics of FANCC and FANCG in familial pancreatic cancer. Cancer Biol Ther 2004;3(2):167–9.

[55] Calin GA, Trapasso F, Shimizu M, et al. Familial cancer associated with a polymorphism in ARLTS1. N Engl J Med 2005;352(16):1667–76.

[56] Schutte M, da Costa LT, Hahn SA, et al. Identification by representational difference analysis of a homozygous deletion in pancreatic carcinoma that lies within the BRCA2 region. Proc Natl Acad Sci USA 1995;92(13):5950–4.

[57] Hahn SA, Greenhalf B, Ellis I, et al. BRCA2 germline mutations in familial pancreatic carcinoma. J Natl Cancer Inst 2003;95(3):214–21.

[58] Martin ST, Matsubayashi H, Rogers CD, et al. Increased prevalence of the BRCA2 poly-morphic stop codon K3326X among individuals with familial pancreatic cancer. Oncogene 2005;24(22):3652–6.

[59] Brand R, Rubinstein C, Lerch MM, et al. Consensus guidelines for counselling patients at risk for developing pancreatic cancer. Pancreatology, in press.

[60] Rulyak SJ, Brentnall TA. Inherited pancreatic cancer: surveillance and treatment strategies for affected families. Pancreatology 2001;1(5):477–85.

[61] Canto MI, Goggins M, Yeo CJ, et al. Screening for pancreatic neoplasia in high-risk individ-uals: an EUS-based approach. Clin Gastroenterol Hepatol 2004;2(7):606–21.

[62] Langer P, Rothmund M, Bartsch DK. Prophylaktische Chirurgie des Pankreas. Chirurg 2006;77:25–32.

ELSEVIER
SAUNDERS

Endocrinol Metab Clin N Am
35 (2006) 431–447

ENDOCRINOLOGY
AND METABOLISM
CLINICS
OF NORTH AMERICA

Endocrine Tumors of the Pancreas

Peter Simon, MD, Elisabeth Spilcke-Liss, MD,
Henri Wallaschofski, MD*

*Department of Gastroenterology, Endocrinology and Nutrition,
Ernst-Moritz-Arndt-University, Friedrich Loeffler Strasse 23A, D-17487 Greifswald, Germany*

Neuroendocrine tumors (NETs) are a heterogeneous group of neoplasms that originate from a common precursor cell population that share a number of antigens with nerve elements, like neuron-specific enolase, chromogranins, and synaptophysin. NETs affect endocrine glands (eg, pituitary gland, parathyroids, or the neuroendocrine adrenal gland) and endocrine islets within glandular tissues (eg, thyroid or pancreatic) and cells dispersed between exocrine cells (digestive or respiratory tract). The pancreatic endocrine tumors (PETs) are rare NETs of the pancreas originating from totipotential stem cells or differentiated mature endocrine cells within the exocrine gland. PETs have been frequently called "islet cell tumors," whereas it is uncertain that they all originate from pancreatic islets. In case of nonfunctioning PETs this name is a misnomer, and in tumors with a typical pattern of hormones (gastrinoma, VIPoma, and so forth) that originate from the gastrointestinal tract outside the pancreas [1,2]. Most patients without typical symptoms are not investigated routinely for the full spectrum of possibly released peptides or hormones and might be miscategorized.

It is commonly assumed that hormone or peptide release influences tumor behavior and outcome. PETs releasing insulin show a lower risk of behaving aggressively than those releasing pancreatic polypeptide, somatostatin, glucagon, adrenocortocotropin hormone, calcitonin, or growth hormone–releasing hormone (Table 1). The diagnosis of NETs mainly relies on the positive assessment of markers of neuroendocrine differentiation by immunohistochemistry. The most commonly used markers are general neuroendocrine markers (applicable to all neuroendocrine cells),

H.W. received payments for services from Novartis (Basel, Switzerland) and Ipsen (Paris, France). Various passages have been adapted from an outstanding review in this field by GA Kaltsas et al [1].

* Corresponding author.
E-mail address: henri.wallaschofski@uni-greifswald.de (H. Wallaschofski).

Table 1
Classification of pancreatic endocrine tumours

Well differentiated neuroendocrine tumor	
Benign behavior	Confined to pancreas
	No angioinvasion
	<20 mm in size
	<2 mitosis per 10 HPF
	<2% Ki-67 proliferation/10 HPF
	Nonfunctioning
	Insulin producing
	Tumors
Uncertain behavior	Confirmed to pancreas
	Angioinvasion
	>20 mm in size
	>2 mitosis per 10 HPF
	>2% Ki-67 proliferation/10 HPF
	Nonfunctioning
	Functioning (gastrin, insulin, VIP, glucagon, somatostatin, ACTH, GH, PTHrP)
Low-grade malignant	Local invasion/metastases
	Angioinvasion/perineural invasion
	2–9 mitosis per 10 HPF
	2%–10% Ki-67 proliferation/10 HPF
	Nonfunctioning
	Functioning (gastrin, insulin, VIP, glucagon, somatostatin, ACTH, GH, PTHrP)
Poorly differentiated neuroendocrine carcinoma	
	High-grade malignant tumours with atypical cells
	Undifferentiated carcinoma
	Prominent angioinvasion
	>10 mitosis per 10 HPF
	>10% Ki-67 proliferation/10 HPF

Abbreviations: ACTH, adrenocorticotropic hormome; GH, growth hormone; HPF, high-power field; PTHrP, parathormone related peptide; VIP, vasoactive intestinal polypeptide.

either in the cytosol, such as neuron-specific enolase and the protein gene product 9.5, or granular markers, such as chromogranin A and synaptophysin [3–7]. Histologic and hormonal features of specific cell types are integrated in a so-called "morphofunctional" classification to predict the natural course of the tumor. Currently, the World Health Organization included both histopathologic and functional parameters into a widely accepted classification [3] of gastroenteropancreatic (GEP) NETs, which is probably applicable to all PETs (see Table 1), respectively. The following types have been recognized:

1. Well-differentiated NETs (benign or low-grade malignant): Most NETs are well-differentiated tumors that are characterized by a solid trabecular or glandular structure; tumor cell monomorphism with absent or low cytologic atypia; and a low mitotic (<2 mitoses/mm^2) and proliferative status ($<2\%$ Ki-67–positive cells).

2. Well-differentiated neuroendocrine carcinoma (low malignancy): Such tumors are slow-growing but can occasionally exhibit more aggressive behavior (>2 mitoses/mm^2 or proliferation index $>2\%$ Ki-67–positive cells). Only in the presence of metastases or invasiveness a tumor is defined as a well-differentiated neuroendocrine carcinoma.

3. Poorly differentiated neuroendocrine carcinoma (highly malignant): Poorly differentiated NETs are invariably malignant tumors and defined as poorly differentiated neuroendocrine carcinomas. They are characterized by a predominantly solid structure with abundant necrosis; cellular atypia with a high mitotic index (≥ 10 mitoses/mm^2); a proliferative status ($>15\%$ Ki-67–positive cells); diffuse reactivity for cytosolic markers; and scant or weak reactivity for granular markers or neurosecretory products.

4. Mixed exocrine-endocrine carcinoma: Mixed exocrine-endocrine carcinomas are epithelial tumors with a predominant exocrine component admixed with an endocrine component comprising at least one third of the entire tumor cell population. Their biologic behavior is essentially dictated by the exocrine component, which may be of acinar or ductal type. It is hoped that, in the future, other factors, such as the angiogenic capacity of tumor cells and specific genetic changes, may prove to be valuable tools in determining prognosis, biologic behavior, and response to therapy.

Clinical aspects

Previously, the incidence of PETs has been estimated about 0.4 to 1 per 100,000 [8]. In autopsy surveys, however, the incidence ranges from 0% to 10%, and in surgical series up to 15% of pancreatic neoplasms have been identified as PETs [9]. Most PETs occur in patients over 30 years of age [10]. They present clinically as functioning or nonfunctioning tumors depending on various clinical signs and symptoms related to peptides or hormone excess but the occurrence is not specific. The absence of typical clinical signs does not reflect an absence of hormone excess. The nonfunctioning PETs are clinically silent until they are detected at an unresectable stage with symptoms caused by the mass effect of the tumor or metastatic disease. They seem to be more common than the functioning tumors like insulinoma and gastrinoma. Functional PETs are named after the predominantly released peptide or hormone (Table 2).

Insulinoma

Most functioning PETs are insulinomas (60%). Unlike other PETs that are often malignant, insulinomas are usually benign. A total of 10% of PETs occur in multiple locations, 10% are malignant, and 4% to 7% might be associated with multiple endocrine neoplasia (MEN)-1. The diagnosis of insulinoma is based on Whipple's triad (symptoms of neuroglycopenia,

Table 2
Frequent pancreatic endocrine tumor syndromes

Name	Peptide/hormone	Clinical feature	Incidence (new cases/ 10^6/y)	Tumor location in %	Malignant in %	Associated with MEN-1 in%	Patients with MEN-1 develop in %
Insulinoma	Insulin	Whipple's triad (plasma glucose of <5 mmol/L neuroglycopenia, relief of symptoms after glucose intake)	1–2	99 pancreas	<10	4–7	20
Gastrinoma	Gastrin	Zollinger-Ellison syndrome, hyperchlorhydria / diarrhea, gastric/duodenal ulcer	0.5–1.5	70 duodenum 25 pancreas 5 other	60–90	20–25	54
VIPoma	Vasoactive intestinal peptide	Watery diarrhea, hypokalemia, achlorhydria	0.05–0.2	80 pancreas 20 other	40–70	9	17
Glucagonoma	Glucagon	Weight loss, rash/necrolytic migratory erythema, cheilosis or stomatitis, diabetes and diarrhea	0.01–0.1	100 pancreas	50–80	5–17	3
Somatostatinoma	Somatostatin	Hyperglycemia, cholelithiasis, steatorrhea diarrhea, hypochlorhydria	Unknown	53 pancreas 47 duodenum	>70	45	Unknown
GRFoma	Growth hormone–releasing hormone	Acromegaly	Unknown	50 lung 30 pancreas 7 jejunum 13 other	>60	16	Unknown
ACTHoma	ACTH	Cushing's syndrome	Unknown	Unknown	>95	Rare	Rare

Abbreviations: ACTH, adrenocorticotropic hormone; MEN, multiple endocrine neoplasia.

plasma glucose of <2.5 mmol/L, and relief of symptoms with sugar intake). If an insulinoma is suspected, the 72-hour fasting test is considered as investigation of choice and capable of detecting hypoglycemia and hypoglycemia-associated inappropriate insulin (>6 µU/mL), proinsulin (>0.2 ng/mL), and C-peptide (>300 pmol/L) concentrations. In equivocal cases the presence of sulfonylurea or related drugs in the urine or plasma should exclude self-induced hypoglycemia. Exogenously administered insulin is associated with raised insulin plasma but low plasma C-peptide levels. Proinsulin levels have been shown to be of diagnostic value, because more than 90% of patients with insulinomas have a plasma proinsulin component of at least 25% of the total immunoreactive insulin. In most series using the fasting test as a diagnostic tool, 30% of patients develop symptoms within 12 hours from the start, 80% within 24 hours, and almost 100% after 72 hours. If hypoglycemia is confirmed rare metabolic syndromes and factitious hypoglycemia and ectopic secretion of pro–insulin growth factor-II by certain tumors should be considered. Malignant insulinomas arise usually singular and large with an average diameter of 6 cm. Affected patients show a median survival of 4 years. Successful excision of a benign lesion is associated with normal life expectancy, whereas a 10-year survival of 29% has been described for malignant insulinomas [11].

Gastrinoma

Gastrinomas are the second most frequent endocrine tumors of the pancreas, which occur either sporadically or in up to 25% in association with MEN-1. They can lead to the Zollinger-Ellison syndrome, which is characterized by hypergastrinemia resulting in hyperchlorhydria and gastric mucosal thickening. In a recent review of 261 patients with Zollinger-Ellison syndrome, the mean age at clinical presentation of the disease was 41 years with a 5.2-year delay between onset of symptoms and time of diagnosis [12]. Ulceration of the upper gastrointestinal mucosa develops in more than 90%. Diarrhea is also a common symptom, developing in 50% to 65% and can precede, parallel, or follow ulcer formation. The presence of Zollinger-Ellison syndrome should always be considered in patients with an unusual ulcer location, with ulcers refractory to treatment, with unexplained diarrhea and weight loss, and with prominent gastric folds on endoscopy. Fasting serum gastrin levels ≥ 1000 pg/mL in combination with a gastric fluid pH ≤ 2.5 define gastrinoma as long as the patient is normocalcemic and free of pyloric obstruction and renal failure. Before measuring serum, gastrin H_2-antagonists or proton pump inhibitors have to be discontinued for a minimum of 1 week or 3 weeks, respectively.

Most gastrinomas are malignant. Tumor size or histologic findings seem not to be associated with biologic behavior or clinical course. Lymph node or liver metastases are present in 70% to 80% at diagnosis. Overall survival in patients with MEN-1–related gastrinomas does not differ from the overall survival in patients with the sporadic form and depends generally on the presence of liver metastases [12].

VIPoma

Most VIPomas occur sporadically. The leading symptom is severe secretory watery diarrhea. About 70% to 80% originate from PETs, usually located in the pancreatic tail. Mostly, the tumors measure more than 2 cm in diameter and pancreatic VIPomas show in 50% to 60% an aggressive behavior with metastasis formation in the liver and lymph nodes at the time of diagnosis. VIPomas can be multifocal in 4% and 9% are associated with MEN-1. The diagnosis is based on the presence of secretory diarrhea associated with elevated fasting vasoactive intestinal polypeptide levels and a pancreatic or other lesion associated with vasoactive polypeptide production [13].

Somatostatinoma

Somatostatinomas are rare. Recently 173 cases have been reported; 92 of these patients showed extrapancreatic localization. Clinical signs are caused by inhibition of exocrine and endocrine secretion. Symptoms related to somatostatin hypersecretion are found in approximately 11% of patients with somatostatinomas: hyperglycemia (95%); cholelithiasis (68%); diarrhea (60%); steatorrhea (47%); and hypochlorhydria (26%). They might be associated with neurofibromatosis-1 and pheochromocytomas, suggesting an inherited endocrinopathy. The diagnosis is established by demonstrating elevated somatostatin levels in patients with a relevant history and the presence of a pancreatic tumor. There is no significant difference in the rate of metastases and malignant tissue invasion between pancreatic and extrapancreatic somatostatinomas. The observed overall postoperative 5-year survival rate is 75.2%, 59.9% in patients with metastases, and 100% in patients without metastases [14]. There is no specific treatment for somatostatinomas besides administration of somatostatin analogues that inhibit somatostatin receptor activation.

Glucagonoma

Glucagonomas are slow-growing tumors that arise from pancreatic α-cells. They are associated with an excessive secretion of glucagon and other peptides. Most of these tumors occur sporadic, whereas 5% to 17% are associated with MEN-1. Patients suffering from sporadic glucagonomas usually present with symptoms in their fifth decade of life, whereas patients with MEN-1 present symptoms at a younger age. Most glucagonomas are located in the tail of the pancreas. Glucagonomas may be more common than suggested by clinical diagnosis, because autopsy series have demonstrated an occurrence of 0.8% of microglucagonomas in adult-onset diabetics. Glucagonomas can be as large as 6 cm, are highly malignant, and over 80% of the sporadic tumors demonstrate hepatic metastases at time of diagnosis. The most common symptoms are weight loss (70%–80%); rash (65%–80%); diabetes (75%); cheilosis or stomatitis (30%–40%); and diarrhea (15%–30%). A skin rash and a necrolytic migratory erythema are rare but characteristic signs. Either lesion typically evolves over 7 to 14 days, beginning as a small erythema in the groin and extending to the perineum, lower extremities, and perioral regions. The diagnosis of glucagonomas is based on fasting plasma glucagon levels ≥ 50 pmol/L in the presence of a pancreatic tumor. Patients without metastases seem to have a good outcome after surgery alone, with an overall postoperative 5-year survival greater than 85%. Thromboembolic events may account for over 50% of all deaths directly attributed to the glucagonoma syndrome [15].

Serotonin- and 5-hydroxyindoleacetic acid–releasing tumors

Primary pancreatic carcinoids (serotonin-producing tumors of the pancreas) are a rare subtype of pancreatic tumors with approximately 100 cases reported [16]. These tumors are relatively large with a high rate of metastasis formation (69%–88.4%) at the time of diagnosis. Pancreatic carcinoid tumors produce high levels of serotoninergic hormones. The typical clinical sign of flush is reported by only 30% of affected patients. The diagnosis is based on a demonstrable pancreatic mass in combination with increased 5-hydroxyindoleacetic acid in the urine, whereas not all tumors show a detectable hyperserotoninemia. Pancreatic carcinoids are associated with a poor prognosis caused by delayed diagnosis, which precludes extensive resection and a good response to other therapeutic modalities. A single reported patient has been associated with MEN-1 [1,16].

Pancreatic polypeptide–releasing tumor

These tumors account for about 20% of all endocrine pancreatic tumors and are not associated with clinical syndromes caused by hormonal hypersecretion [17,18]. They are most often diagnosed in the fifth to sixth decade of life and are mainly located in the pancreas rather than in the duodenum [1]. Their clinical quiescence may be related to inactive hormonal production, cosecretion of peptide inhibitors, or down-regulation of peripheral receptors. They are usually large and diagnosed either as an incidental finding, because of symptoms caused by an expanding mass or because of metastases. Approximately two thirds are truly malignant. Overall 5- and 10-year survival rates of 65% and 49%, respectively, have been described.

Adrenocortocotropin hormone–, growth hormone releasing
factor (GRF)-, calcitonin-, parathormone related peptide
(PTHrP)-releasing tumor

These tumors are rare. Most prevalent are ACTHomas (approximately 110 cases reported). GRFomas can be associated with acromegaly (approximately 50 cases); neurotensinomas (approximately 50 cases); and parathyrinomas (approximately 35 cases) [19]. Very rarely, pancreatic tumors secreting calcitonin, enteroglucagon, cholecystokinin, gastric inhibitory peptide, leutinizing hormone, gastrin-releasing peptide, and ghrelin have also been described [7].

Nonfunctioning pancreatic endocrine tumors

Nonfunctioning PETs are defined by a lack of symptoms or signs and the absence of a detectable hormonal secretion. Most tumors are diagnosed in the disease-course by abdominal pain, weight loss, or a palpable mass. Usually the tumors are large and metastases are already present. The differentiation from pancreatic adenocarcinoma or serous cystadenoma is often difficult [20].

Molecular pathogenetic aspects

PETs may occur sporadically or in a familial context of autosomal-dominant inherited diseases, such as MEN and tuberous sclerosis. Overall, approximately 1% of patients with NETs have a positive family history in first-degree relatives. A family history is associated with a threefold increased relative risk, and this increases further when both parents are affected [1].

Noninherited forms (sporadic pancreatic endocrine tumors)

In contrast to nonendocrine tumors of the pancreas sporadic PETs, as opposed to the inherited varieties, show no consistent association to common oncogenes or tumor suppressor genes [21]. Up to now their molecular pathogenesis is poorly understood. Various chromosomal alterations have been documented in sporadic PETs. The most consistent alteration is a loss of chromosome 11q, including the MEN-1 gene. Recent studies demonstrated MEN-1 gene mutations (27%–39%) or a loss of heterozygosity (93%) in sporadic PETs or gastrinoma, respectively [19,22]. These data imply that MEN-1 gene alterations play an important role in the pathogenesis of at least one third of noninherited PETs [7]. In various sporadic PETs some further genetic markers like K-ras, PTEN (phosphatase and tensin homolog deleted on chromosome 10), or p16 have been identified without specificity for diagnostic or therapeutic approach. K-ras mutations have also been frequently found in insulin-producing tumors. The loss of heterozygosity of PTEN, a dual-phosphatase tumor suppressor gene, might be associated only with malignant PETs. Moreover, it has been suggested that the progression of NETs might be influenced by overexpression of various growth factors triggering cell proliferation of endocrine or endothelial tissues. Especially, the overexpression of vascular endothelial growth factor, which has been detected in some PETs, could promote the growth of these tumors.

Inherited forms of pancreatic endocrine tumors

Four major MEN syndromes (MEN-1, von Hippel-Lindau disease, neurofibromatosis, and tuberous sclerosis) represent forms of inherited PETs with a variable but high penetrance in various neuroendocrine tissues. MEN-1 is an autosomal-dominant syndrome with high penetrance characterized mainly by hyperplasia or multiple tumors of the parathyroid, endocrine pancreas, anterior pituitary, foregut-derived neuroendocrine tissues, and adrenocortical glands. Mostly, MEN-1 families suffer from heterogenous germline mutations of the MEN-1 gene, including chromosomal loss with duplication, mitotic recombination, or point mutations. The MEN-1 tumor suppressor gene is located on chromosome 11q13. The molecular alterations lead to a loss of function of the tumor suppressive protein menin, which plays an important role in DNA repair and in synthesis of DNA or transcription factors [1,23].

PETs have been detected in more than 60% of MEN-1–affected individuals. There seems to be no correlation between genotype and phenotype. In clinical practice, the genetic analysis is useful to assess the diagnosis of MEN-1 but the syndrome cannot be excluded with certainty if a mutation cannot be detected [8]. The clinical screening of patients remains a prerequisite for genetic analysis. Knowledge of the particular genetic defects in a MEN-1 family is essential for early screening and counseling of unaffected family members.

Von Hippel-Lindau disease is an autosomal-dominant disease caused by alterations of a tumor suppressor gene located on chromosome 3p25.5. The most common clinical presentations are retinal and central nervous system hemangioblastomas and cystic formations in the kidney (often clear cell renal cell carcinomas); epididymis; and liver or lung pheochromocytomas. Pancreatic von Hippel-Lindau disease–related lesions include benign cysts or serous adenomas (papillary cystadenomas), which occur in 35% to 70% of von Hippel-Lindau disease patients. PETs have been reported with much lower frequency (12% to 25%) of affected patients and are mostly nonfunctional. The incidence of specific tumors depends on the phenotypic class of von Hippel-Lindau disease, of which four have been described (type 1 and types 2A, 2B, and 2C). Von Hippel-Lindau disease protein seems to be involved in the regulation of angiogenetic factors and in the cell cycle [1].

Less commonly, PETs have been observed in phacomatoses, such as neurofibromatosis type 1 with inactivating somatic mutations and tuberous sclerosis. Diagnostic criteria for neurofibromatosis type 1 include cutaneous or subcutaneous neurofibromas; café-au-lait spots appearing early in life; optic glioma; benign iris hamartomas (Lisch nodules); and specific dysplastic bone lesions.

Imaging

Recently, several prospective studies have investigated the relative usefulness of currently available techniques and helped to establish a diagnostic work-up on evidence-based information. Because of its high sensitivity and its ability to obtain whole-body images, scintigraphy with ^{111}In-octreotide is considered the initial imaging procedure of choice for GEP tumors because it is more sensitive than any other single imaging method for localizing a gastrinoma or identifying hepatic metastases. Up to 30% of gastrinomas ultimately detected on surgical exploration are diagnostically missed by scintigraphy. In another prospective study, ^{111}In-octreotide altered the management in many patients with gastrinomas by successfully locating the primary tumor and by clarifying equivocal localization results obtained by other imaging modalities. Imaging with ^{123}I-MIBG has a poor sensitivity in identifying islet cell tumors and should not generally be used in cases with negative ^{111}In-octreotide scintigraphy. Positron emission tomography using ^{11}C-5-HTP produces very good tumor visibility because of selective uptake in tumor tissue compared with surrounding tissue. It can be used for the examination of both the thorax and abdomen and has been shown on several occasions to be superior to scintigraphy with ^{111}In-octreotide. The lack of general availability and the high cost limits its use. Intraoperative radionucleid imaging can be used to help define the exact location of a biochemically proved NET and improves its complete resection [24,25].

Transabdominal ultrasound exhibits a detection rate for insulinomas and gastrinomas between 25% and 30%, respectively. Detection rates are better in lesions greater than 3 cm in diameter and are relatively poor in lesions smaller than 1 cm. Endoluminal ultrasound allows the positioning of a high-frequency (7.5–10 MHz) transducer in close proximity to the pancreas for detection of lesions as small as 5 mm. Although there is a potential blind-spot at the splenic hilum, sensitivities as high as 79% to 82% have been obtained [26,27]. A recent single-center prospective study revealed a sensitivity of 93% and a specificity of 95% in localization of intrapancreatic lesions [28]. Endoluminal ultrasound detected all tumors visualized by any other conventional technique (excluding scintigraphy with ^{111}In-octreotide), calling into question the necessity for these other imaging modalities.

Intraoperative ultrasound also allows direct high-resolution examination of the pancreas. The combination of intraoperative ultrasound and surgical palpation has led to 97% cure rates in patients with benign insulinomas. The overall sensitivity for gastrinomas is 100% of intrapancreatic lesions detected in large series. Dual-face helical CT scan allows multiphase imaging during a single bolus of contrast administration and can achieve sensitivities of 82% to 92% [29]. Reviewing most recently published series using T1-weighted fat suppression images, MRI identified 71 of 78 lesions, a 91% sensitivity in 57 islet cell tumors [9,30]. A comparative study showed that the sensitivity of T1-weighted MRI is equivalent to delayed dynamic CT.

MRI is considered the most sensitive technique for demonstrating liver and bone metastases in patients with NETs and is recommended for the monitoring of response to therapy.

Therapy

Before applying any kind of therapy, the possibility of an MEN-1 syndrome should always be considered in patients with PETs. Such an approach is important because there is considerable difference in the management of these tumors when they occur as part of the MEN syndromes [1]. Surgery remains the treatment of choice and the only approach that can achieve a cure in patients with PETs [31–33]. Recently, the surgical approach has become more aggressive, including wide resections of metastases together with enucleation of liver metastases or hepatic artery embolization with adjuvant chemotherapy or focal hepatic ablation techniques.

Medical treatment should always be considered as an adjuvant to surgery, unless either the general condition of the patient or other contraindications preclude surgery. Patients are reviewed at 3- to 6-month intervals. Review assessment comprises clinical, biochemical, and radiologic evaluation. The rationale for applying further treatment at these time intervals is contingent on the relative prolonged replication period of these tumors. If surgical intervention is not possible, treatment should be guided according to currently established classification systems and prognostic factors. Well-differentiated and slow-growing GEP tumors should be treated with somatostatin analogues or interferon (IFN)-α alone or in combination, although the preference is to use somatostatin analogues at an early stage and rarely the addition of IFN-α is needed. Systemic medical treatment of GEP tumors includes treatment with biologic agents, somatostatin, IFN-α, and chemotherapy. Somatostatin analogues can reliably control hormone-mediated symptoms, may exert an antiproliferative effect, and control tumor growth. They can also have modulatory effects on the vascular and immune system [34–36]. Somatostatin analogues are the gold standard for management of clinical symptoms from hormone-producing PETs.

A controversial area concerns the therapy of patients with nonfunctioning endocrine tumors. Somatostatin analogues are poor tumoricidal agents but may show tumoristatic effects and retard further NET growth, resulting in tumor stabilization. Regular octreotide at a daily dose of 200 to 450 μg is associated with a median 60% symptomatic, 70% biochemical, and 5% to 11% tumoral response [37–39]. There is no direct evidence that treatment with somatostatin analogues prolongs survival in patients with GEP tumors. A retrospective comparison with a cohort of patients treated with chemotherapy has shown that octreotide was associated with a threefold improved survival [40]. It has been suggested that high-dose treatment (> 3000 μg/day) can produce additional antiproliferative effects in patients failing on standard doses, but the costs of high-dose somatostatin analogues can be prohibitive. In a recent review, doses of octreotide up to 30 (60) mg every 3 to 4 weeks has been recommended [41]. The accepted indications for the somatostatin therapy include peptide and amine-induced syndromes with clinical symptoms, progressive metastatic disease even without hormone-induced syndrome, and perioperative prevention of a carcinoid crisis.

INF-α has been used either alone or in combination with chemotherapy and somatostatin analogues in various but mainly carcinoid and endocrine tumors [1,38,39]. The antitumor action of INF-α includes stimulation of natural killer cell function affecting proliferation, apoptosis, differentiation, and angiogenesis [39]. INF-α also exerts an immunomodulatory effect and induces fibrosis in metastatic, particularly hepatic lesions. In patients with low proliferative endocrine pancreatic tumors, a biochemical response rate of approximately 50% and a tumor reduction of up to 15%, lasting for more than 2 years has been observed [1,39]. There seems to be no clear dose-response relationship and higher doses were not associated with an improved response [1]. Retrospective data suggest a prolongation of survival. There are only a few randomized control studies demonstrating a better outcome of patients treated with INF-α compared with patients treated with chemotherapy or somatostatin analogues [39]. In another randomized study, discontinuation of successful INF-α therapy was associated with shortening of life expectancy [42].

In a study with progressive carcinoid or PETs, the combination of somatostatin analogues and INF-α was associated with significant symptomatic and biochemical improvement, inhibition of tumor growth, and probably prolongation of survival in the responder group [43]. The combination of recombinant INF-α and chemotherapy with streptozotocin (STZ) and doxorubicin or 5-fluorouracil in randomized controlled trials was not associated with a synergistic effect, although considerable toxicity was encountered [44].

Chemotherapy should be considered for poorly differentiated and progressive GEP tumors. Therapy with radionuclides, ^{131}I-MIBG for chromaffin cell tumors and treatment with radiolabeled SS analogues for other NETs, may be used for tumors exhibiting uptake on a diagnostic scan either after surgery to eradicate microscopic residual disease or later if conventional treatment or biotherapy fails.

Chemotherapy for pancreatic endocrine tumors

In general, NETs are not highly chemosensitive and if they do respond, any improvements may be slow to appear. This may be caused by NETs' generally low rate of mitosis, the target of many cytotoxic drugs, and also by their biologic properties. NETs show a high expression of the antiapoptotic gene Bcl-2, which may contribute further to the intrinsic resistance to chemotherapy agents. Chemotherapy has to be weighed against potential side effects but may be the only alternative, particularly in poorly differentiated tumors. Patients with functioning tumors respond better than those with nonfunctioning tumors [1]. Nevertheless, the response to treatment may be limited because of potential toxicity.

Currently, chemotherapy is considered for progressive well-differentiated tumors and fast proliferating tumors (Ki-67 > 10%). The combination of streptozotocin and doxorubicin has demonstrated significant benefit with a 69% objective response rate and might be superior to other regimens, mainly streptozotocin and 5-fluorouracil with response rate of 45% (Table 3) [42–49]. In cases where the use of doxorubicin is limited because of its potential cumulative cardiotoxicity, the traditional combination of streptozotocin and 5-fluorouracil can be used as an alternative. It is considered that the use of systemic chemotherapy for well-differentiated GEP tumors is beneficial when the general condition of the patient is sufficiently well and after an observational period to appreciate the rate of tumor growth. Antitumor efficacy should be evaluated after 6 months unless further clinical tumor progression has already occurred [1]. Patients who respond may also be good candidates for secondary surgical excision. There are also anecdotal reports of the use of thalidomide, an antiangiogenic agent, and of antagonists to the epidermal growth factor for the therapy of NETs [1].

^{131}I-MIBG therapy for malignant neuroendocrine tumors

Potential advantages of MIBG therapy are that it represents a systemic treatment targeting both primary tumors and distant metastases. It has

Table 3
Chemotherapy for pancreatic endocrine tumours

Author	Year	N	Therapy	Phase	Survival months	Tumor response in %	Ref.
Broder and Canter	1973	52	STZ	II	42	42	44
Moertel et al	1980	84	STZ	III		36	43
			STZ + 5-Fu			63	
Moertel et al	1992	36	STZ + adriamycin	III	18	69	41
		33	STZ + 5-FU	II	14	45	
		33	Chlorozotocin		17	30	
Bukowski et al	1992	44	Chlorozotocin and adriamycin	II	11	36	45
Erikson and oberg	1993	31	STZ + 5-FU	II	23	35	42
Bajetta et al	1998	15	5-FU + dacarbazine + epirubicin	II	15	27	46
Rivera and Ajani	1998	11	Doxorubicin + STZ + 5-FU	II	21	54	47
Cheng and Saltz	1999	16	Doxorubicin + STZ	II	No data	6	48
Kaltsas et al	2002	5	Lomustine + 5-FU	II	24	40	49

Abbreviations: 5-FU, 5-fluoroacil; STZ, streptozotocin.

a preferential radiation delivery to tumoral lesions with relative sparing of healthy tissues (mainly β-emission with only a 10% γ-emission contribution) and it has little pharmacologic toxicity [50,51]. Most of the patients treated so far had no other therapeutic options or were refractory to conventional treatment strategies with only a few prospective trials incorporating treatment-naive patients. Very few cases of ^{131}I-MIBG treatment in PETs have been reported, reflecting the poor uptake of MIBG in these tumors. Radionuclide therapy is feasible and safe and significantly defers the occurrence of fatal and nonfatal events in patients clinically uncontrolled by conventional therapy [51]. In a current review the ^{131}I-MIBG treatment showed symptomatic response in about 60% and a hormonal response without a significant reduction of tumor mass in about 12.5% [1]. Furthermore, an additive antitumor effect for the combination of MIBG with chemotherapy has been demonstrated. Controlled studies are needed to clarify the benefit for patients and patient selection.

Supportive therapy for endocrine active pancreatic endocrine tumors

Insulinomas are least sensitive to treatment with somatostatin analogues. Only around 50% of patients with insulinomas respond to treatment with somatostatin analogues, which may relate to the lack of somatostatin receptor subtype 2 in many of these tumors or to the presence of tumors with no or atypical β-granules. Diazoxide at doses of 50 to 300 mg/d (but up to 600 mg/d) usually decreases insulin secretion and it is the most effective drug for controlling hypoglycemia. It can cause marked edema, renal impairment, and hirsutism. Verapamil, glucocorticoids, and phenytoin have also been used, although less effectively. In refractory cases, glucocorticoids might be effective.

In gastrinomas, proton pump inhibitors are currently the therapeutic agents of choice for short- and long-term control of gastric acid secretion. Gastric acid secretion is best controlled by a mean morning dose of 40 to 80 mg of omeprazole or an equivalent dose of other similar compounds. If higher doses are required (>240 mg per 24 hours have been used), they should be given every 12 hours. Glucagonomas and vipomas respond to somatostatin infusion irrespective of alterations in hormone levels. Because surgical resection may be considered even if the tumor is metastatic, it is important to correct hypoaminoacidemia and mineral deficiency, to control diabetes, and to administer low-dose heparin for decreasing the risk of thrombosis. Somatostatin analogues preoperatively have also been advocated [1].

The increasing number of investigative and therapeutic options and procedures of NETs might be managed best by a multidisciplinary approach. Such an interdisciplinary team should include pathologists, endocrinologists, gastroenterologists, interventional radiologists, surgeons, oncologists, and a nuclear medicine expert. Because of the relative rarity of such tumors, optimum management should be performed in centers with considerable experience and expertise. Because most of these tumors are slow growing and even patients with disseminated disease may have prolonged survival, early involvement in palliative programs is helpful. Patients with metastatic disease may still show prolonged survival. The improvement in quality of life should be weighted against the potential side effects of any systemic treatment.

References

[1] Kaltsas GA, Besser GM, Grossman AB. The diagnosis and medical management of advanced neuroendocrine tumors. Endocr Rev 2004;25:458–511.

[2] Rindi G, Villanacci V, Ubiali A, et al. Endocrine tumors of the digestive tract and pancreas: histogenesis, diagnosis and molecular basis. Expert Rev Mol Diagn 2001;1:323–33.

[3] Solcia E, Kloppel G, Sobin LH. Histological typing of endocrine tumours. 2nd edition. Heidelberg: World Health Organization; 2000.

[4] Rindi G, Villanacci V, Ubiali A. Biological and molecular aspects of gastroenteropancreatic neuroendocrine tumors. Digestion 2000;62(Suppl 1):19–26.

[5] Lack EE, Lloyd RV, Carney JA, et al. Recommendations for reporting of extra-adrenal paragangliomas. Mod Pathol 2003;16:833–5.

[6] Kloppel G. Classification of neuroendocrine tumors. Verh Dtsch Ges Pathol 1997;81:111–7.

[7] Gumbs AA, Moore PS, Falconi M, et al. Review of the clinical, histological, and molecular aspects of pancreatic endocrine neoplasms. J Surg Oncol 2002;81:45–53.

[8] Wick MR, Graeme-Cook FM. Pancreatic neuroendocrine neoplasms: a current summary of diagnostic, prognostic, and differential diagnostic information. Am J Clin Pathol 2001;115: S28–45.

[9] Owen NJ, Sohaib SA, Peppercorn PD, et al. MRI of pancreatic neuroendocrine tumours. Br J Radiol 2001;74:968–73.

[10] Oberg K, Eriksson B. Endocrine tumours of the pancreas. Best Pract Res Clin Gastroenterol 2005;19:753–81.

[11] Service FJ, McMahon MM, O'Brien PC, et al. Functioning insulinoma–incidence, recurrence, and long-term survival of patients: a 60-year study. Mayo Clin Proc 1991;66:711–9.

[12] Roy PK, Venzon DJ, Shojamanesh H, et al. Zollinger-Ellison syndrome: clinical presentation in 261 patients. Medicine (Baltimore) 2000;79:379–411.

[13] Soga J, Yakuwa Y. Vipoma/diarrheogenic syndrome: a statistical evaluation of 241 reported cases. J Exp Clin Cancer Res 1998;17:389–400.

[14] Soga J, Yakuwa Y. Somatostatinoma/inhibitory syndrome: a statistical evaluation of 173 reported cases as compared to other pancreatic endocarcrinomas. J Exp Clin Cancer Res 1999;18:13–22.

[15] Chastain MA. The glucagonoma syndrome: a review of its features and discussion of new perspectives. Am J Med Sci 2001;321:306–20.

[16] Mao C, el Attar A, Domenico DR, et al. Carcinoid tumors of the pancreas: status report based on two cases and review of the world's literature. Int J Pancreatol 1998;23:153–64.

[17] Venkatesh S, Ordonez NG, Ajani J, et al. Islet cell carcinoma of the pancreas: a study of 98 patients. Cancer 1990;65:354–7.

[18] Mignon M. Natural history of neuroendocrine enteropancreatic tumors. Digestion 2000; 62(Suppl 1):51–8.

[19] Zhuang Z, Vortmeyer AO, Pack S, et al. Somatic mutations of the MEN1 tumor suppressor gene in sporadic gastrinomas and insulinomas. Cancer Res 1997;57:4682–6.

[20] Plockinger U, Wiedemann B. Diagnosis of non-functioning neuro-endocrine gastroenteropancreatic tumours. Neuroendocrinology 2004;80(Suppl 1):35–8.

[21] Weber HC, Venzon DJ, Lin JT, et al. Determinants of metastatic rate and survival in patients with Zollinger-Ellison syndrome: a prospective long-term study. Gastroenterology 1995;108: 1637–49.

[22] Wang EH, Ebrahimi SA, Wu AY, et al. Mutation of the MENIN gene in sporadic pancreatic endocrine tumors. Cancer Res 1998;58:4417–20.

[23] Akerstrom G, Hessman O, Hellman P, et al. Pancreatic tumours as part of the MEN-1 syndrome. Best Pract Res Clin Gastroenterol 2005;19:819–30.

[24] Kaltsas G, Rockall A, Papadogias D, et al. Recent advances in radiological and radionuclide imaging and therapy of neuroendocrine tumours. Eur J Endocrinol 2004;151:15–27.

[25] Kaltsas GA, Mukherjee JJ, Grossman AB. The value of radiolabelled MIBG and octreotide in the diagnosis and management of neuroendocrine tumours. Ann Oncol 2001;12(Suppl 2): S47–50.

[26] Rosch T, Lightdale CJ, Botet JF, et al. Localization of pancreatic endocrine tumors by endoscopic ultrasonography. N Engl J Med 1992;326:1721–6.

[27] Glover JR, Shorvon PJ, Lees WR. Endoscopic ultrasound for localisation of islet cell tumours. Gut 1992;33:108–10.

[28] Anderson MA, Carpenter S, Thompson NW, et al. Endoscopic ultrasound is highly accurate and directs management in patients with neuroendocrine tumors of the pancreas. Am J Gastroenterol 2000;95:2271–7.

[29] Legmann P, Vignaux O, Dousset B, et al. Pancreatic tumors: comparison of dual-phase helical CT and endoscopic sonography. AJR Am J Roentgenol 1998;170:1315–22.

[30] Semelka RC, Cumming MJ, Shoenut JP, et al. Islet cell tumors: comparison of dynamic contrast-enhanced CT and MR imaging with dynamic gadolinium enhancement and fat suppression. Radiology 1993;186:799–802.

[31] Arnold R, Frank M. Control of growth in neuroendocrine gastro-enteropancreatic tumours. Digestion 1996;57(Suppl 1):69–71.

[32] Arnold R, Hiddemann W. Therapy of metastatic endocrine tumors of the gastrointestinal tract. Dtsch Med Wochenschr 1996;121:1346–7.

[33] Norton JA, Fraker DL, Alexander HR, et al. Surgery to cure the Zollinger-Ellison syndrome. N Engl J Med 1999;341:635–44.

[34] Arnold R, Frank M. Gastrointestinal endocrine tumours: medical management. Baillieres Clin Gastroenterol 1996;10:737–59.

[35] Arnold R, Simon B, Wied M. Treatment of neuroendocrine GEP tumours with somatostatin analogues: a review. Digestion 2000;62(Suppl 1):84–91.

[36] Aparicio T, Ducreux M, Baudin E, et al. Antitumour activity of somatostatin analogues in progressive metastatic neuroendocrine tumours. Eur J Cancer 2001;37:1014–9.

[37] Oberg K. Interferon in the management of neuroendocrine GEP-tumors: a review. Digestion 2000;62(Suppl 1):92–7.

[38] Jacobsen MB, Hanssen LE, Kolmannskog F, et al. Interferon-α 2b, with or without prior hepatic artery embolization: clinical response and survival in mid-gut carcinoid patients. The Norwegian Carcinoid Study. Scand J Gastroenterol 1995;30:789–96.

[39] Oberg K. Advances in chemotherapy and biotherapy of endocrine tumors. Curr Opin Oncol 1998;10:58–65.

[40] Oberg K, Kvols L, Caplin M, et al. Consensus report on the use of somatostatin analogs for the management of neuroendocrine tumors of the gastroenteropancreatic system. Ann Oncol 2004;15:966–73.

[41] Moertel CG, Lefkopoulo M, Lipsitz S, et al. Streptozocin-doxorubicin, streptozocin-fluorouracil or chlorozotocin in the treatment of advanced islet-cell carcinoma. N Engl J Med 1992;326:519–23.

[42] Eriksson B, Oberg K. An update of the medical treatment of malignant endocrine pancreatic tumors. Acta Oncol 1993;32:203–8.

[43] Moertel CG, Hanley JA, Johnson LA. Streptozocin alone compared with streptozocin plus fluorouracil in the treatment of advanced islet-cell carcinoma. N Engl J Med 1980;303:1189–94.

[44] Broder LE, Carter SK. Pancreatic islet cell carcinoma. II. Results of therapy with streptozo-
     tocin in 52 patients. Ann Intern Med 1973;79:108–18.
[45] Bukowski RM, Tangen C, Lee R, et al. 1992 Phase II trial of chlorozotocin and fluorouracil
     in islet cell carcinoma: a Southwest Oncology Group study. J Clin Oncol 1992;10:1914–8.
[46] Bajetta E, Rimassa L, Carnaghi C, et al. 5-Fluorouracil, dacarbazine, and epirubicin in the
     treatment of patients with neuroendocrine tumors. Cancer 1998;83:372–8.
[47] Rivera E, Ajani JA. Doxorubicin, streptozocin, and 5-fluorouracil chemotherapy for
     patients with metastatic islet-cell carcinoma. Am J Clin Oncol 1998;21:36–8.
[48] Cheng PN, Saltz LB. Failure to confirm major objective antitumor activity for streptozocin
     and doxorubicin in the treatment of patients with advanced islet cell carcinoma. Cancer
     1999;86:944–8.
[49] Kaltsas GA, Mukherjee JJ, Isidori A, et al. Treatment of advanced neuroendocrine tumours
     using combination chemotherapy with lomustine and 5-fluorouracil. Clin Endocrinol (Oxf)
     2002;57:169–83.
[50] Troncone L, Rufini V. Nuclear medicine therapy of pheochromocytoma and paragangli-
     oma. Q J Nucl Med 1999;43:344–55.
[51] Nguyen C, Faraggi M, Giraudet AL, et al. Long-term efficacy of radionuclide therapy in
     patients with disseminated neuroendocrine tumors uncontrolled by conventional therapy.
     J Nucl Med 2004;45:1660–8.

ELSEVIER
SAUNDERS

Endocrinol Metab Clin N Am
35 (2006) 449–468

ENDOCRINOLOGY
AND METABOLISM
CLINICS
OF NORTH AMERICA

Index

Note: Page numbers of article titles are in **boldface** type.

0889-8529/06/$ - see front matter © 2006 Elsevier Inc. All rights reserved.
doi:10.1016/S0889-8529(06)00026-0

endo.theclinics.com

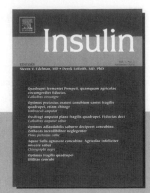

Changing Your Address?

Make sure your subscription changes too! When you notify us of your new address, you can help make our job easier by including an exact copy of your Clinics label number with your old address (see illustration below.) This number identifies you to our computer system and will speed the processing of your address change. Please be sure this label number accompanies your old address and your corrected address—you can send an old Clinics label with your number on it or just copy it exactly and send it to the address listed below.

We appreciate your help in our attempt to give you continuous coverage. Thank you.

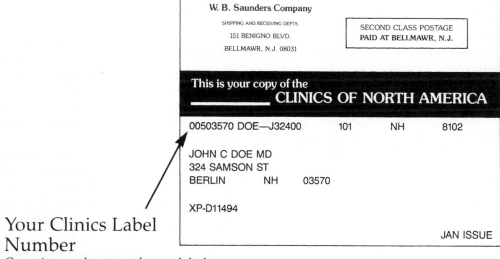

W. B. Saunders Company

SHIPPING AND RECEIVING DEPTS.
151 BENIGNO BLVD.
BELLMAWR, N.J. 08031

SECOND CLASS POSTAGE
PAID AT BELLMAWR, N.J.

This is your copy of the
_____ **CLINICS OF NORTH AMERICA**

00503570 DOE—J32400   101   NH   8102

JOHN C DOE MD
324 SAMSON ST
BERLIN   NH   03570

XP-D11494

JAN ISSUE

Your Clinics Label Number
Copy it exactly or send your label
along with your address to:
Elsevier Periodicals Customer Service
6277 Sea Harbor Drive
Orlando, FL 32887-4800
Call Toll Free 1-800-654-2452

Please allow four to six weeks for delivery of new subscriptions and for processing address changes.

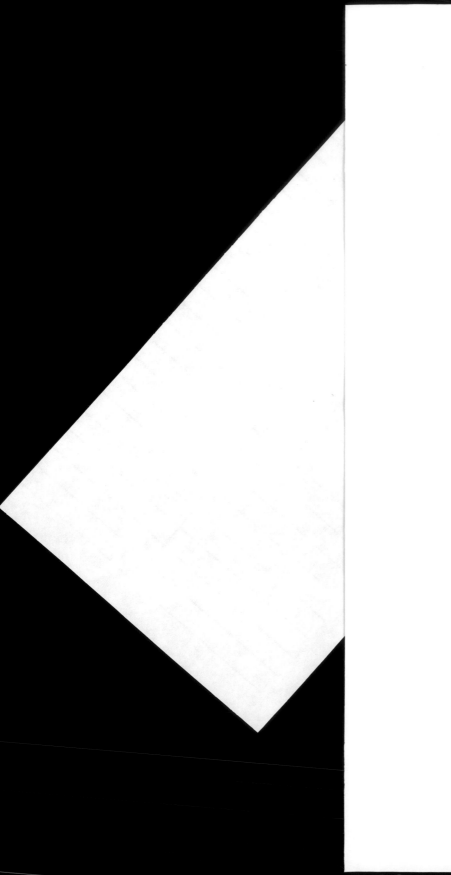

This volume may circulate for 1 week.

Renewals may be made in person or by phone
X6-6050; from outside dial 746-6050
renewals please. Fines are ch~
~ms. Please renew p~

item   Date Due

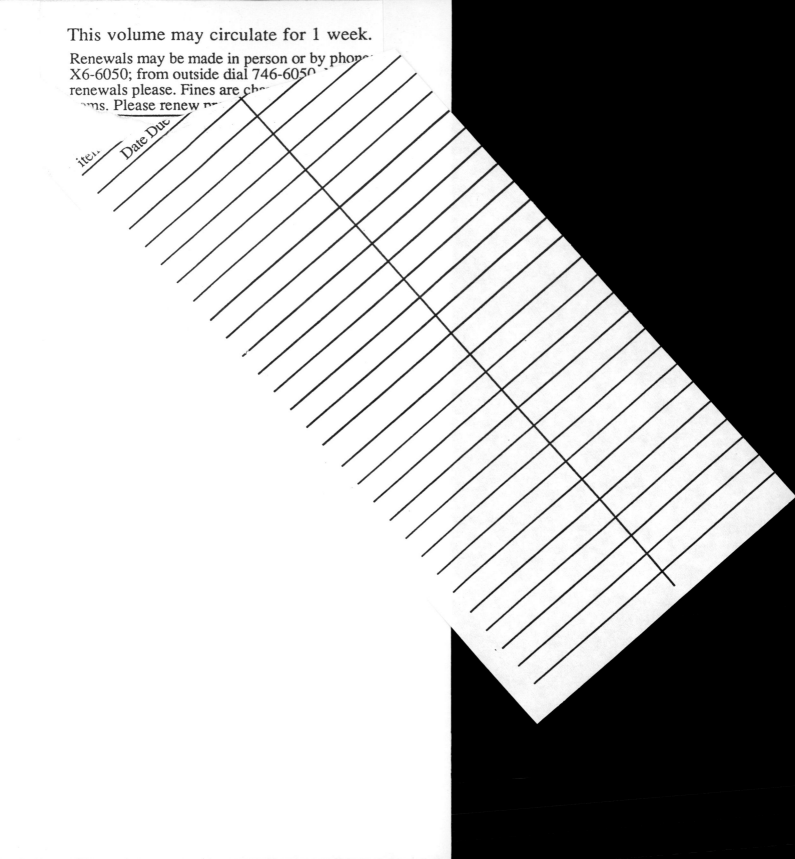